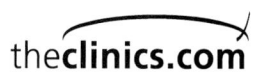

PRIMARY CARE: CLINICS IN OFFICE PRACTICE

Behavioral Pediatrics

GUEST EDITORS
Donald E. Greydanus, MD
Helen D. Pratt, PhD, and
Dilip R. Patel, MD

June 2007 • Volume 34 • Number 2

SAUNDERS

An Imprint of Elsevier, Inc.
PHILADELPHIA LONDON TORONTO MONTREAL SYDNEY TOKYO

W.B. SAUNDERS COMPANY
A Division of Elsevier Inc.

1600 John F. Kennedy Boulevard, Suite 1800 • Philadelphia, PA 19103-2899

http://www.theclinics.com

PRIMARY CARE: CLINICS IN OFFICE PRACTICE　　　　　　Volume 34, Number 2
June 2007　　　　　　　　　　　　　　　　　　　　　　　　　ISSN 0095–4543
Editor: Barbara Cohen-Kligerman　　　　　　　　　　ISBN-13: 978-1-4160-4360-7
　　　　　　　　　　　　　　　　　　　　　　　　　　　ISBN-10: 1-4160-4360-8

Copyright © 2007 Elsevier Inc. All rights reserved. No part of this publication may be reproduced or transmitted in any form or by any means, electronic or mechanical, including photocopy, recording, or any information storage and retrieval system, without written permission from the publisher.

Single photocopies of single articles may be made for personal use as allowed by national copyright laws. Permission of the publisher and payment of a fee is required for all other photocopying, including multiple or systematic copying, copying for advertising or promotional purposes, resale, and all forms of document delivery. Special rates are available for educational institutions that wish to make photocopies for non-profit educational classroom use. Permission may be sought directly from Elsevier's Global Rights Department in Oxford, UK: phone: 215-239-3804 or +44 (0)1865 843830, fax +44 (0) 1865 853333, email healthpermissions@elsevier.com. Requests may also be completed online via the Elsevier home page (http://www.elsevier.com/permissions). In the USA, users may clear permissions and make payments through the Copyright Clearance Center, Inc., 222 Rosewood Drive, Danvers, MA 01923, USA; phone: (978) 750-8400, fax: (978) 750-4744, and in the UK through the Copyright Licensing Agency Rapid Clearance Service (CLARCS), 90 Tottenham Court Road, London WIP 0LP, UK; phone: (+44) 171 436 5931; fax: (+44) 171 436 3986. Other countries may have a local reprographic rights agency for payments.

The ideas and opinions expressed in the *Primary Care: Clinics in Office Practice* do not necessarily reflect those of the Publisher. The Publisher does not assume any responsibility for any injury and/or damage to persons or property arising out of or related to any use of the material contained in this periodical. The reader is advised to check the appropriate medical literature and the product information currently provided by the manufacturer of each drug to be administered to verify the dosage, the method and duration of administration, or contraindications. It is the responsibility of the treating physician or other health care professional, relying on independent experience and knowledge of the patient, to determine drug dosages and the best treatment for the patient. Mention of any product in this issue should not be construed as endorsement by the contributors, editors, or the Publisher of the product or manufacturers' claims.

Primary Care: Clinics in Office Practice (ISSN: 0095–4543) is published quarterly by Elsevier Inc., 360 Park Avenue South, New York, NY 10010-1710. Months of issue are March, June, September, and December. Business and Editorial Offices: 1600 John F. Kennedy Blvd., Suite 1800, Philadelphia, PA 19103-2899. Customer Service Office: 6277 Sea Harbor Drive, Orlando, FL 32887–4800. Periodicals postage paid at New York, NY and additional mailing offices. Subscription prices are $151.00 per year (US individuals), $249.00 (US institutions), $76.00 (US students), $184.00 (Canadian individuals), $286.00 (Canadian institutions), $113.00 (Canadian students), $216.00 (foreign individuals), $286.00 (foreign institutions), and $113.00 (foreign students). Foreign air speed delivery is included in all *Clinics* subscription prices. All prices are subject to change without notice. POSTMASTER: Send address changes to *Primary Care: Clinics in Office Practice*, Elsevier Periodicals Customer Service, 6277 Sea Harbor Drive, Orlando, FL 32887–4800. **Customer Service: 1-800-654-2452 (US). From outside the United States, call 1-407-345-4000. E-mail: hhspcs@wbsaunders.com.**

Reprints. For copies of 100 or more, of articles in this publication, please contact the Commercial Reprints Department, Elsevier Inc., 360 Park Avenue South, New York, New York 10010-1710. Tel. (212) 633-3813, Fax: (212) 462-1935, email: reprints@elsevier.com.

Primary Care: Clinics in Office Practice is covered in *Index Medicus* and *EMBASE/Excerpta Medica*, *Current Contents/Clinical Medicine*, and *ISI/BIOMED*.

Printed in the United States of America.

BEHAVIORAL PEDIATRICS

GUEST EDITORS

DONALD E. GREYDANUS, MD, Professor, Pediatrics and Human Development, Department of Pediatrics, College of Human Medicine, Michigan State University, East Lansing; Director, Pediatrics Program, Michigan State University/Kalamazoo Center for Medical Studies, Kalamazoo, Michigan

HELEN D. PRATT, PhD, Licensed Psychologist, Behavioral and Developmental Pediatrics Division, Michigan State University/Kalamazoo Center for Medical Studies, Kalamazoo; Professor, Pediatrics and Human Development, Department of Pediatrics, College of Human Medicine, Michigan State University, East Lansing, Michigan

DILIP R. PATEL, MD, Professor, Pediatrics and Human Development, Department of Pediatrics, College of Human Medicine, Michigan State University, East Lansing, Michigan

CONTRIBUTORS

ROGER W. APPLE, MA, Behavioral and Developmental Pediatrics Division, Pediatrics Program, Michigan State University, Kalamazoo Center for Medical Studies, Kalamazoo, Michigan

JOSEPH L. CALLES, Jr., MD, Clinical Associate Professor of Psychiatry, College of Human Medicine, Michigan State University, East Lansing, Michigan; Director, Child and Adolescent Psychiatry, Psychiatry Residency Training Program, Michigan State University/Kalamazoo Center for Medical Studies, Kalamazoo, Michigan

JAMES E. CARR, PhD, Associate Professor of Psychology, Department of Psychology, Western Michigan University, Kalamazoo, Michigan

HELENA FONSECA, MD, Assistant Professor of Pediatrics, Faculty of Medicine, University of Lisbon, Lisbon, Portugal

MARK G. GOETTING, MD, Clinical Associate Professor, College of Human Medicine, Michigan State University, Portage, Michigan

DONALD E. GREYDANUS, MD, Professor, Pediatrics and Human Development, Department of Pediatrics, College of Human Medicine, Michigan State University, East Lansing; Director, Pediatrics Program, Michigan State University/Kalamazoo Center for Medical Studies, Kalamazoo, Michigan

SREENIVAS KATRAGADDA, MD, Fellow in Child and Adolescent Psychiatry, Department of Psychiatry, Dartmouth-Hitchcock Medical Center, Lebanon, New Hampshire

LINDA A. LEBLANC, PhD, Associate Professor of Psychology, Department of Psychology, Western Michigan University, Kalamazoo, Michigan

ASIAH MASON, PhD, Coordinator for Emotional Intelligence, National Mission Initiatives, Laurent Clerc National Deaf Education Center, Gallaudet University, Washington, DC

MATTHEW MASON, PhD, Clinical Psychologist, Norbel School, Columbia, Maryland

JACK W. MILLER, MD, Medical Director and Developmental-Behavioral Pediatrician, Tanner Behavioral Services, Child and Adolescent Partial Hospitalization Program, Carrollton, Georgia

KANAKO OTSUI, PhD, Department of Integrated Psychological Science, Kwansei Gakuin University, Uegahara, Nishinomiya City, Japan

DILIP R. PATEL, MD, Professor, Pediatrics and Human Development, Department of Pediatrics, College of Human Medicine, Michigan State University, East Lansing, Michigan

BRIAN PLAISIER, MD, Trauma Program, Bronson Healthcare Group, Bronson Methodist Hospital, Kalamazoo, Michigan

BRANDY M. PRATT, MA, Consultant, Programs and Youth Development, Pratt & Associates, Kalamazoo, Michigan

HELEN D. PRATT, PhD, Licensed Psychologist, Behavioral and Developmental Pediatrics Division, Michigan State University/Kalamazoo Center for Medical Studies, Kalamazoo; Professor, Pediatrics and Human Development, Department of Pediatrics, College of Human Medicine, Michigan State University, East Lansing, Michigan

JORI REIJONEN, PhD, Licensed Psychologist, Sleep Health: Comprehensive Sleep Medicine, Portage, Michigan

MILA SACKETT, Honors College, Western Michigan University, Kalamazoo, Michigan

NISHANI SAMARAWEERA, MA, Department of Psychology, Western Michigan University, Kalamazoo, Michigan

HOWARD SCHUBINER, MD, Clinical Professor, Departments of Internal Medicine, Pediatrics, and Psychiatry and Behavioral Neurosciences, Wayne State University School of Medicine, Detroit; and Department of Internal Medicine, Providence Hospital, Southfield, Michigan

ANTONIO C. SISON, MD, Clinical Associate Professor, Department of Psychiatry, University of the Philippines, Philippine General Hospital, Malate, Manila, Philippines

THERESA SOUZA, MA, Department of Psychology, Western Michigan University, Kalamazoo, Michigan

C. RICHARD SPATES, PhD, Professor of Psychology, Department of Psychology, Western Michigan University, Kalamazoo, Michigan

ARTEMIS K. TSITSIKA, MD, PhD, Pediatrics–Adolescent Medicine, Adolescent Health Unit, Second Department of Pediatrics, University of Athens, P&A Kiriakou Children's Hospital, Athens, Greece

BEHAVIORAL PEDIATRICS

CONTENTS

Preface xiii
Donald E. Greydanus, Helen D. Pratt, and Dilip R. Patel

**Screening Children for Developmental Behavioral
Problems: Principles for the Practitioner** 177
Jack W. Miller

> Behavioral and developmental problems are commonly seen in children who are cared for by primary care clinicians. This article discusses practical screening tools that can be used by clinicians to screen for these problems and make appropriate referrals to consultants for behavioral and developmental disorders of children.

**Fetal, Childhood, and Adolescence Interventions Leading
to Adult Disease Prevention** 203
Helen D. Pratt and Artemis K. Tsitsika

> Lifestyle choices result in the development and increased severity of many adult diseases that can cause death (eg, heart disease, stroke, cancer, obesity). Most health-damaging behaviors are learned during childhood and adolescence, making that time period a critical window of opportunity to teach health-promoting behaviors. Primary care physicians can implement their overall commitment to providing comprehensive health care to patients and their families by following the anticipatory guidelines of their discipline (eg, pediatrics, family and internal medicine) and by educating patients and their families about the recommendations included on the Web sites of the Centers for Disease Control and Prevention Office of Women's Health and Office of Strategy and Innovation.

Youth Survival: Addressing the Role of Promoting the Acquisition of the Prosocial Triad and Other Survival Skills in Youth 219
Helen D. Pratt, Brandy M. Pratt and Mila Sackett

> This article addresses the issue of teaching youth skills that will help them to maximize opportunities and positive consequences and minimize exposure to negative consequences in their lives. These skills will allow them to mature into mentally healthy, productive members of society. Essential skills that are critical to allow this maturational process include developing prosocial skills; the ability to recognize, discriminate the level of threat, and use strategies to avoid danger; and the ability to adapt to the changing demands of his or her environment.

Cross-Cultural Assessment and Management in Primary Care 227
Helen D. Pratt and Roger W. Apple

> The increasing number of culturally diverse patients in primary care and the demands to provide culturally sensitive health care make it essential that physicians provide care that is responsive to a culturally diverse population. Physicians must use cross-cultural techniques in their assessment and management practices. The cross-culturally competent physician has the potential to increase his or her ability to provide effective and culturally responsive treatment to a wider spectrum of patients, resulting in more positive treatment outcomes.

Depression in Children and Adolescents 243
Joseph L. Calles, Jr.

> Primary care physicians are often the first health care providers to have contact with depressed children and adolescents. This article discusses the epidemiology, clinical features, comorbid conditions, risk and protective factors, treatment modalities, and clinical course of early-onset depression.

Suicide in Children and Adolescents 259
Donald E. Greydanus and Joseph L. Calles, Jr.

> The tragedy of suicide in children and adolescents is considered a national and global phenomenon. There are approximately 900,000 suicides in the world each year, including as many as 200,000 adolescents and young adults. Suicide rates vary from country to country depending on local factors, including reporting methods. Causes of suicide include depression; abuse; loss of friends (including boyfriend or girlfriend); academic failure; social isolation; and substance abuse. The link between use of antidepressants and suicidal ideation is discussed, and concepts of management are also considered.

Sexuality in the Child, Teen, and Young Adult: Concepts for the Clinician 275
Helena Fonseca and Donald E. Greydanus

> This article discusses basic concepts of sexuality in children, adolescents, and young adults based on development stages. Sexual behavior of adolescents is a common phenomenon, leading to sexually transmitted diseases (STDs) and unwanted pregnancy. Clinicians should provide anticipatory guidance to help with healthy sexuality development while reducing negative aspects of human sexuality. Comprehensive sexuality education should be provided, with emphasis on avoiding unwanted sexual advances (including Internet dangers), bullying, pregnancy, and STDs. Clinicians can teach sexually active patients to use effective contraception and condoms for STD protection. Ensuring full immunization with the hepatitis B vaccine and the human papillomavirus vaccine also is important.

Deconstructing Adolescent Same-Sex Attraction and Sexual Behavior in the Twenty-First Century: Perspectives for the Clinician 293
Antonio C. Sison and Donald E. Greydanus

> The adolescent with same-sex attraction in the twenty-first century straddles ambivalent cultural and religious attitudes regarding gay, lesbian, bisexual, or transgender (GLBT) issues; rapid technologic advances that provide easy access to information on sex and sex partners; and the clinician's sensitivity about GLBT issues and his or her awareness of how adolescents can use technology for sex-seeking behavior. It is necessary to deconstruct these factors into defined frameworks. Three checklists, the Clinician's Framework Guide Questions for the GLBT Adolescent, Clinician Reaction to GLBT Issues Checklist, and Global GLBT Checklist for Biopsychosocial Risk Factors, may aid the clinician in acquiring an appreciation of the global dynamics between the gay adolescent, the clinician, and the impact of current social realities.

The Adolescent Sexual Offender 305
Helen D. Pratt, Donald E. Greydanus, and Dilip R. Patel

> Although the research on adolescent sexual offenders is limited, what we do know is sobering. Adolescents less than 18 years of age account for 20% of arrests for all sexual offenses (excluding prostitution). These youth reside in urban and rural areas and may be brought into the physician's office by their parents for help with addressing this maladaptive behavior. Family physicians may also get involved during a sexual abuse investigation, and may be called on to facilitate initial evaluation and coordination of services. Physicians who are aware of adolescent sexual offending can increase their ability to detect adolescents who have aberrant or deviant sexual behavior patterns allowing for early referral and intervention.

ADHD in Children, Adolescents, and Adults
Sreenivas Katragadda and Howard Schubiner

317

> Attention-deficit–hyperactivity disorder (ADHD) is a commonly occurring, heritable neurobehavioral disorder distributed worldwide that does not typically resolve after childhood. The significant impact of ADHD on an individual's family, relationships, educational performance, and performance at work is now well established. Medical treatment of ADHD is effective, not only alleviating symptoms but also improving overall functioning. It is imperative that primary care physicians be well versed in this disorder and its clinical features across the age groups. The primary care physician should be able to screen, diagnose, educate, and initiate medication management in patients with uncomplicated ADHD.

Autism Spectrum Disorders in Early Childhood: An Overview for Practicing Physicians
James E. Carr and Linda A. LeBlanc

343

> Autism spectrum disorders (ASDs) affect approximately 1 in 166 children in the United States, making it likely for the average physician to encounter patients with ASDs in his or her practice. In particular, pediatricians and developmental neurologists play a critical role in early identification, resource referrals, and management of a variety of comorbid physical and medical concerns. This article reviews the current literature on ASDs and provides recommendations for practice in areas critical to the provision of medical services.

Learning Disorders in Children and Adolescents
Helen D. Pratt and Dilip R. Patel

361

> Findings indicate that students with severe learning disabilities can profit from instruction geared toward abstract higher-order comprehension when it is designed according to their particular instructional requirements. Early intervention improves outcomes for most children with disorders of learning, attention, and cognition. Impairments in the physical, language, sensory, or mental domains are usually harder to diagnose before a child's entry into school system, but they are easier to treat if caught early. Children with above-average intellectual abilities often have the ability to compensate or master appropriate coping mechanisms that greatly minimize their overall negative outcomes. Parental attitudes and commitment, availability of resources, and the presence of an associated neurologic deficit or medical disorder can also significantly impact outcomes.

Intellectual Disability (Mental Retardation) in Children and Adolescents 375
Helen D. Pratt and Donald E. Greydanus

> Mental retardation or MR (current term, *intellectual disability* [ID]) is a label used to describe a constellation of symptoms that includes severe deficits or limitations in an individual's developmental skills in several areas or domains of function: cognitive, language, motor, auditory, psychosocial, moral judgment, and specific integrative adaptive (ie, activities of daily living). This article reviews concepts of ID in children and adolescents useful for the primary care clinician who cares for these individuals. The majority of youth with ID can live independent or semi-independent lives as adults if they have received the appropriate personalized support over a sustained period of their lives, especially during the formative years.

Psychological Impact of Trauma on Developing Children and Youth 387
C. Richard Spates, Nishani Samaraweera, Brian Plaisier, Theresa Souza, and Kanako Otsui

> All too often, children and adolescents are exposed to traumatic events that lead to physical injury in many cases, psychological perturbation in most cases, and enduring psychological reactions, notably posttraumatic stress disorder, in a minority of individuals. This sequence of events can affect later development, learning, emotions, and behavior. In the process of caring for the physical injury, it is important for the primary care practitioner (PCP) to correctly interpret these presentations and anticipate the need for specific assessments, immediate intervention, referral, and follow-up. This report provides the foundation for such actions on the part of the PCP.

Psychologic Impact of Deafness on the Child and Adolescent 407
Asiah Mason and Matthew Mason

> The purpose of this article is to provide a brief overview of the psychologic impact (stimuli and events that influence cognitive, social, and emotional development) of deafness on children and adolescents. In addition, methods for connecting with families to provide information, support, and resources to enhance deaf children's development are described.

Pediatric Insomnia: A Behavioral Approach 427
Mark G. Goetting and Jori Reijonen

> This article discusses the two common causes of insomnia in children, behavioral insomnia of childhood and delayed sleep phase syndrome. Both of these conditions are primarily treated with behavioral interventions that can be initiated and managed by the primary care provider. A review of these behavioral interventions is provided.

Index 437

FORTHCOMING ISSUES

September 2007
Mental Health
Ralph A. Gillies, PhD, and
J. Sloan Manning, MD, *Guest Editors*

December 2007
Diabetes Management
Jeffrey Unger, MD, *Guest Editor*

March 2008
Allergy, Asthma, and Immune Deficiency
Rohit Katial, MD, *Guest Editor*

RECENT ISSUES

March 2007
Evidence-Based Approaches to Common Primary Care Dilemmas, Part II
William F. Miser, MD, MA, and
John R. McConaghy, MD, *Guest Editors*

December 2006
Evidence-Based Approaches to Common Primary Care Dilemmas, Part I
William F. Miser, MD, MA, and
John R. McConaghy, MD, *Guest Editors*

September 2006
Emergency Medicine
Robert L. Rogers, MD, and
Joseph P. Martinez, MD, *Guest Editors*

THE CLINICS ARE NOW AVAILABLE ONLINE!

Access your subscription at:
http://www.theclinics.com

Preface

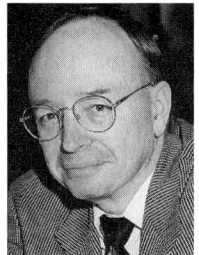
Donald E. Greydanus, MD

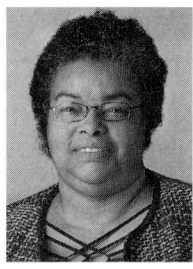
Helen D. Pratt, PhD
Guest Editors

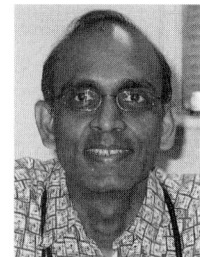
Dilip R. Patel, MD

> The boundary between biology and behavior is arbitrary and changing. It has been imposed not by the natural contours of disciplines but by lack of knowledge.
>
> —Kandel [1]

Our children have many complex challenges as they go through a myriad of developmental phases from birth and infancy (ab incunabulis) to adulthood. Parents often turn to their primary care clinician when behavioral problems arise and they also expect that their family doctor will identify the problems parents cannot yet comprehend. Indeed, many pediatric patients in these offices have either nonmedical (ie, behavioral) dilemmas or have medical problems complicated by behavioral influences [2,3]. Behavioral Pediatrics has been defined as "what the clinician does to diagnose, to treat, and most importantly, to *prevent* mental illness in children and adolescents" [4]. The term was derived in the early 1970s by Dr. Robert Haggerty and his colleagues at the University of Rochester (Rochester, New York) who were looking at mental health problems of children from the viewpoint of non-psychiatrists [4]. Dr. Stanford Friedman defined Behavioral Pediatrics as a field "...which focuses on the psychological, social, and learning problems of children and adolescents" [5].

It was in the nineteenth century that specific attention was focused on children (versus adults) based on the then gradually emerging concept that children were not simply small adults and thus needed separate study regarding their health [6]. Before the twentieth century, clinicians dealing with children were focusing on preventing morbidity and mortality from uncontrollable infections [7–10]. Advancements in pediatric infectious diseases in the twentieth and the twenty-first centuries have allowed clinicians more opportunity to deal with other issues, including the mental health of these children and adolescents. More impetus was developed by the unfolding of child psychiatry in the 1920s and 1930s, the emergence of family therapy as a management tool in the 1950s, and the advancement of psychopharmacology for all ages in the latter part of the twentieth century [2,3]. The major shortage of child psychiatrists and other mental heath specialists who are available to deal with emotional disorders in children and adolescents has required increased attention to these issues from primary care clinicians.

The twenty-first century view of child development has emerged from the nineteenth and twentieth century models of evolution (with Charles Darwin), the organismic model (with Jean Piaget and G. Stanley Hall), the psychoanalytic model (with Sigmund Freud), the mechanistic model (with B.F. Skinner), and the contextualistic model (with William James) [2,3]. The proposed link between mental health and criminal behavior began centuries ago and only now is slowly receding. Perhaps the sine qua non of Behavioral Pediatrics is attention-deficit-hyperactivity disorder (ADHD), a condition linked in England in 1902 with "defects of moral control" [11]. Today ADHD is understood as a genetic, neurobehavioral disorder with complex neurotransmitter dysfunction and many emerging subtypes [12].

Research in the neurobiologic model of mental illness has resulted in an explosion of psychopharmacologic agents available to the clinician for management of mental illness in pediatrics, further expanding the realm of behavioral pediatrics [13,14]. Rapidly developing research can also be confusing to those on the front lines of care, however. For example, the recent Food and Drug Administration's warnings linking potential suicidality and the use of antidepressants has led to a decrease by primary care clinicians in the use of these medications [15–17]. More education in these important areas is constantly needed, because translational research with monumental impact on our children occurs in the primary care clinician's office and not just in the laboratory or halls of academia.

It is within this crucial context that our issue of *Primary Care: Clinics in Office Practice* presents a potpourri of articles that fit within the rubric of Behavioral Pediatrics. This issue explores various elements in the wide and fascinating world of pediatric mental illness that present to the primary care clinician. We look at screening tools useful to detect developmental-behavioral problems of children, identify behavioral interventions in childhood with the hope of preventing adult diseases, present methods of teaching self control, and comment on the role of cross-cultural issues in primary care. We also look at classic examples of behavioral pediatrics, such as depression, suicidality, ADHD, autism, learning disorders, and mental retardation (intellectual disability). Every day headlines in the media remind us of the exposure our children have to violence in our society, and thus we look at psychologic aspects of trauma. This issue also addresses deafness and insomnia. Finally, any discussion of behavioral pediatrics should acknowledge the importance of human sexuality; thus we look at general aspects of childhood sexuality, same-sex attractions, and the adolescent sexual offender.

The editors of this issue are indebted to the many outstanding experts who gave of their valuable time to prepare these articles. We also thank Karen Sorensen for her wonderful professional help and encouragement in the development of this issue on Behavioral Pediatrics. Finally, we sincerely hope that this collection of articles will prove useful to you, the reader of this journal, in your quest to improve the lives of the children and adolescents in your practice. This work is dedicated to you with much respect and admiration (ab imo pectore) for the wonderful work you do every day on the front lines of health care in the United States.

> Who loves not knowledge? Who shall rail
> Against her beauty? May she mix
> With men and prosper! Who shall fix
> Her pillars? Let her work prevail.
>
> —*In Memoriam, CXIV,* Tennyson [18]

Donald E. Greydanus, MD
Helen D. Pratt, PhD
Dilip R. Patel, MD
Pediatrics & Human Development
Michigan State University College of Human Medicine
Pediatrics Program
Michigan State University/Kalamazoo Center for Medical Studies
1000 Oakland Drive
Kalamazoo, MI 49008-1284, USA

E-mail address: greydanus@kcms.msu.edu

References

[1] King A: " Adolescence." In: Child and adolescent psychiatry. A comprehensive textbook, 3rd edition. Ed: M. Lewis, Philadelphia: Lippincott Williams & Wilkins; 2002. p. 332–42.
[2] Greydanus DE, Pratt HD, Patel DR. Behavioral pediatrics, part I. Pediatr Clin North Am 2003;50(4):741–961.
[3] Greydanus DE, Pratt HD, Patel DR. Behavioral pediatrics, part II. Pediatr Clin North Am 2003;50(5):963–1231.
[4] Haggerty RJ. Foreword to behavioral pediatrics. In: Greydanus DE, Patel DR, Pratt HD, editors. Behavioral pediatrics. 2nd edition. iUniverse Publishers; 2006. p. xxiii.
[5] Friedman SB. Introduction: behavioral pediatrics. Pediatr Clin North Am 1975;22:55.
[6] Stern AM, Markel H. Formative years: children's health in the United States, 1880–2000. Ann Arbor (MI): University of Michigan Press; 2002. p. 320.
[7] R Von Rosenstein: The diseases of children and their remedies. London. Cadell, 1776. p. 31.

[8] Eberle J. Treatise on the diseases and physical education of children. Philadelphia: Grigg and Elliot; 1837. p. 489.
[9] Scudder NJM. The eclectic practice of diseases of children. Cincinnati (OH): American Publishing Co.; 1869. p. 19.
[10] Radbill SX. The first treatise on pediatrics. Am J Dis Child 1971;122:369–76.
[11] Still G. The Coulstonian lectures on some abnormal physical conditions in children. Lancet 1902;1:1163–8.
[12] Greydanus DE, Pratt HD, Patel DR. Attention deficit hyperactivity disorder across the lifespan. Dis Mon 2007;53(2):65–132.
[13] Werry JS, Zametkin A, Ernst M: Brain and behavior. [chapter 8], In: Child and adolescent psychiatry. A comprehensive textbook, 3rd edition. Ed: M Lewis, Philadelphia: Lippincott Williams & Wilkins; 2002. p. 120–5.
[14] Greydanus DE, Calles J, Patel DR: Pediatric and adolescent psychopharmacology: principles for the practitioner. Cambridge, England: Cambridge University Press, 350 pages, 2007.
[15] Nemeroff CB, Kalali A, Keller MB, et al. Impact of publicity concerning pediatric suicidality data on physician practice patterns in the United States. Arch Gen Psychiatry 2007;64: 466–72.
[16] Bridge JA, Iyengar S, Salary CB, et al. Clinical response and risk for reported suicidal ideation and suicide attempts in pediatric antidepressant treatment. A meta-analysis of randomized controlled trials. JAMA 2007;297:1683–96.
[17] Roy-Byrne P. Antidepressants in pediatric patients: benefits might outweigh risks. J Watch Psychiatry 2007;1. Available at: http://psychiatry.jwatch.org/cgi/content/full/2007/417/1. Accessed April 20, 2007.
[18] Osler W. Aequ animitas. Philadelphia: The Blakiston Co; 1904. p. 75.

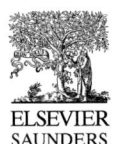

Screening Children for Developmental Behavioral Problems: Principles for the Practitioner

Jack W. Miller, MD

Tanner Behavioral Services, Child and Adolescent Partial Hospitalization Program, 100 Professional Park, Suite 104, Carrollton, GA 30117, USA

The practice of medicine has changed dramatically for those caring for children. The recent past has seen primary care evolve from treating infectious diseases, trauma, ingestions, dehydration, and other acute care pediatric medicine to a near revolution of successful preventive care measures that have improved the health and outlook of children and created the expectation of longer, safer lives.

As these problems were conquered or reduced to smaller or even insignificant numbers, the demographics of what began to appear in the primary care clinician's office also changed. The advent of Salk's polio vaccine in 1954 eventually resulted in the eradication of poliomyelitis in the Western Hemisphere. In a few short years after *Haemophilus influenzae* vaccine was first administered in 1985, there followed a dramatic drop in *H influenzae* meningitis cases in tertiary care pediatric hospitals from an average of prevaccine days of 63 per year to zero. In exponential numbers the very existence of many infectious diseases was either severely limited or eradicated altogether. The result was a mostly pleasant change in lifestyle for those practitioners providing primary care for children.

What followed was a mandate for practice styles with more focus on success in other realms of life including school, family dynamics, and the nonconquered disease and genetic milieu, and caring for those born premature. Just saving a child from a dreaded prior scourge was no longer the standard of care.

Evaluating developmental status and advocating for optimal nurturing environments became the charge of those caring for children. Communication with other disciplines was the rule and multidisciplinary evaluations

E-mail address: jmbehave@bellsouth.net

common. New specialties and subspecialties sprouted (ie, developmental-disability, neurodevelopmental, and developmental-behavioral pediatrics); each approached this new field from various points of view and widely heterogeneous backgrounds and training.

Their expertise ranged from treating *high-severity*, *low-frequency* developmental problems to *high-frequency*, relatively *low-severity* issues. This distribution exists today in combination with various mental health specialists including child and adolescent psychiatrists, various therapists, speech and language specialists, occupational and physical therapists, physiatrists, social workers, and a multitude of psychologists and school learning specialists. They all provide a wide range of help but also some confusion for parents and primary care clinicians as to when and where to refer a child with developmental behavioral problems.

In addition, until recently training for clinicians only allocated minimal time for learning to manage these frequently difficult and always complex problems. There were numerous and not always proven approaches and not enough reliable studies for proved effective treatments. For example, tricyclic antidepressants were approved after a study involving fewer than 24 subjects. In the early days of proprietary formulas there were no controlled studies regarding how much of which ingredients were better nutritionally for bone growth height; the studies merely mimicked human breast milk more or less in their own way. Fortunately, current studies are generally better designed to answer these and other important questions.

Need for developmental behavioral screening tools

If the clinician sees children and provides well-child care, one can expect about 40% to 50% of office visits to involve behavioral, psychosocial, or educational problems. In addition, approximately 75% of children with psychiatric disturbances are first seen in primary care settings, further emphasizing the need to screen using brief yet effective tools that are available and are noted in this article.

Screening and surveillance

It is important to understand why screening for developmental disabilities and behavioral problems is necessary, and determine which screening tools are most efficient in the office setting (Box 1). The American Academy of Pediatrics recommends routine standardized developmental and behavioral screening. These tools can identify the likelihood of a disability and assist in establishing a working differential diagnosis that can focus on referrals; however, these tools do not provide a specific diagnosis.

Early identification and intervention increases the outcomes and ultimate chances for success for these children, leading to higher graduation rates,

Box 1. Why screen for developmental disabilities

- 12% to 22% of children in the United States have developmental or behavioral disorders
- Many options now exist to tailor the screening to what works in specific practice situations
- Services are available to children with developmental delays starting from birth
- Outcomes are better for those children who are screened and become participants

reduced teenage pregnancy, better employment rates, decreased criminal behavior, and reduced violent crime. The overall cost savings to society is considerable and the availability of services is much better than in the past. According to Lavigne, 80% of children with mental health problems are not identified if there are no screening tests. Most mental health problems of children can be detected by appropriate screening tests. According to Glascoe, most overreferrals on standardized screens were children with below-average development and psychosocial risk factors who also benefited from intervention. Reasons (myths) for clinicians not performing screening tests are listed in Box 2.

The answer to these issues involves using newer, more accurate, and briefer screening tools for developmental and behavioral issues. The administration of these tools involves using the parents or professionals. Parents can be an accurate source of information. Screens using parent report are as accurate as other methods. Tests are designed to correct for overreporting and underreporting of information.

Some tests require specialized training and expertise to use effectively. Many practices do not have access to such personnel; screening instruments

Box 2. Reasons why clinicians do not perform screening tests

- My practice is too busy and these tests are too long
- Many are too difficult or complex to administer
- It seems like whenever I try, the child always becomes uncooperative
- Reimbursement is limited or nonexistent
- The dog chasing a fire truck dilemma: what to do after identification with unfamiliar referral sources or uneven availability
- Some of the older screening tools did not seem to be very helpful for various reasons, such as too many false-negatives

must be user friendly and have few false-negatives and false-positives. The Denver-II has been the gold standard over the years; however, its poor sensitivity and specificity has been recognized. Others that have been used include PDQ; Early Screening Profile; ELM; DIAL-III; Early Screening Inventory; and Gesell (another of the older gold standards). These all have problems with validation, were normed on referral patients, and have poor sensitivity and specificity or poor predictive value. This is true for all screening instruments and psychologic tests. There are some screening tests for clinicians to consider that are more physician friendly, as noted in Box 3.

Appendix 1 provides comments about each screening test. Appendix 2 provides more details on the tests using a chart complied by Glascoe, who notes that these tests meet standards for screening test accuracy, identifying correctly at least 70% of children with disabilities and also correctly identifying at least 70% of children without disabilities. All tests were standardized on national samples and validated against a range of measures. They can be administered efficiently and many have questionnaires that can be filled out in the waiting room using less professional time (see Box 3).

More accurate and more helpful developmental screens are now available. Nonmedical care providers play an important role in administering these screening tools. Very detailed screening and other diagnostic evaluations can be provided through schools and preschools by the Individuals with Disabilities Education Act, so that a wide range of talented and available help is available.

It is ideal for clinicians to establish a relationship with medical and nonmedical consultants. These professionals may be school psychologists or heads of special education; local mental health workers including counselors, therapists, and psychiatrists; the local Individuals with Disabilities Education Act coordinator; and pediatricians (especially developmental pediatricians).

Parents view well visits mostly as an opportunity to see how their child is doing and to ask questions. What standardized screens are showing is that little is left to the chance of false reassurance and the research behind the

---

Box 3. Currently recommended screening tests

- Parents' Evaluation of Developmental Status (PEDS), for use 0 through 8 years
- Child Development Inventories (CDIs), for use 0 through 6 years
- Ages and Stages, 0 through 6 years
- Pediatric Symptom Checklist (PSC), 4 through 18 years
- Brigance Screens, 0 through 8 years
- Safety Word Inventory and Literacy Screener (SWILS), 6 through 14 years

measures shows that when a problem is identified (whether it be a milestone not being met or a behavioral issue), most of the time one or both of the parents had some awareness of the problem. Nevertheless, it turns a well visit into potentially stressful visit. This is all the more reason to have tools to rely on and avoid the pitfalls of the "wait and see" approach. Ironically, a standardized screen takes less time in most cases than premature reassurance and provides a source of information for referral sources and a guide for ongoing observation of the child and improved communication with the family.

Barriers to developmental screening

A survey of pediatricians by the American Academy of Pediatrics (794 responding) noted the following:

- 94% of the surveyed medical doctors thought is was important to inquire about development
- 80% felt confident in their own ability to advise parents on developmental issues
- 65% reported inadequate training in developmental assessment
- 64% reported insufficient time to conduct developmental assessment
- Physicians with more than 50% of their patients on public insurance were significantly more likely to cite lack of confidence, time, training, and staff as barriers to conducting developmental assessments

How does one adapt to screening in a busy office? There are a multitude of very helpful resources to assist in setting up or improving an existing office screening procedure.

Behavioral screens

There are a number of behavioral screening tests that the clinician can use (Box 4). One can seek assistance from nonmedical behavioral health professionals, who can provide additional help and insight regarding the use of these tests. The M-CHAT is an important focused special screen for all primary care physicians. It is a brief and very helpful screening tool that needs to be administered on any child who is not displaying age-appropriate expressive language. In most cases this includes youngsters who fail the language portion of other screens, but it can also be administered separately to unusually quiet children or if the parent or professional has any concern about the child's speech development.

The M-CHAT takes a few minutes to perform and is done at the 18- or 24-month visit. It is in the public domain and is available on more than one Web site, including www.austism.org. The results are divided into possible autistic spectrum disorder, speech delay, or global delay. If a family comes in with a 30-month-old child who is not "talking yet," it is acceptable to do

Box 4. Behavioral screening tests

1. Child Behavioral Checklist
- Multiple domains to identify mental health conditions
- Teacher and parent forms good, screener less valuable for following treatment
- Scored in multiple areas including internalizing, externalizing, somatic complaints, aggressive behaviors, and attention

2. Pediatric Symptom Checklist
- Evaluates children 0 to 8 years
- Screens for mental health and behavioral problems
- Presents parents with a list of problematic behaviors
- Produces four distinct factors: (1) internalizing (depressed, withdrawn, anxious); (2) externalizing (conduct, negative or problematic behavior); (3) attention (impulsivity, distractibility, and so forth); (4) academic and global
- Takes about 7 minutes for parents to complete
- Takes 4 to 5 minutes to score various factors
- Available in English, Spanish, and Chinese

3. NICHQ Vanderbilt assessment
- Detailed questions about behavior to assess attention, opposition, conduct, anxiety, depression, and performance
- Helpful for breakdown into diagnoses
- Very high sensitivity and specificity: >94% when collateral assessments with both parent and teacher forms

4. Connors
- Specific tool for attention deficit–hyperactivity disorder with high sensitivity and specificity (>90%)
- Subtypes of inattentive and hyperactive (slated to be changed with *Diagnostic and Statistical Manual V*)
- Does not determine cause, nor should it be used in isolation
- Must rule out other or additional underlying conditions (MR, LD, anxiety, hearing, vision, and so forth)
- Available in Spanish editions
- Can be used for assistance in monitoring medications

this even though the child is older because if he or she fails, it makes referral even more appropriate (see Box 4).

Internalizing child

A commonly overlooked population in primary care practices that need referral for behavioral services is the internalizing child. Most children come

> **Box 5. Signs of internalizing behavior**
>
> - Isolating himself or herself from family and peers
> - Sleep disturbances
> - Appetite change (in either direction with unexplained weight loss or gain)
> - Signs of self-injury
> - Assessing self-injury

to the attention of their parents, teachers, or physicians through externalizing behavior that is disruptive, offensive, or dangerous. There is a group of young people who are disturbed and in pain, however, but they act "in" instead if acting "out." This subgroup is difficult to assess and often remains under the radar of medical professionals. Moreover, even the behavioral scales and assessment tools are not constructed completely to evaluate these types of children and youth. The difficulty in assessing them becomes even more problematic when one considers that these children are often at higher risk for self-injury and suicide ideation (and attempts) than their more externalizing peers.

Do not assume that a child is just shy or "nervous" if they do not make eye contact or actively engage in conversation. Certainly, physicians' offices can be intimidating places, but it is wise and helpful to ask the caretaker or guardian if this is their normal behavior or social pattern. The clinician can assess for signs of internalizing behavior as listed in Box 5. Although it is disturbing for professionals who take care of these children to be confronted with self-effacing behavior, it is not uncommon for behavioral specialists to see the same child or youth multiple times for evaluation and treatment of self-inflicted injuries. Box 6 lists concepts to keep in mind when evaluating children or youth with self-injury.

> **Box 6. Issues to consider in dealing with children with self-injures**
>
> 1. Self-injury is almost never present without a coexisting psychiatric condition.
> 2. Not all self-injuries are suicide attempts; most are not.
> 3. Ask the patient if they were trying to hurt or kill themselves; in many cases they will give the clinician a positive response in this regard.
> 4. Ask to see the injury for evaluation. Ask: "may I see the cut or check for infection or bleeding." One can explain it is our job to look at the site. Ask about other injuries. A nonjudgmental approach is important.
> 5. Seek assistance from a behavioral health professional.

Learning difficulties

A youngster who is struggling with academics or who has an unrecognized learning disability may present with more than poor grades. He or she may exhibit externalizing behavior or it may be disguised as underlying symptoms (ie, depression). Typically, unidentified learning problems are dealt with in school with an *Individual Education Plan* (IEP). If you suspect trouble in the learning environment, ask if the youngster has an Individual Education Plan in place and if it is being implemented.

A lot of help is available for clinicians, not only to assist in the appropriate referral but also to set up an office for screening, detecting, and addressing developmental or behavioral problems. Appendix 3 provides a list of Web sites that provide excellent and well-organized information to help in this regard.

Two other valuable sources for practical assistance with evaluating these issues are *The Classification of Child and Adolescent Mental Diagnoses in Primary Care: Diagnostic and Statistical Manual for Primary Care (DSM-PC) Child and Adolescent Version* and *Bright Futures in Practice: Mental Health—Vol II*. Another excellent source is the model that the Illinois chapter of the American Academy of Pediatrics put together for learning, organizing, and teaching screening in the office. The STEPPS program is available on-line as a power point presentation but may be available for about 3 hours of continuing medical education, is open to mid-level providers, and can save invaluable time in one's practice.

Another helpful resource is *Collaborating with Parents.* Copyright-free handouts are also available to help organize offices for detecting and addressing developmental and behavioral problems, and as sources for patient education material. These handouts are available on-line. Appendix 2 provides a summary of screening tests as compiled by Glascoe. Fig. 1 provides a flowchart that the clinician can use in pediatric developmental screening.

Referral and follow-up care

A physician or midlevel provider can even use one of the behavioral screens when the visit is not well care and the presenting problem is a behavior or developmental one. The screening tool can provide guidance before or during the interview, save time, and provide valuable decision-making information for referral. In cases where referral is resisted it provides the needed information for the parent or caretaker to be educated in the importance of such help much in the same way a radiograph or laboratory value does in other conditions.

Clinicians sometimes worry about the phenomenon of overreferral. This concern should not lead the clinician to hesitate in referral of a patient. The worst that will happen is a reassuring second opinion by someone who is experienced with the complex, multifaceted, and frequently uncertain nature

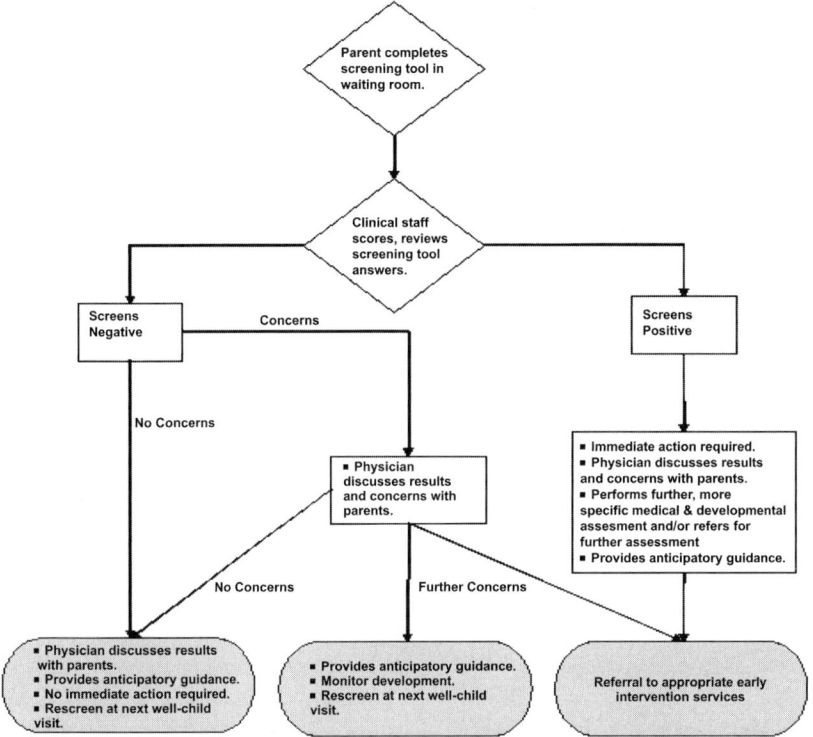

Fig. 1. Pediatric developmental screening flowchart. (*From* Department of Health and Human Services Centers for Disease Control and Prevention. Developmental screening for health care providers. Available at: http://www.cdc.gov/ncbddd/child/screen_provider.htm. Accessed July 10, 2007.)

of these problems. An occasional overreferral is still far better than premature reassurance. Parent follow-up interviews have been heavily weighted with more discontent with physician delay and hesitation that usually comes in the form of the platitudes known too well: "he'll grow out of it" or "oh, he is just a boy!"

Summary

Well-child care is much improved if behavioral and developmental problems are screened as early as possible with appropriate referral of identified problems. It is very helpful to back up one's clinical impression of a problem with an appropriate screen. One should not exceed one's comfort level, and when in doubt or in need of more help. Referral to nonmedical behavioral colleagues is often helpful to the patient, the family, and the clinician. Identifying and addressing developmental and behavioral problems can be very rewarding in one's practice.

Appendix 1. Recommended screening tests

Parents' Evaluation of Developmental Status (PEDS)

- For children up to age 8
- Available in English, Spanish, and Vietnamese
- Takes 2 minutes to score
- Elicits parents' concerns
- Sorts children into high-, moderate-, or low-risk categories for developmental and behavioral problems
- Presented at fourth to fifth grade reading level so greater than 90% of parents can complete it independently
- Score and interpretation form printed front and back and is used longitudinally
- PEDS' Evidenced Based Decisions: Helps with all of the following with a much higher degree of accuracy than the wait and see approach:
    When and where to refer (eg, mental health services, speech and language specialists, developmental pediatricians or school psychologists, and so forth)
    When to screen further or refer
    When to offer developmental promotion
    When behavioral guidance is needed
    When to observe vigilantly
    When reassurance and routine monitoring are sufficient
- Other advantages:
    It has actually been shown to reduce the "oh by the way" concerns because the common ones are addressed proactively
    Shortens visit length by focusing each visit
    Facilitates patient flow in this regard
    Improves patient and parent satisfaction and reinforces positive parenting practices
    Improves confidence in decision making by physician and other medical caretakers

Child development inventories

- There are three screenings for children 0 to 6 years
    Infant Development Inventory, 0 to 18 months
    Early Child Development Inventory, 18 to 36 months
    Preschool Developmental Inventory, 36 to 72 months
- The summary of each screen has 60 items; all are short descriptions of child behavior and development
- Takes about 10 minutes for parents to complete; parents mark yes or no to each question
- Written at the ninth grade level

- Takes about 2 minutes to score
- Infant screen shows strengths and weaknesses in each domain
- Scores for older children provide a single cutoff score
- Available in English and Spanish

Ages and Stages Questionnaire (ASQ)

- One of two most common screening tools
- A different three- to four-page form for each visit
- 30 to 35 items per form describing skill
- Forms include helpful illustrations
- Completed by parent report
- Taps major domains of development
- Takes about 15 minutes to complete, and 5 minutes to score
- ASQ-Social-Emotional: operates similarly and measures behavior, temperament, and so forth

Brigance screens

- Takes 10 to 15 minutes of professional time
- Produces a range of scores across domains
- Detects children who are delayed and advanced
- Nine separate forms across 0- to 8-year age range; similar format to Denver II
- Each produces 100 points and is compared with an overall cutoff
- Available in multiple languages
- Widely used by schools and practices with PNPs
- Computer scoring software, on-line version forthcoming
- Strong predictive validity
- Separate cutoffs for children at psychosocial risk who have recently entered intervention programs (to minimize unnecessary referrals for dx services)

Safety Word Inventory and Literacy Screen (SWILS)

- 29 common signs and safety words
- Child given credit for correct pronunciation
- Number correct is compared with a cutoff for age
- Performance correlates with reading and math
- For use from 6 to 14 years of age
- Takes 1 to 5 minutes to administer
- In the public domain
- Can serve as possible lead to injury-prevention counseling

Appendix 2. Test details compiled by Glascoe

Developmental screens relying on information from parents

	Age range	Description	Scoring	Accuracy	Time frame/Costs
Parents' Evaluations of Developmental Status (PEDS) (1997). Ellsworth & Vandermeer Press, PO Box 68164, Nashville, TN 37206. Phone: 615-226-4460; fax: 615-227-0411. Available at: http://www.pedstest.com ($30). PEDS is also available online together with the Modified Checklist of Autism in Toddlers for electronic records at: support@forepath.org	Birth–8 y	Ten questions eliciting parents' concerns in English, Spanish, and Vietnamese. Written at the 5th grade level. Determines when to refer; provide a second screen; provide patient education; or monitor development, behavior-emotional, and academic progress. Provides longitudinal surveillance and triage.	Identifies children as low, moderate, or high risk for various kinds of disabilities and delays.	Sensitivity ranging from 74%–79% and specificity ranging from 70%–80% across age levels.	About 2 minutes (if interview needed).
Ages and Stages Questionnaire (formerly Infant Monitoring System) (2004). Paul H. Brookes Publishing, PO Box 10624, Baltimore, MD 21285. Phone: 1-800-638-3775 ($190).	4–60 mo	Parents indicate children's developmental skills on 25–35 items (four to five pages) using a different form for each well visit. Reading level varies across items from third to twelfth grade.	Single pass-fail score for developmental status.	Sensitivity 70%–90% at all ages except the 4-month level; specificity 76%–91%.	Print materials ~$.31 Admin. ~$.88 Total = ~$1.19 About 15 minutes (if interview needed).

DEVELOPMENTAL BEHAVIORAL PROBLEMS 189

Available at: http://www.pbrookes.com		Can be used in mass mail-outs for child-find programs. In English, Spanish, and French.		Materials ~$.40 Admin. ~$4.20 Total = ~$4.60
Infant-Toddler Checklist for Language and Communication (1998). Paul H. Brookes Publishing, PO Box 10624, Baltimore, MD 21285. Phone: 1-800-638-3775. (Part of CSBS-DP) Available at: http://www.pbrookes.com ($99.95 with CD-ROM).	6–24 mo	Parents complete the Checklist's 24 multiple-choice questions in English. Reading level is sixth grade. Based on screening for delays in language development as the first evident symptom that a child is not developing typically. Does not screen for motor milestones. The Checklist is copyrighted but remains free for use at the Brookes Web site, although the factor scoring system is complicated and requires purchase of the CD-ROM.	Manual table of cutoff scores at 1.25 standard deviations below the mean or an optional scoring CD-ROM.	Sensitivity 78%; specificity 84%.	About 5 to 10 minutes	Materials ~$.20 Admin. ~$3.40 Total ~$3.60

(continued on next page)

Appendix 2 (*continued*)

Developmental screens relying on information from parents	Age range	Description	Scoring	Accuracy	Time frame/ Costs
PEDS- Developmental Milestones (PEDS-DM) (December 2006, in press) Ellsworth & Vandermeer Press, PO Box 68164, Nashville, TN 37206. Phone: 615-226-4460; fax: 615-227-0411. Available at; http://www.pedstest.com, to be online at www.forepath.org	0–8 y	PEDS-DM is a validated checklist of milestones, consisting of six to eight items at each age level (spanning the well visit schedule). Each item taps a different domain (fine-gross motor, self-help, academics, expressive-receptive language, social-emotional). It can be used to complement PEDS or stand alone. Administered by parent report or directly. Written at the second grade level.	Cutoffs tied to performance above and below the sixteenth percentile for each item and its domain.	Sensitivity (75%–87%); specificity (71%–88%) to performance in each domain. Sensitivity (70%–94%); specificity (77%–93%) across age.	About 3 minutes

Behavioral and emotional screens relying on information from parents

Eyberg Child Behavior Inventory/Sutter-Eyberg Student Behavior Inventory. Psychological Assessment Resources, PO Box 998, Odessa, FL 33556. Phone: 1-	2–16 y	The ECBI/SESBI consists of 36–38 short statements of common behavior problems. More than 16 suggests the referrals for behavioral interventions. Fewer than 16 enables the	Single refer-nonrefer score for externalizing problems, conduct, aggression, and so forth.	Sensitivity 80%, specificity 86% to disruptive behavior problems.	Materials ~$.20 Admin. ~$1.00 Total ~$1.20 About 7 minutes (if interview needed).

800-331-8378 ($120). Available at: http://www.parinc.com measure to function as a problems list for planning in-office counseling, selecting handouts, and monitoring progress.				
Pediatric Symptom Checklist. Jellinek MS, Murphy JM, Robinson J, et al. Pediatric Symptom Checklist: screening school age children for academic and psychosocial dysfunction. J Pediatr 1988;112:201–209 (the test is included in the article). Also can be freely downloaded at: http://psc.partners.org/or with factor scores at www.pedstest.com The Pictorial PSC, useful with low-income Spanish-speaking families, can be downloaded freely at: www.dbpeds.org (included in the PEDS:DM)	4–16 y	Thirty-five short statements of problem behaviors including both externalizing (conduct) and internalizing (depression, anxiety, adjustment, and so forth). Ratings of never, sometimes, or often are assigned a value of 0, 1, or 2. Scores totaling 28 or more suggest referrals. Factor scores identify attentional, internalizing, and externalizing problems. Factor scoring is available for download at: http://www.pedstest.com/links/resources.html	Single refer-nonrefer score.	All but one study showed high sensitivity (80%–95%) but somewhat scattered specificity (68%–100%).	Materials ∼$.30 Admin. ∼$2.38 Total = ∼$2.68 About 7 minutes (if interview needed).

(continued on next page)

Appendix 2 (*continued*)

Developmental screens relying on information from parents	Age range	Description	Scoring	Accuracy	Time frame/Costs
Parents' Evaluations of Developmental Status (PEDS) (1997). Ellsworth & Vandermeer Press, PO Box 68164, Nashville, TN 37206. Phone: 615-226-4460; fax: 615-227-0411. Available at: http://www.pedstest.com ($30). PEDS is also available on-line and for electronic medical records. Contact support@forepath.org	Birth–9 y	Ten questions eliciting parents' concerns in English, Spanish, Vietnamese, Arabic, and Somali. Written at the 4th grade level. Determines when to refer, provide a second screen, provide patient education, or monitor development, behavior-emotional, and academic progress. Provides longitudinal surveillance and triage.	Identifies children as low, moderate, or high risk for various kinds of disabilities and delays.	Sensitivity 74%–79% and specificity 70%–80% across age levels.	Materials ~$.10 Admin. ~$2.38 Total = ~$2.48 About 2 minutes (if interview needed).
Ages & Stages Questiomnaires: Social-Emotional (ASQ:SE). Paul H. Brookes, Publishers, PO Box 10,624, Baltimore, MD 21285. Phone: 1-800-638-	6–60 mo	Designed to supplement the ASQ, the ASQ SE consists of 30 item forms (four to five pages long) for each of eight visits between 6 and 60 months. Items	Single cutoff score indicating when a referral is needed.	Sensitivity 71%–85%. Specificity 90%–98%.	Print materials ~$.31 Admin. ~$.88 Total = ~$1.19 10–15 minutes if interview needed.

3775 ($125). Available at: http://www.pbrookes.com		focus on self-regulation, compliance, communication, adaptive functioning, autonomy, affect, and interaction with people.		Materials ~$.40 Admin. ~$4.20 Total = ~$4.40 5–7 minutes
Brief-Infant-Toddler Social-Emotional Assessment (BITSEA). Harcourt Assessment, 19500 Bulverde Road, San Antonio, TX 78259. Phone: 1-800-211-8378 ($99). Available at: harcourtassessment.com	12–36 mo	Forty-two item parent-report measure for identifying social-emotional and behavioral problems and delays in competence. Items were drawn from the assessment level measure, the ITSEA. Written at the fourth to sixth grade level. Available in Spanish, French, Dutch, and Hebrew.	Cut-points based on child age and gender show presence or absence of problems and competence.	Sensitivity (80%–85%) in detecting children with socioemotional-behavioral problems, and specificity 75%–80%.	Materials ~$1.15 Admin. ~$.88 Total ~$2.03

(continued on next page)

Appendix 2 (*continued*)

Developmental screens relying on information from parents	Age range	Description	Scoring	Accuracy	Time frame/Costs
PEDS- Developmental Milestones (PEDS-DM) (December,2006, in press) Ellsworth & Vandermeer Press, PO Box 68164, Nashville, TN 37206. Phone: 615-226-4460; fax: 615-227-0411. available at: http://www.pedstest.com, to be on-line at www.forepath.org	0–8 y	The PEDS-DM is a validated checklist of milestones, consisting of six to eight items at each age level (spanning the well visit schedule). Each item taps a different domain (fine-gross motor, self-help, academics, expressive-receptive language, social-emotional). Administered by parent report or directly. Written at the second grade level.	Cutoffs tied to performance above and below the sixteenth percentile for each item and its domain.	Sensitivity (75%–87%); specificity (71%–88%) to performance in each domain. Sensitivity (70%–94%); specificity (77%–93%) across age.	About 3 minutes

Family screens

| Family Psychosocial Screening. Kemper KJ, Kelleher KJ. Family psychosocial screening: instruments and techniques. Ambulatory Child Health. 1996;4:325-339. The measures are included in the article and downloadable at: http:// | Screens parents and best used along with the above screens | A two-page clinic intake form that identifies psychosocial risk factors associated with developmental problems including a four-item measure of parental history of physical abuse as a child, a six-item measure of parental substance abuse, | Refer-nonrefer scores for each risk factor. Also has guides to referring and resource lists. | All studies showed sensitivity and specificity to larger inventories greater than 90%. | Materials ~$.20 Admin. ~$1.00 Total ~$1.20 About 15 minutes (if interview needed). |

www.pedstest.com (included in the PEDS:DM)		and a three-item measure of maternal depression.		Materials ~$.20 Admin. ~$4.20 Total = ~$4.40

Developmental screens relying on eliciting skills directly from children

Brigance Screens-II (2005). Curriculum Associates, 153 Rangeway Road. North Billerica, MA 01862. Phone: 1-800-225-0248 ($501). Available at: http://www.curriculumassociates.com	0–90 mo	Nine separate forms, one for each 12-month age range. Taps speech-language, motor, readiness, and general knowledge at younger ages and also reading and math at older ages. Uses direct elicitation and observation. In the 0–2 year age range, can be administered by parent report.	Cutoff, quotients, percentiles, age equivalent scores in various domains and overall.	Sensitivity and specificity to giftedness and to developmental and academic problems are 70%–82% across ages.	10–15 minutes	Materials ~$1.53 Admin. ~$10.15 Total = ~$11.68

(continued on next page)

Appendix 2 (continued)

Developmental screens relying on information from parents	Age range	Description	Scoring	Accuracy	Time frame/Costs
Bayley Infant Neurodevelopmental Screen (BINS) (1995). The Psychological Corporation, 555 Academic Court, San Antonio, TX 78204. Phone: 1-800-228-0752 ($265). Available at: http://www.psychcorp.com	3–24 mo	Uses 10–13 directly elicited items per 3–6 month age range. Assess neurologic processes (reflexes and tone); neurodevelopmental skills (movement and symmetry); and developmental accomplishments (object permanence, imitation, and language).	Categorizes performance into low, moderate, or high risk by cut scores. Provides subtest cut scores for each domain.	Specificity and sensitivity are 75%–86% across ages.	10–15 minutes
Battelle Developmental Inventory Screening Test –II (BDIST)–2 (2006). Riverside Publishing Company, 8420 Bryn Mawr Avenue, Chicago, IL 60631. Phone: 1-800-323-9540 ($239). Available at: www.riversidepublishing.com	0–95 mo	Items (20 per domain) use a combination of direct assessment, observation, and parental interview. A high level of examiner skill is required. Well standardized and validated. Scoring software including a PDA application is	Age equivalents and cutoffs at 1, 1.5, and 2 standard deviations below the mean in each of five domains.	Sensitivity (72%–93%) to various disabilities; specificity (79%–88%). Accuracy information across age ranges is not available.	Materials ~$.30 Admin. ~$10.15 Total = ~$10.45 10–30 minutes

available. Available in English and Spanish.

Materials ~$1.65
Admin. ~$20.15
Total = ~$21.80

Academic screens

Comprehensive Inventory of Basic Skills-Revised Screener (CIBS-R Screener) (1985). Curriculum Associates, 153 Rangeway Road, North Billerica, MA 01862. Phone: 1-800-225-0248 ($224). Available at: http://www.curriculumassociates.com

1st–6th grade

Administration involves one or more of three subtests (reading comprehension, math computation, and sentence writing). Timing performance also enables an assessment of information processing skills, especially rate.

Computerized or hand-scoring produces percentiles, quotients, cutoffs.

70%–80% accuracy across all grades.

Takes 10–15 minutes.

Materials ~$.53
Admin. ~$10.15
Total = ~$10.68

(continued on next page)

Appendix 2 (*continued*)

Developmental screens relying on information from parents	Age range	Description	Scoring	Accuracy	Time frame/Costs
Safety Word Inventory and Literacy Screener (SWILS). Glascoe FP. Clin Pediatr 2002. Items courtesy of Curriculum Associates. The SWILS can be freely downloaded at: http://www.pedstest.com	5–14 y	Children are asked to read 29 common safety words (eg, high voltage, wait, poison) aloud. The number of correctly read words is compared with a cutoff score. Results predict performance in math, written language, and a range of reading skills. Test content may serve as a springboard to injury prevention counseling.	Single cutoff score indicating the need for a referral.	78%–84% sensitivity and specificity across all ages.	About 7 minutes. (if interview needed).

Narrow-band screens for autism and attention deficit–hyperactivity disorder

| Modified Checklist for Autism in Toddlers (M-CHAT) (1997). Free download at the First Signs Web site: http://www.firstsigns.org/downloads/m-chat.PDF. On-line for parents and EMRS at www.forepath.org | 18–60 mo | Parent report of 23 questions modified for American usage at fourth to sixth grade reading level. Available in English and Spanish. Uses telephone follow-up for concerns. The M-CHAT is copyrighted but | Cutoff based on two of three critical items or any three from checklist. | Initial study shows sensitivity at 90%; specificity at 99%. Future studies are needed for a full picture. Promising tool. | Materials ~$.30 Admin. ~$2.38 Total = ~$2.68 About 5 minutes. |

($1) (also included in the PEDS:DM)			remains free for use on the First Signs Web site. The full text article appeared in the April 2001 issue of the *Journal of Autism and Developmental Disorders*.	Print materials ~$.10 Admin. ~$.88 Total = ~$.98 About 20 minutes.
Connors Rating Scale-Revised (CRS-R). Multi-Health Systems, PO Box 950, North Tonawanda, NY 14120-0950. Phone: 1-800-456-3003 or 1-416-492-2627; fax 1-888-540-4484 or 1-416-492-3343 ($193). Available at: http://www.mhs.com/	3–17 y	Although the CRSR can screen for a range of problems, Several subscales specific to attention deficit–hyperactivity disorder are included: DSM-IV symptom subscales (inattentive, hyperactive-impulsive, and total); global indices (restless-impulsive, emotional lability, and total); and an attention deficit–hyperactivity disorder index. The GI is useful for treatment monitoring. Also available in French	Cutoff tied to the ninety-third percentile for each factor.	Sensitivity 78%–92%; specificity 84%–94%	Materials ~$.2.25 Admin. ~$20.15 Total = ~$22.40

From Glascoe FP. Collaborating with parents. Ellsworth & Vandermeer Press: Nashville (TN); 2006; with permission.

Appendix 3. Web sites for screening developmental-behavioral problems

www.cdc.gov/ncbddd/childscreen_provider.htm
http://dbpeds.org
http://www.medicalhomeinfo.org

Referral resources

- http://www.nectac.org for locating state, regional, and local early intervention programs and testing services for young children requiring or suspected of needing intervention
- http://www.ehsnrc.org/ for assistance with head start programs
- http://naeyc.org to assist in locating quality preschool programs
- http://www.patnc.org for help with locating parenting programs
- http://www.mentalheallth.org for help in locating mental health services
- http://www.firstsigns.org for services and information about autism spectrum disorders
- http://www.aap.org, www.dbpeds.org and www.pedstest.com all have excellent patient education materials and good links to other sites
- http://www.Firstsigns.org

Further readings

American Academy of Pediatrics. Periodic survey of fellows, division of health policy research. Elk Grove Village (IL); American Academy of Pediatrics; 2000.

American Academy of Pediatrics. American pediatrics: milestones at the millennium. Pediatrics 2001;107(6):1482–91.

American Academy of Pediatrics. Diagnostic and statistical manual of mental disorders. 4th (revised) edition. Washington, DC: American Psychiatric Association; 2000:85–93.

Bernal P. Hidden morbidity in pediatric primary care. Pediatr Ann 2003;32:413–8.

Costello EJ, Pantino T. The new morbidity: who should treat it? J Dev Behav Pediatr 1987;8: 288–91.

Fredericks EM, Opipari-Arrigan L. Behavioral assessment. In: Greydanus DE, Patel DR, Pratt HD, editors. Behavioral pediatrics. 2nd edition. New York: iUniverse Publishers; 2006. p. 651–69.

Glascoe FP. Early detection of developmental and behavioral problems. Pediatr Rev 2000;21(8): 272–80.

Glascoe FP. Collaborating with parents: using parents' evaluations of developmental status to detect and address developmental and behavioral problems. Nashville (TN): Ellsworth & Vandermeer Press, Ltd.; 1998:2006.

Jellinek MS, Patel BP, Froehle MC, editors. Bright futures in practice: mental health. Arlington (VA): National Center for Education in Maternal and Child Health; 2002.

Lavigne JV, Binns HJ, Christoffel KK, et al, Pediatric Practice Research Group. Behavioral and emotional problems among preschool children in pediatric primary care: prevalence and pediatricians' recognition [Pediatric Practice Research Group]. Pediatrics 1993;91(3):649–55.

Mahnke CB. The growth and development of a specialty: the history of pediatrics. Clin Pediatr (Phila) 2000.

Williams J, Burwell S, Capri GF, et al. Addressing behavioral health issues during well child visits by pediatric residents. Clin Pediatr (Phila) 2006;45:734.

Wolraich ML, Felice ME, Drotar D, editors. The classification of child and adolescent mental diagnoses in primary care: diagnostic and statistical manual for primary care (DSM-PC) child and adolescent version. Elk Grove Village (IL): American Academy of Pediatrics; 1996.

Wolraich ML. Addressing behavior problems among school-aged children: traditional and controversial approaches. Pediatr Rev 1997;18:266–70.

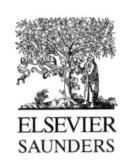

Fetal, Childhood, and Adolescence Interventions Leading to Adult Disease Prevention

Helen D. Pratt, PhD[a],*, Artemis K. Tsitsika, MD, PhD[b]

[a]Behavioral and Developmental Pediatrics Division, Michigan State University/Kalamazoo Center for Medical Studies, 1000 Oakland Drive, Kalamazoo, MI 49048, USA
[b]Pediatrics-Adolescent Medicine, Adolescent Health Unit, Second Department of Pediatrics, University of Athens, P&A Kiriakou Children's Hospital, Mesogion 24, Athens 11527, Greece

Primary care physicians have an overall commitment to (1) providing comprehensive health care to patients and their families; (2) understanding which interventions are most effective; and (3) educating parents, teachers, and other authority figures about the critical nature of modeling, facilitating, and encouraging health-promoting behaviors. Although genetics and environmental causes for disease and death are significant factors, lifestyle choices can exacerbate their severity and quicken their onset. Unhealthy lifestyle choices have a significant impact on the course of the disease process and can hasten death. Therefore, physicians must provide guidelines and suggestions for helping patients and their parents to make decisions that can improve their health status, minimize or prevent disease, and eliminate lethal but preventable causes of death. The role of primary care physicians who treat pregnant mothers, infants, children, and adolescents emerges as a critical role.

The focus of this article is on presenting interventions that address the leading causes of mortality and morbidity for adults in the United States. Focusing on these causes is important, because most of the impairment, costs, and lethality are attributable to preventable causes or lifestyle choices. Many of these health-damaging behaviors have their foundations during childhood and adolescence.

---

* Corresponding author.
E-mail address: pratt@kcms.msu.edu (H.D. Pratt).

Mortality

The leading causes of death among adults in the United States are as follows: diseases of the heart; malignant neoplasms (cancer); cerebrovascular diseases; chronic lower respiratory disease; unintentional injuries; diabetes mellitus; influenza and pneumonia; Alzheimer's disease; nephritis, nephrotic syndrome, and nephrosis; and septicemia. The rank order of these causes shifts slightly for women as compared with men and for minorities [1,2]. Such diseases as HIV for African-American women, American Indian or Alaska Native women, Hispanic-American men, and Asian or Pacific Islander men; chronic liver disease for Hispanic-American women; and tuberculosis for Asian or Pacific Islander women emerge as leading causes of death [2]. Conditions that contribute to theses deaths include hypertension, type 2 diabetes, cancer, and osteoporosis. These diseases are largely the result of lifestyle choices (ie, smoking, obesity, lack of exercise) and contribute to morbidity and mortality [2].

Morbidity

Americans in the United States have an increased life expectancy; however, this also means that there is an increasing prevalence of chronic diseases and conditions that are associated with aging and lifestyle choices. Some diseases (ie, high serum cholesterol, hypertension, type 2 diabetes, overweight or obesity, polycystic ovary disease) produce cumulative damage and death if not properly treated [3–9]. The impact risk of adult morbidity begins with maternal body composition, conditions during pregnancy, and low birth weight (BW). Other conditions (eg, having a mother who was obese during pregnancy, being a low-BW infant, leading a sedentary life style) increase the individual's risk of obesity and type 2 diabetes. Brief discussions of key diseases that increase the risk of morbidity are presented next.

Maternal body composition at pregnancy plays an important role in the outcome of offspring. Risk factors for becoming an overweight adult can begin in the womb. Maternal fatness is associated with the development of coronary heart disease (CHD) and polycystic ovary disease in offspring during adulthood, whereas low body weight at pregnancy may predict elevated blood pressure (BP) of future adults [10–13]. The protective effect of breast-feeding on the development of obesity and hypertension in childhood has been reported in several studies. This effect may be associated with the beneficial results of long-chain polyunsaturates in breast milk [14].

Low BW is associated with an elevated risk of death and disability in infants. In 2004, the low-BW rate (less than 2500 g, or 5.5 lb, at birth) increased to 8.1%, up from 7.0% in 1990. Various epidemiologic studies have demonstrated the association between low BW attributable to intrauterine growth retardation (IUGR) and an increased risk of CHD [3–9]. Premature neonates are also small at birth, but their intrauterine growth has not been undermined as a result of negative fetal environment [15]. Thus, premature infants do not present with significantly higher possibilities for developing adult diseases [15]. Some studies have proved that high BW also leads to greater adult obesity and chronic disease, whereas macrosomia in newborns raises the risk for BW-related problems [16].

Problems associated with low BW can possibly be explained by considering the diminished capacity of several organs in the human body attributable to a fetal growth restriction process. The adverse intrauterine situation leads to a reduced number or smaller size of tissue cells of trunk organs (eg, pancreas, kidney, liver), leading to metabolic (type 2 diabetes), BP (hypertension), and biochemical (hyperlipidemia) alterations, especially if accelerated postnatal growth takes place, maximizing demands. Type 2 diabetes may also occur at higher rates in neonates weighing 4.5 kg or greater at birth [13]. The fetus may be influenced in different critical gestational periods. When affected early in gestation, the fetus is symmetrically small in all parameters (height, weight, and head circumference). After birth, these children do not "catch up" to their normal weight and height for age and gender. When affected later in gestation, the neonate is nonsymmetric, with a normal head circumference but affected height and weight. In this case, the number of tissue cells is normal but their size is smaller as an adaptive response to the adverse intrauterine environment. These neonates present with catch-up growth and are at risk for adult obesity, CHD, type 2 diabetes, and hyperlipidemia. Conversely, the symmetric type is more at risk for elevated adult BP [4,5]. Based on these findings, maternal nutrition during pregnancy as well as maternal body composition, substance use, and psychosocial stress status should be areas of intervention so as to achieve the optimum in utero environment and to minimize the prevalence of common adult diseases. The potential health benefits from a reduction in the prevalence of overweight and obesity are of significant public health importance. Physicians who care for pregnant mothers must continue to stress the need for good nutrition and healthy lifestyles and monitor for symptoms of eclampsia and other causes of prematurity.

High blood cholesterol is a major risk factor for narrowing of the arteries, heart disease, and other complications [17,18]. Eating patterns and genetics affect blood cholesterol levels and CHD risk. Elevated cholesterol levels early in life have been identified as having a role in the development of atherosclerosis in adults, which begins in childhood and progresses slowly into adulthood, potentially leading to CHD [17–19]. Knapp [20] offered that although there are no long-term studies showing the relation of blood cholesterol levels measured in childhood to CHD in later life, it can be concluded that the relation is inferred, partially because youth in the United States have higher cholesterol levels and higher rates of CHD than their counterparts in other countries. Furthermore, they eat more foods that have saturated fatty acids and cholesterol [20].

Suggestions from the American Heart Association (AHA) [19] state that prevention includes encouraging youth to never start or to quit smoking tobacco, engage in regular aerobic exercise, and maintain a healthy weight as well as diagnosing and treating high BP and diabetes mellitus.

High BP in childhood is another major risk factor for hypertension in early adulthood and adult heart disease [21]. Lowering BP by changes in lifestyle or by medication can lower the risk of heart disease and heart attack. Hypertension and prehypertension have become significant health issues in the young because of the strong association of high BP with overweight and the marked increase in the prevalence of overweight children in the United States [21–23]. As one's body mass index (BMI) increases, so does the prevalence of primary hypertension in children. Children and adolescents with primary hypertension are frequently overweight and frequently have some degree of insulin resistance (a prediabetic condition). Overweight and high BP pressure are also components of the insulin resistance syndrome, or metabolic syndrome, a condition of multiple metabolic risk factors for CHD as well as for type 2 diabetes. Secondary hypertension is more common in children than in adults. Because overweight is strongly linked to hypertension, weight reduction is the primary therapy for obesity-related hypertension [19,21–23].

Recommendations for prevention also include family-based interventions, such as loss of excess or abnormal weight, engaging in regular physical activity, and implementing dietary modifications to support good nutrition [18,21–24].

Heart disease and stroke are the first and third leading causes of death for men and women in the United States and are major causes of disability [24]. Heart disease is the leading cause of death for American Indians and Alaska Natives, blacks, Hispanics, and whites. Two major independent risk factors for heart disease and stroke are high BP and high blood cholesterol. Other important risk factors include diabetes, tobacco use, physical inactivity, poor nutrition, and being overweight or obese [18].

Because most adolescents who have high BP have no disease causing the problem, prevention depends on lifestyle changes. These changes include having an appropriate weight for one's height, reasonable sodium intake, and moderate aerobic physical activity; reducing stress levels; and having good sleep hygiene [21].

Recommendations for lowering one's risk of stroke include controlling high BP and cholesterol, avoiding alcohol, maintaining a healthy weight, eating a healthy diet, engaging in regular physical activity, not smoking, and effectively managing heart disease and other chronic conditions [25].

Cancer

Cancer is the second leading cause of death and is responsible for one of every four deaths in the United States [1,2,12,18]. For Asians and Pacific Islanders, cancer is the leading cause of death (accounting for 26.1% of all deaths) and heart disease is a close second (accounting 26.0% of all deaths) [18]. Cancer disease is associated with higher BW, whereas catch-up or accelerated growth generally has negative health effects [16]. Studies of diet and cancer do not prove direct causal relations between dietary fat and cancer; however, increased energy intake and body size in childhood as well as low dietary fiber contribute to earlier age at menarche (<12 years), which is associated with a stronger risk for breast cancer [26]. Low dietary fiber, low fruit and vegetable consumption, and high red meat consumption are associated with colon cancer and other cancers. If these dietary patterns begin in early life years, there may be an increase in age-specific rates of colon cancer in adult life. The risk may be reversed with a later dietary change, however [27]. Children and adolescents may be targets of dietary intervention so as to establish dietary trends that may prevent cancer later in life. Dietary interventions that begin at younger ages are significant, leading to an opportunity to prevent adult-onset cancer. Improvement in dietary knowledge and practices of young people through school-based and other intervention models is an undisputable need for ameliorating chances of reaching the previously mentioned goal [28].

Recommendations for cancer prevention include adopting healthier lifestyles; for example, avoiding tobacco use, increasing physical activity, achieving a healthy weight, improving nutrition, and avoiding sun overexposure can significantly reduce a person's risk for cancer. Early cancer screening (especially for breast, cervical, and colorectal cancer), information, and referral services should be made available and accessible to parents and youth.

Type 2 diabetes (non–insulin-dependent diabetes) increased in prevalence for all age groups in the United States. Minorities are disproportionately affected, and most of the youth are overweight and have decreased energy expenditure. Prevention requires a complex set of behavioral changes in individuals, their families, schools, and communities [25,29–31].

Osteoporosis is mainly genetically determined (70%); however, peak bone mass acquisition can be helped by altering modifiable influencing factors, including nutrition, exercise, hormonal status, and substance use [20]. Smoking and alcohol are influencing factors, the avoidance of which can ameliorate results. Sex hormones (estrogens and testosterone) play an important role in maintaining bone mass. Although osteoporosis is thought to be a disease of the elderly, it has been recognized recently as preventable by interventions in childhood and adolescence. These are crucial periods for prevention, because bone mass increases during this time; bone formation exceeds bone resorption until early adulthood [32,33]. Most of the peak bone mass is acquired in adolescence (40%–60%), determining future bone health [33]. After adolescence, bone mass stops increasing and remains at a steady state for years until bone resorption starts exceeding formation and bone loss takes place (at an older age >40 years). Severe estrogen deficiency in adolescent girls with eating disorders (eg, anorexia nervosa, bulimia nervosa) or in elite adolescent athletes (athlete triad) has devastating life course effects on bone health.

Overweight prevalence doubled for children (6–11 years of age) during the past 30 years and tripled for adolescents (12–19 years of age). Currently, 19% of children and 17% of adolescents are overweight. Overall, the prevalence of being overweight is greater among African Americans, Hispanics, and Native Americans than among whites [34].

Obesity is associated with higher low-density lipoprotein (LDL; "bad") cholesterol and triglyceride levels and with lower high-density lipoprotein (HDL; "good") cholesterol as well as with a higher risk for developing severe cardiovascular disease, type 2 non–insulin-dependent diabetes, some types of cancer (breast, bowel, and prostate cancer), hypertension, arthritis, syndrome X, polycystic ovary disease, arthritis, and other musculoskeletal problems [1,17,24,25,35] The effects of the increasing prevalence of obesity on the cardiovascular health of children and adolescents remain unclear [24]. The level of risk for adult CHD occurs for youth who were obese as children and for those who were of normal weight but became obese as adults. Therefore, some researchers contend that we really do not have sufficient data to determine the independent relation of childhood weight status to morbidity attributable to CHD. The researchers concluded that more analysis needs to be done for primary and secondary prevention [36].

Polycystic ovary syndrome is also combined with obesity (50% of patients with polycystic ovary syndrome are obese), and it often leads to infertility problems, psychologic distress, and psychosocial problems. The combination of obesity, type 2 (non–insulin-dependent) diabetes, hypertension, and hyperlipidemia is globally known as syndrome X [5,6].

Impact of having multiple diagnoses of chronic diseases

Multiple diagnoses of chronic illness (three or more conditions, including hypertension, heart disease, stroke, emphysema, diabetes, cancer, arthritis, or asthma as a chronic condition) significantly limit a person's ability to perform his or her adult daily living skills or to have independent movement. Approximately 34.1 million persons (12%) are limited in their usual activities because of having one or more chronic health conditions. This includes 6% of children younger than the age of 12 years [1,37]. These conditions impair one's ability to perform self-care and other activities independently [1]. Arthritis and other musculoskeletal conditions were the leading cause of activity limitation among working-age adults 18 to 64 years old [1].

Lifestyle choices that decrease health status and increase morbidity and mortality

Cigarette smoking

Smoking is the main preventable cause of death in the United States; more than 430,000 Americans die from causes related to smoking every year [26]. Tobacco consumption is highly addictive because of nicotine, and most smokers (>90%) start the habit as adolescents (more than 3,000,000 adolescents smoke in the United States). Adult diseases related to smoking are numerous; there is a significantly increased risk of heart disease, heart attack, lung cancer, chronic lung diseases (eg, emphysema, laryngeal carcinoma), other cancers, mucosal keratosis, and atherosclerosis as well as increased levels of blood clotting factors (eg, fibrinogen). Nicotine raises BP, and carbon monoxide reduces the amount of oxygen that blood can carry. Exposure to other people's smoke can increase the risk of heart disease, even for nonsmokers [1].

Nearly one fifth of women (10% of pregnant women) and one quarter of men smoke cigarettes. Maternal smoking is also associated with elevated BP of offspring in adulthood [38]. Smoking during pregnancy contributes to elevated risk of miscarriage, premature delivery, and having a low-BW infant [1]. The Youth Risk Behavior Surveillance (YRBS) conducted in 2005 reported that more than half (54.3%) of high school students nationwide stated that they had not tried cigarette smoking (even one or two puffs during the 30 days preceding the survey), 13.4% had smoked at least one cigarette every day for 30 days, 23.0% had smoked cigarettes more than one time, 23.0% reported current cigarette use, and 10.7% had smoked more than 10 cigarettes a day. Use of smokeless tobacco was reported by 8.0% (eg, chewing tobacco, snuff, dip); 14.0% had smoked cigars, cigarillos, or little cigars more than one time; and 28.4% reported current cigarette, smokeless tobacco, or current cigar use (ie, current tobacco use) [34].

Adolescence is the critical period of prevention and intervention through educational programs, counseling, and peer-delivered information [26]. Motivational interviewing and tobacco therapy programs are applied for smoking youth. Results can be surprisingly positive, because most adolescents want to quit smoking and the cessation process can be intriguing for them [26,39].

Poor dietary habits

Several aspects of dietary patterns have been linked to heart disease and related conditions. These include diets high in saturated fats and cholesterol, which raise blood cholesterol levels and promote atherosclerosis. High salt or sodium in the diet causes raised BP levels. Nationwide, 20.1% of high school students reported that they had eaten fruits and vegetables five or more times a day during the 7 days preceding the survey, and only 16.2% said they had had three or more glasses of milk a day [34].

Lack of physical exercise

Regular physical activity is associated with increased health benefits, which include reduced risks of premature mortality, CHD, diabetes, colon cancer, hypertension, and osteoporosis. Regular physical activity also improves symptoms associated with musculoskeletal conditions and mental health conditions, such as depression and anxiety. In addition, physical activity can enhance physical functioning and aid in weight control. Physical inactivity is related to the development of heart disease, and almost 38% of adults do not exercise [19]. It also can have an impact on other risk factors, including obesity, high BP, high triglycerides, a low level of HDL cholesterol, and diabetes. Regular physical activity can improve risk factor levels [19].

The YRBS 2005 results showed that, nationwide, slightly more than one third (35.8%) of students had been physically active doing any kind of physical activity that increased their heart rate and made them breathe hard some of the time for a total of at least 60 minutes each day on 5 or more of the 7 days preceding the survey (ie, met currently recommended levels of physical activity). A little more than two thirds had participated in at least 20 minutes of vigorous physical activity (ie, physical activity that made them sweat and breathe hard) on 3 or more days of the same period [34].

Sexual behaviors that contribute to unintended pregnancy and sexually transmitted diseases, including HIV infection

Sexually active adolescents are at increased risk for sexually transmitted diseases (STDs) because of various reasons (high sexual activity rates, multiple sex partners, use of sex and drugs concomitantly, immature female cervix, magical thinking of adolescence [ie, no harm can come to them despite high risk behavior], and difficulty in dealing with the medical system for treatment). Although the incidence of STDs has been gradually declining during the past several years, adolescents and young adults present with increasing trends and have higher disease levels than any other age group [40,41]. Some of these diseases can be silent or asymptomatic and are associated with pelvic inflammatory disease and future infertility. Cervical dysplasia and cancer are conditions associated with types 16 and 18 of human papilloma virus (HPV), which is the most common sexually acquired viral disease [41].

Although most youth experience intercourse for the first time during adolescence, a small number (6.2%) reported experiencing sexual intercourse for the first time before the age of 13 years. A total of 46.8% of high school students reported that they had experienced sexual intercourse, 7.5% said that they had been physically forced to have sexual intercourse when they did not want to, 33.9% had had sexual intercourse with one or more partners during their lifetime, and 14.3% had had sexual intercourse with four or more partners during their lifetime [34]. Among the 33.9% of currently sexually active students nationwide, 62.8% reported that they or their partner had used a condom during last sexual intercourse, 23.3% had drunk alcohol or used drugs before last sexual intercourse, and 17.6% reported that they or their partner had used birth control pills to prevent pregnancy. Nationwide, 87.9% of students had ever been taught in school about AIDS or HIV infection and 11.9% of students had been tested for HIV [34].

Substance abuse

Most youth begin drinking alcohol after the age of 13 years, and three quarters of them had had at least one drink of alcohol on more than 1 day during their lifetime. Nationwide, 43.3% of students had had at least one drink of alcohol on more than 1 of the 30 days preceding the survey (ie, current alcohol use), and 25.5% had five or more drinks of alcohol in a row (ie, within a couple of hours) on 1 or more of the 30 days preceding the survey (ie, episodic heavy drinking) [34].

In 2005, 30% of high school students in grades 11 and 12 reported binge drinking and 22% reported marijuana use in the past 30 days preceding the YRBS survey. Binge drinking and marijuana use among high school students have serious consequences. Alcohol use has been related to academic difficulties, social problems, risky sexual behavior, and motor vehicle accidents [34]. Some studies have found that high school students who use marijuana get lower grades and are less likely to graduate than students who do not use marijuana [34]. Excessive alcohol use leads to an increase in BP and increases the risk for heart disease. It also increases blood levels of triglycerides, which contributes to atherosclerosis [34,36].

The YRBS results also show that nationwide, 8.7% of students had tried marijuana for the first time before the age of 13 years. Nationwide, 38.4% of students had used marijuana one or more times during their life (ie, lifetime marijuana use), and 20.2% were current marijuana users during the survey period; 7.6% had used any form of cocaine (eg, powder, crack, or freebase) one or more times during their life (ie, lifetime cocaine use), and 3.4% had used any form of cocaine (eg, powder, crack, or freebase) one or more times during the 30 days preceding the survey [34].

Nationwide, the survey showed that students reported lifetime rates of use one or more times for the following substances: 2.1% had used a needle to inject any illegal drug into their body; 12.4% had sniffed glue, breathed the contents of aerosol spray cans, or inhaled any paints or sprays to get high; 4.0% had taken steroid pills or shots without a doctor's prescription; 2.4% had used heroin (also called smack, junk, or China white); 8.5% had used hallucinogenic drugs (eg, lysergic acid diethylamide [LSD], acid, phencyclidine [PCP], angel dust, mescaline, mushrooms); 6.2% had used methamphetamines (also called speed, crystal, crank, or ice); and 6.3% had used 3,4-methylenedioxy methamphetamine (MDMA; also called ecstasy) [34].

Box 1. Interventions for health promotion and disease elimination, reduction, or prevention.

1. Infants and toddlers, aged 0 to 3 years
Main goal: start strong
- Increase the number of infants and toddlers who have a strong start for healthy and safe lives.
- Promote healthy pregnancy and birth outcomes (eg, preconception care).
- Promote healthy lifestyle choices by mothers (including weight management).
- Reduce infectious diseases and other preventable conditions and their consequences among infants and toddlers (eg, acute respiratory infection, diarrheal disease, fetal alcohol syndrome, pregnancy-associated infections, sudden infant death syndrome [SIDS], vaccine-preventable disease).
- Prevent injury and violence and their consequences among infants and toddlers (eg, child maltreatment, drowning, motor vehicle injury).
- Promote optimal development among infants and toddlers (eg, language and communications skills, motor abilities).
- Increase early identification, tracking, and follow-up of infants and toddlers with special health care and developmental needs.
- Increase the number of infants and toddlers who live in social and physical environments that support their health, safety, and development (eg, increase the number of infants and toddlers who live in lead-safe housing; increase the number of infants and toddlers who have access to and receive quality, comprehensive, pediatric health services, including dental services).
- Improve risk and protective factors for future disease among infants and toddlers (eg, environmental tobacco smoke, nutrition [including breastfeeding]).

2. Children, aged 4 to 11 years
Main goal: grow safe and strong
- Increase the number of children who grow up healthy, safe, and ready to learn.
- Improve risk and protective factors for future disease among children (eg, inactivity, bad nutrition, overweight).
    a. Elementary school–aged children should exercise 30 to 60 minutes in developmentally appropriate physical activity from a variety of activities on all or most days of the week.

b. A change of school environment (dietary education and providing school canteens with healthy snacks) and promotion of better nutrition and increased opportunities to exercise and learn about healthy lifestyles should be encouraged [46].
  c. Children should be educated about the hazards of substance use and abuse and sexual activity at this age.
3. Adolescents, aged 12 to 19 years

Main goal: achieve health independence

- Increase the number of adolescents who are prepared to be healthy, safe, independent, and productive members of society.
- Increase the number of adolescents who live, learn, work, and play in social and physical environments that are accessible; support health, safety, and development; and promote healthy behaviors.
- Osteoporosis prevention: educate parents and youth that calcium is an essential element for achieving full potential peak bone mass, and, thus, it is important for adolescents to meet their calcium dietary reference intake (DRI for calcium: 1300 mg daily), comprising at least three portions of milk products daily (eg, milk, yogurt, hard yellow cheese). Unfortunately, less than 16% of adolescent girls in the United States meet their DRI for calcium [47]. Exogenous calcium administration (supplements) does not have the same positive effect on bone increase as dietary calcium does. Certain types of exercise (eg, running, basket ball, tennis) promote bone formation by applying mechanical force to the skeleton and are highly recommended during adolescence [33].
- Early detection of eating disorders and atypical cases that do not meet all the diagnostic criteria (eating disorders not otherwise specified [EDNOS]) seems to ameliorate intervention results and offers chances for better skeleton status [48].
- Decreasing cigarette smoking among adolescents and adults is a major public health objective for the nation. Preventing smoking among teenagers and young adults is critical, because smoking usually begins in adolescence.
- Increase the number of adolescents who receive recommended effective evidence-based preventive and health care services. Prevent HIV, STDs, and unintended pregnancies and their consequences among adolescents. Prevention of STDs: sexual education and appropriate

> vaccination in adolescence may (to some extent) prevent STDs in sexually active adolescents. Annual screening tests (eg, *Chlamydia* testing, pap smear cytology) in sexually active adolescents may lead to better chances for early and successful intervention, and thus avoidance of adult infertility or other forms of genitourinary system dysfunction [27]. Physicians may encourage abstinence until late adolescence (at least); many adolescents meet their developmental goals and become fit for realistic and functional relationships before entering adulthood. Those adolescents who have had their virginity taken or who have previously engaged in sexual intercourse can be encouraged to embrace secondary virginity (abstinence). If adolescents choose to be sexually active, they should be well informed about protection methods (eg, condom use), STD symptoms, and the obligation to visit an expert when symptomatic. Other areas of focus are the obligation to inform their partner for testing and treatment (when needed) and to avoid intercourse at the time of an active STD. Sexual activity requires responsibility, and this is an area for education, school programming, and demonstration [41].
> - Promote healthy activity and nutrition behaviors and prevent overweight and its consequences among adolescents. Prevent substance use, including tobacco, alcohol, and other drugs, among adolescents [42].

Interventions

Interventions to prevent and reduce the onset or severity of morbidity and mortality risk factors for youth are presented by group and by risk factor. General recommendations are for all age groups but are listed under the age group or developmental stage at which unhealthy behaviors generally emerge (Box 1). These recommendations also include some of the recommendations listed on the Center for Disease Control and Prevention (CDC) Office of Women's Health's Web site entitled "ABCs of raising safe and healthy kids: steps to staying safe and healthy" (2007) and the CDC Office of Strategy and Innovation's (OSI's) Web site entitled "Healthy people in every stage of life. Health protection goals: criteria and objectives" (2007) [17,42–45].

Summary

The time to address prevention and to eliminate or reduce adult morbidity and mortality is during childhood and adolescence. Genetics and environmental exposure do determine many risk factors for developing chronic diseases that lead to limitations of daily functioning and to death during adulthood. Lifestyle choices result in the development and increased severity of many diseases that can cause death, however. Most adults learned their dietary, exercise, and smoking habits as well as the consumption of any substances (including alcohol) as young people. This makes the periods of childhood and adolescence critical windows of opportunity to teach health promotion behaviors. Primary care physicians have an overall commitment to providing comprehensive health care to their patients and their families by implementing the anticipatory guidelines of their discipline (eg, pediatrics, family and internal medicine), educating their patients and their parents about the recommendations included on the following Web sites: the CDC Office of Women's Health's Web site entitled "ABCs of raising safe and healthy kids: steps to staying safe and healthy" (2007) and the CDC OSI's Web site entitled "Healthy people in every stage of life. Health protection goals: criteria and objectives (2007). [17,42].

References

[1] National Center for Health Statistics. Health, United States, 2006 with chartbook on trends in the health of Americans. Hyattsville (MD) 2006. Available at: http://www.cdc.gov/nchs/data/hus/hus06.pdf. Accessed April 7, 2007.
[2] Anderson RN, Smith BL. Deaths: leading causes for 2002. Division of Vital Statistics Health and Human Services, Centers for Disease Control and Prevention, National Center for Health Statistics 2005;53(17). Available at: www.cdc.gov/nchs/data/nvsr/nvsr53/nvsr53_17.pdf. Accessed April 7, 2007.
[3] Godfrey KM, Barker DJP. Fetal nutrition and adult disease. Am J Clin Nutr 2000; 71(Suppl):1344S–52S.
[4] Barker DJP. Fetal origins of coronary heart disease. BMJ 1995;311:171–4.
[5] Barker DJP. Mothers, babies and health in later life. Edinburgh (UK): Harcourt Brace & Co Ltd; 1998.
[6] Barker DJP, Hales CN, Fall CHD, et al. Type 2 (non insulin dependent) diabetes mellitus, hypertension and hyperlipidemia (syndrome X): relation to reduce fetal growth. Diabetologia 1993;36:62–7.
[7] Rose G. Familial patterns in ischaemic heart disease. Br J Prev Soc Med 1964;18:75–80.
[8] Forsdahl A. Are poor living conditions in childhood and adolescence an important risk factor for arteriosclerotic heart disease? Br J Prev Soc Med 1977;31:91–5.
[9] Osmond C, Barker DJP, Winter PD, et al. Early growth and death from cardiovascular disease in women. BMJ 1993;307:1519–24.
[10] Clark PM, Atton C, Law CM, et al. Weight gain in pregnancy, triceps skin fold thickness and blood pressure in the offspring. J Obstet Gynaecol 1998;91:103–7.
[11] Godfrey KM, Forrester T, Barker DJP, et al. Maternal nutritional status in pregnancy and blood pressure in childhood. Br J Obstet Gynaecol 1994;101:398–403.
[12] Stein CE, Fall CHD, Kumaran K, et al. Fetal growth and coronary heart disease in South India. Lancet 1996;348:1269–73.
[13] Cresswell JL, Barker DJP, Osmond C, et al. Fetal growth, length of gestation, and polycystic ovaries in adult life. Lancet 1997;350:1131–5.
[14] Whincup PH, Cook DG, Shaper AG. Early influences on blood pressure: a study of children aged 5-7 years. BMJ 1989;299:587–91.

[15] Barker DJP, Osmond C, Simmonds SJ, et al. The relation of small head circumference and thinness at birth to death from cardiovascular disease in adult life. BMJ 1993;306:422–6.
[16] Krone B, Kolmel KF, Grange JM, et al. Impact of vaccinations and infectious diseases on the risk of melanoma—evaluation of an EORTC case-control study. Eur J Cancer 2003; 39(16):2372–8.
[17] Centers for Disease Control and Prevention, Office of Women's Health. ABCs of raising safe and healthy kids: steps to staying safe and healthy. Atlanta: Office of Women's Health, Centers for Disease Control and Prevention.
[18] US Department of Health and Human Services and Centers for Disease Control and Prevention. Profiling the leading causes of death in the United States heart disease. Stroke, and Cancer 2006. Available at: http://www.cdc.gov/nccdphp/publications/factsheets/ChronicDisease/pdfs/00_ChronicDiseaseAllStates.pdf. Accessed April 7, 2007.
[19] American heart Association. Cholesterol and atherosclerosis in children 2007. Available at: http://americanheart.org/presenter.jhtml?identifier=4499. Accessed April 7, 2007.
[20] Knapp R. Blood cholesterol levels in children and adolescents. Available at: http://www.rogerknapp.com/medical/cholesterol.htm. Accessed April 7, 2007.
[21] Massachusetts General Hospital and Harvard Medical School. High blood pressure 2007. Available at: http://www.mgh.harvard.edu/children/adolescenthealth/articles/aa_high_blood_pressure.aspx. Accessed April 7, 2007.
[22] Update on the 1987 task force report high blood pressure in children and adolescents: a working group report from the National High Blood Pressure Education Program. Pediatrics 1996;98(4):649–59.
[23] National High Blood Pressure Education Program Working Group on High Blood Pressure in Children and Adolescents. The fourth report on the diagnosis, evaluation, and treatment of high blood pressure in children and adolescents. Pediatrics 2004;114(Suppl Pt 3):555–76.
[24] Ford ES, Mokdad AH, Ajani UA. Trends in risk factors for cardiovascular disease among children and adolescents in the United States. Pediatrics 2004;114(6):1534–44.
[25] Center for Disease Control and Prevention. Stroke. Department of Health and Human Services 2007. Available at: http://www.cdc.gov/stroke/. Accessed April 7, 2007.
[26] Mettlin C. Dietary cancer prevention in children. Cancer 1993;71(Suppl 10):3367–9.
[27] Johnson J. Sexually transmitted diseases in the adolescent. In: Grydanus DE, Patel DR, Pratt HD, editors. Essential adolescent medicine. New York: McGraw-Hill; 2006.
[28] Samaras TT, Elrick H, Storms LH. Birthweight, rapid growth, cancer, and longevity: a review. J Natl Med Assoc 2003;95(12):1170–83.
[29] Gale EAM. Is there really an epidemic of type 2 diabetes? Lancet 2003;362(9383):503–4.
[30] National Diabetes Education Program. An update on type 2 diabetes in youth. Pediatrics 2004;114(1):259–63.
[31] Type 2 diabetes in children and adolescents. Pediatrics 2000;105(3):671.
[32] Golden NH. Osteoporosis prevention: a pediatric challenge. Arch Pediatr Adolesc Med 2000;154:542–3.
[33] Katzman DK, Bachrach LK, Carter DR, et al. Clinical and anthropometric correlates of bone mineral acquisition in healthy adolescent girls. J Clin Endocrinol Metab 1991;73: 1332–9.
[34] Centers for Disease Control and Prevention. Youth risk behavior surveillance—United States, 2005. MMWR Surveill Summ 2006;55:SS-5. Available at: http://www.cdc.gov/mmwr/PDF/SS/SS5505.pdf. Accessed April 7, 2007.
[35] Kohn M, Booth M. The worldwide epidemic of obesity in adolescents. Adolescent Medicine: State of the Art Reviews 2003;14(1):1–10.
[36] Freedman DS, Khan LK, Dietz WH, et al. Relationship of childhood obesity to coronary heart disease risk factors in adulthood: the Bogalusa Heart Study. Pediatrics 2001;108(3): 712–8.

[37] Adams PF, Dey AN, Vickerie JL. Summary health statistics for the U.S. population: National Health Interview Survey, 2005. National Center for Health Statistics. Vital Health Stat 2007;10(233):1–104.
[38] Blake KV, Gurrin LC, Evans SF, et al. Maternal cigarette smoking during pregnancy, low birth weight and subsequent blood pressure in early childhood. Early Hum Dev 2000;57: 137–47.
[39] Law M. Dietary fat and adult diseases and the implications for childhood nutrition: an epidemiologic approach. Am J Clin Nutr 2000;72(Suppl 5):1291S–6S.
[40] Lawson MA, Blythe MJ. Pelvic inflammatory disease in adolescents.Pediatr Clin North Am 1999;46:767–82.
[41] Buchan H, Vessey M, Goldacre M, et al. Morbidity following pelvic inflammatory disease. Br J Obstet Gynaecol 1993;100:558–62.
[42] Office of Strategy and Innovation (OSI), Centers for Disease Control and Prevention (CDC). Healthy people in every stage of life. Health protection goals: criteria and objectives. Atlanta (GA). Available at: http://www.cdc.gov/about/goals. Accessed April 7, 2007.
[43] Office of Strategy and Innovation (OSI), Centers for Disease Control and Prevention (CDC). Healthy people in every stage of life. Health protection goals: criteria and objectives. Atlanta (GA). Available at: http://www.cdc.gov/osi/goals/people/people0to3.html. Accessed April 7, 2007.
[44] Office of Strategy and Innovation (OSI), Centers for Disease Control and Prevention (CDC). Healthy people in every stage of life. Health protection goals: criteria and objectives. Atlanta (GA). Available at: http://www.cdc.gov/osi/goals/people/people4to11.html. Accessed April 7, 2007.
[45] Office of Strategy and Innovation (OSI), Centers for Disease Control and Prevention (CDC). Healthy people in every stage of life. Health protection goals: criteria and objectives. Atlanta (GA). Available at: http://www.cdc.gov/osi/goals/people/people12to19.html. Accessed April 7, 2007.
[46] Dietz WH. Health consequences of obesity in youth. Childhood predictors of adult disease. Pediatrics 1998;101(15):518–25.
[47] Albertson AM, Tobelmann RC, Marquart L. Estimated dietary calcium intake and food sources for adolescent females: 1980–1992. J Adolesc Health 1997;20:20–6.
[48] Golden NH, Shenker IR. Amenorrhea in anorexia nervosa: etiology and implications. Adolesc Med 1992;3:503–18.

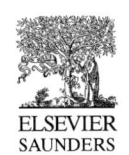

Youth Survival: Addressing the Role of Promoting the Acquisition of the Prosocial Triad and Other Survival Skills in Youth

Helen D. Pratt, PhD[a],*, Brandy M. Pratt, MA[b], Mila Sackett[c]

[a]*Behavioral and Developmental Pediatrics Division, Michigan State University/Kalamazoo Center for Medical Studies, 1000 Oakland Drive, Kalamazoo, MI 49048, USA*
[b]*Pratt & Associates, 2988 N. 30th Street, Kalamazoo, MI 49048, USA*
[c]*Western Michigan University, Kalamazoo, MI 49008, USA*

The journey from childhood to adulthood can present many obstacles to youth along the way. Adolescents will make mistakes in their quest to learn, experience, and grow. The literature on adolescent criminals, delinquents, and adolescents with serious mental and behavioral health issues generally focuses on interventions that include teaching youth problem-solving, social, assertiveness, anger management, empathy, perspective-taking, and self-control skills [1–6]. Some theorists offer that youth who are competent, flexible, and have good self-control are more likely to be successful and experience more positive relationships with parents, teachers, and peers.

The family physician sees a number of children and adolescents in the office who present with emotional or behavior problems that range from mild to severe. The ability to recognize and encourage their parents and teachers to focus on teaching these youth prosocial skills will give parents and teachers an opportunity to help these youth maximize rewards and experience fewer problems.

This article addresses the issue of teaching youth skills that will help them to maximize opportunities and positive consequences and minimize exposure to negative consequences in their lives. These skills will allow them to mature into mentally healthy productive members of society.

---

* Corresponding author.
E-mail address: pratt@kcms.msu.edu (H.D. Pratt).

Essential skills that are critical to allow this maturational process include developing prosocial skills; the ability to recognize, discriminate the level of threat, and use strategies to avoid danger; and the ability to adapt to the changing demands of his or her environment [1–6].

Defining the prosocial triad

The prosocial triad consists of a set of skills that, from a developmental perspective, is the attainment of developmental milestones that indicates that the individual is able to experience and exhibit altruism, empathy, and self-control. The ability to master this prosocial triad can contribute significantly to a person's success at initiating and maintaining intimate personal relationships, accessing positive responses from others, and being able to manage one's emotions and behaviors; consequently, these teens are more likely to manage their own lives successfully. For this discussion, altruism, empathy, and self-control are considered subsets of behavior under the classification of prosocial skills.

Issues that predict low prosocial behavior and high victimization in youth include poverty, multiple household moves, low level of mother's education, predicted increases in emotional problems, and disadvantaged school experience. Children who have prosocial behaviors have increased social competence, and those with greater school disadvantage have decreased social competence [7]. Children who live in environments in which they are victimized and not taught prosocial skills learn that the world is a hostile place and that they must fight for what they want.

Altruism

Altruism is the act of performing selfless acts with the best interests and welfare of someone else in mind. The focus is on the needs of the other person instead of on oneself. Often, altruistic acts are portrayed as potentially self-destructive because the performer overlooks his or her personal health, safety, or best interests; this action is not the form of altruism suggested by the authors of this article. Developmentally, altruism requires the ability to engage in abstract thinking, to see another's point of view, and to know what values his or her family embraces with respect to helping others; this skill is most likely developing well during middle adolescence (ages 11–13 years) [8–10].

For example, Mary (age 12) notices that there is a new kid at her school. [Acceptance, especially in the middle school adolescent years, is extremely important to a child's sense of self-worth.] The "new kid" is not wearing the "right clothes" and has not had a chance to meet anyone in the school. Mary's friends dress a certain way and have shunned other youth who did not meet their grooming and clothing standards. Regardless of these circumstances, Mary notices that the new person has no friends and sits alone at lunch; Mary decides that she should go over and befriend this person. She considers the ramifications if one of her friends or classmates were to see this behavior and tell her "clique." Mary knew from past experience that her friends might denounce her for such an act.

She felt strongly that the new person was lonely and needed a friend; despite the risk to herself and her reputation, she goes and sits with the new kid. This act of kindness was done to help another and not Mary. Although Mary may have felt good for engaging in the act, her behavior would not benefit her socially. Such bold action could damage her friendships with her "clique." Mary was able to overlook the possibility of a detrimental effect on her own life because the welfare of the new kid was at the forefront of her concerns.

Empathy

Empathy is the ability to understand what another person is feeling by putting oneself in his/her position. Empathy goes beyond simply feeling sorry for a person in an unfortunate or trying situation. It is actually being able to relate to and understand how the person feels in relation to what they are experiencing. Empathy is an understanding of someone else's feelings from the inside looking out—as opposed to sympathy, which is given from the outside looking in. If one is able to take another person's perspective, he or she will be more likely to understand the other person's experience and feelings.

This skill usually is not present in children until about 10 years of age; the complexity of this skill expands as the individual matures [4,8–12]; however, by the age of 2 years, children normally begin to display the fundamental behaviors of empathy by having an emotional response that corresponds with another person [13]. Even earlier, at 1 year of age, infants have some rudiments of empathy, in the sense that they grasp the intentions of other people. Sometimes, toddlers will comfort others or show concern for them as early as 24 months of age. Also, during the second year, toddlers play games of falsehood or "pretend" in an effort to fool others, and this requires that the child knows what others believe before he or she can manipulate those beliefs [13].

A helpful example to better understand empathy in adolescence is when two adolescents have a shared experience and are able to alter their actions based on their ability to empathize with the other adolescent. Take, for example, a child who was physically abused at some time in his or her life and who witnesses another child suffering from some form of abusive behavior. Normally, George is a bully; he is often mean to other youth who are clumsy and not good at sports. One day on the school playground, George encountered a child who was being bullied by three children. The teachers broke up the actions; the abused child went to another part of the playground and sat down, alone, and looked sad. George thought about how he felt when he was being hurt. His understanding and compassion for this other person was more complicated than just feeling sorry for that person. George walked over to the child and said "Hi." He sat down and told his story to the other child, who was happy for George's friendship and began to talk about his pain. The two individuals found that they had a lot in common, and each believed that the other "understood" his plight. Each child could relate to the other's feelings through first-hand experience. They were able to put themselves in the position of the other and thoroughly experience how he was feeling.

Self-control

Self-control is the ability to regulate the expression of one's desires, impulses, emotions, and actions. It is to be in total command of oneself to the point that one can control directly if and how one's actions are performed and how one's desires, impulses, and emotions are manifested. Self-control involves restraining oneself from acting instinctively, and it often is the difference between being "reactive" and being "proactive" [8-10].

Fighting presents the opportunity for displaying self-control, and it arises often during adolescent years. Obeying an impulse is when an adolescent, for whatever reason, punches another adolescent. The impulse for the adolescent who was assaulted is to respond physically, perhaps returning the punch. Retaliation may be the desired response; however, if that adolescent makes a conscious decision not to act on that impulse and seeks another means of resolving the situation (eg, telling a responsible adult or simply walking away), this child is exhibiting self-control. Individuals learn self-control through recognizing the demands and expectations of a particular situation and then behaving in a manner that will not endanger one's safety or get one into trouble with authority figures.

Youth who cannot learn self-control skills are at increased risk for experiencing personal distress in compromised social functioning; youth who exhibit externalizing (anger and aggression directed at self or others) problems respond well to empathy. Concern for their emotions and needs help them reduce or inhibit antisocial behavior towards others [2].

Defining recognition, discrimination, and danger-avoidance skills

Recognition/detection/avoidance skills

To learn new skills and avoid danger, youth must learn to recognize and evaluate the nature of the situation they are facing. Many youth get into situations that can cause them problems with parents or teachers. They do not know how to get out of the situation or when to exit. One example is the child who is playing with a group of friends on the floor of the classroom; the teacher has stepped out of the room and the children are supposed to be at their desks reading. The teacher walks back toward the classroom and stands outside of the door talking with another person. She places her hand on the doorknob. Paul hears the teacher's voice coming closer to the classroom and sits back at his desk. He touches his friend and looks toward the door. His friend sits back at his desk and resumes working. Alex hears the teacher touch the doorknob and follows suit. Ronnie and Eddie continue to play. The teacher opens the door and Ronnie turns, sees the teacher, and runs to his seat. Eddie is the last "man standing" and gets caught. The teacher yells "What are you doing out of your seat?"; the game is on.

Children like Eddie often repeatedly get in to trouble at school and in group situations. Once teachers become frustrated with a child's behavior problems, parents will be asked to seek a medical evaluation for treatment of the externalizing behaviors. Parental frustration with their child's misbehavior or interference with academic progress may also result in a visit to their family physician to have their child evaluated for the presence of ADHD or other disruptive behavior disorders.

Learning to recognize the characteristics of a situation, detect the changes in that situation, and identify the changes in behavior that are required may allow the child or adolescent to avoid getting into trouble or putting him or herself in a dangerous situation.

Adaptive/flexibility skills

To get ready to learn the next set of requisite skills essential to their success, they must (a) learn how to adapt to the changing conditions within which they must operate, and (b) be willing to work with others, compromise, and be flexible. Research on resilient children supports these skills as being invaluable (Box 1) [14].

Intervention programs

In response to the myriad of social issues regarding youth, many intervention programs have been developed as proactive and reactive measures to combat negative behaviors in youth [15,16]. Most programs eventually focus specifically on promoting prosocial behavior in youth. Often, youth workers in these programs are trained by organizations such as the National Training Institute for Community and Youth Work at the Academy of Education. They are taught youth-development techniques that advance successful youth outcomes. The outcomes are the knowledge, skills, and abilities that youth need to become well-adjusted young adults. Although intervention programs come in all shapes and sizes, more often than not they are centered on schools and other educational institutions because that is where the children are.

> **Box 1. Resilient youth**
>
> Youth who seem to resist peer pressure, violence, drugs, and juvenile delinquency share the following characteristics:
> - They have strong support systems.
> - They have consistent living and educational conditions.
> - They are socially competent.
> - They are responsive.
> - They have caring attitudes.
> - They have good problem solving skills.
> - They are flexible.
> - They have good abstract-thinking skills.
> - They have well-developed conceptual and intellectual-thinking skills.
> - They have good communication skills.
> - They have a sense of humor.
> - They have a positive sense of autonomy and independence.
> - They have high self-esteem.
> - They have impulse control.
> - They have good planning and goal-setting skills.
> - They have a future orientation.
> - They have hope.
>
> ---
>
> *Data from* Resnick MD, Bearman PS, Blum RW, et al. Protecting adolescents from harm: findings from the National Longitudinal Study on Adolescent Health. JAMA 1997;278(10):823–32.

There are five types of intervention programs: home-based programs, community-based programs, state programs, federal programs, and private programs. Although each category has its own venue, expertise, and desired outcome, they have learned to collaborate and integrate their services in response to the often interrelated problem behaviors that are seen in youth [15]. Federal funding is another motivator for collaboration; most new funding opportunities require cooperation among the five types of programs as well as parental and youth involvement. In recent years, faith-based initiatives have resulted in many grants requiring the participation of the faith-based community [16].

Summary

Youth who learn to understand their neighbors will be less likely to become aggressive toward those people or engage in any antisocial behavior (eg, stealing, fighting, name calling or other aggressive acts). There is strong evidence that early problem behavior is linked to later adolescent delinquency and serious adult criminality.

References

[1] Espelage DL, Swearer SM. Research on school bullying and victimization: what have we learned and where do we go from here? School Psych Rev 2003;32(3):365–83.
[2] Liew J, Eisenberg N, Losoya SH, et al. Children's physiological indices of empathy and their socioemotional adjustment: does caregivers' expressivity matter? J Fam Psychol 2003;17(4): 584–97.
[3] Eamon MK, Mulder C. Predicting antisocial behavior among Latino young adolescents: an ecological systems analysis. Am J Orthopsychiatry 2005;75(1):117–27.
[4] Eisenberg N. Empathy-related emotional responses, altruism, and their socialization. In: Davidson RJ, Harrington A, editors. Visions of compassion: Western scientists and Tibetan Buddhists examine human nature. London: Oxford University Press; 2002. p. 131–64.
[5] Valiente C, Nancy Eisenberg N, Fabes RA, et al. Reduction of children's empathy-related responding from their effortful control and parents' expressivity. Dev Psychol 2004;40(6): 911–26.
[6] Chaiken M, Huizinga D, American Society of Criminology Task Force Reports. Criminal justice issues: early prevention of and intervention for delinquency and related problem behavior. Washington, DC: U.S. Department of Justice. Office of Justice Programs National Institute of Justice 1–10 NCJ 158837.
[7] Hoglund WL, Leadbeater BJ. The effects of family, school, and classroom ecologies on changes in children's social competence and emotional and behavioral problems in first grade. Dev Psychol 2004;40(4):533–44.
[8] Soukhanov AH, Ellis K, Severynese M, editors. The American heritage dictionary of the English language. 3rd edition. Boston: Houghton Mifflin Company; 1992. p. 56, 603, 1636.
[9] Myers T, editor. Mosby's dictionary of medicine, nursing and health professionals. St. Louis: Mosby Elsevier; 2006. p. 73, 636.
[10] Knoff H. The assessment of child and adolescent personality. New York: Guilford Press; 2003. p. 364.
[11] Batson CD. Why act for the public good? Four answers. Pers Soc Psychol Bull 1994;20: 603–10.
[12] Hoffman ML. The contribution of empathy to justice and moral judgment. In: Eisenberg N, Strayer J, editors. Empathy and its development. Cambridge (MA): Cambridge University Press; 1987. p. 47–80.
[13] Feldman RS. Development across the life span. Upper Saddle River (NJ): Prentice Hall; 1997.
[14] Resnick MD, Bearman PS, Blum RW, et al. Protecting adolescents from harm: findings from the National Longitudinal Study on Adolescent Health. JAMA 1997;278:823–32.
[15] Morley E, Rossman SB. Helping at-risk youth: lessons from community-based initiatives. Washington, DC: The Urban Institute 1997.
[16] Holder HD, Gruenewald PJ, Ponicki WR, et al. Effect of community-based interventions on high-risk drinking and alcohol-related injuries. JAMA 2000;284:2341–7.

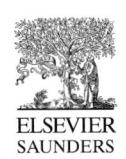

Cross-Cultural Assessment and Management in Primary Care

Helen D. Pratt, PhD*, Roger W. Apple, MA

Behavioral and Developmental Pediatrics Division, Michigan State University/Kalamazoo Center for Medical Studies, 1000 Oakland Drive, Kalamazoo, MI 49048, USA

The shifting demographics in the population of the United States are contributing to the increasing demands for a medical care delivery system that is more responsive to the needs of multicultural groups. Currently, European Americans comprise approximately 67% of the US population; however, in some areas of the West and East Coasts and along the Mexican border, European Americans no longer represent the majority [1]. It is expected that by the year 2030, approximately 40% of the American population is likely to be composed of racial and ethnic minority groups. By the year 2050, Latinas and Latinos are projected to be the largest minority group, consisting of more than 100 million persons [1,2].

Despite significant medical advances made over the past century to improve health outcomes among the overall population, ethnic minority populations have not benefited from such improvements, as evidenced by their dramatically shorter life spans, higher morbidity rates, and continued lack of access to quality care [3]. This article addresses the background terminology helpful in understanding "cross-cultural" assessment and management in primary care. Techniques for providing cross-cultural assessment and management skills are introduced, along with a list of additional resources (Box 1).

Terminology

Ethnicity

The terms or labels *ethnicity* and *ethnic group* are not actually based on scientific biologic classifications or active religious practices [4]. Such terms

---

* Corresponding author.
  E-mail address: pratt@kcms.msu.edu (H.D. Pratt).

> **Box 1. Additional resources for increasing cross-cultural competence**
>
> 1. Brittingham A, de la Cruz GP. Ancestry 2000. Washington (DC): United States Census Bureau; 2004.
> 2. Department of Health and Human Services. Mental health: culture, race, and ethnicity—a supplement to mental health: a report of the surgeon general. Rockville (MD): US Department of Health and Human Services, Substance Abuse and Mental Health Services Administration, Center for Mental Health Services; 2001. SMA-01-3613. Available at: http://www.mentalhealth.org/cre/toc.asp.
> 3. Martin P, Midgley E. Immigration: shaping and reshaping America. Revised and updated 2nd edition. Population bulletin 61(4). Washington (DC): Population Reference Bureau; 2006.
> 4. University of Massachusetts Medical School, Office of Community Programs. Physician toolkit and curriculum: resources to implement cross-cultural clinical practice guidelines for Medicaid practitioners. Washington (DC): US Department of Health and Human Services, Office of Minority Health; 2004.
> 5. US Government Accountability Office (GAO). American community survey: key unresolved issues. Washington (DC): US Government Printing Office; 2004. Available at: www.gao.gov/new.items/d0582.pdf. Accessed August 20, 2005.
> 6. The Annie E. Casey Foundation and the Population Reference Bureau. Kids count census 2000. Available at: http://www.prb.org/pdf05/ChildrenInImmigrant.pdf. Accessed January 10, 2005.

or classifications as *race*, *ethnic group*, and *class* are social myths because their existence depends largely on imaginary and unidentifiable themes. For purposes of clarifying for the reader how these terms are used, however, a discussion follows.

In the United States, the term *ethnicity* refers to characteristics that distinguish individuals from most other people in the same society. These individuals are said to be members of an ethnic group. The members have ties of ancestry, culture, language, nationality, race, religion, or a combination of these things [4]. The term *ethnic group* is used especially to refer to nationality groups that have immigrated to America since approximately 1840. The groups include individuals who are of the following ancestry: African, Chinese, German, Greek, Irish, Italian, Japanese, Mexican, and Polish. Other groups include (1) Native Americans (who were in this country when the Europeans arrived), Pacific Islanders (eg, Hawaiians, Samoans), and Alaskan Indians. Some researchers label individuals of Jewish, Roman Catholic, and Protestant faiths as ethnic groups. All "ethnic groups" are said to share a common background or speech or to have a tradition of having spoken a common language [4].

Ethnocentric

A person who holds an ethnocentric view believes that his or her own culture is superior to all other cultures and groups. This belief system can result in those individuals developing prejudicial attitudes toward others, rejecting ideas from other cultures, and even persecuting individuals or groups who are different from their culture or group [5]. Ethnocentricism is the practice of this belief, and a Eurocentric view is often thought of as meeting this definition [5].

Eurocentric

The term *Eurocentric* is defined as "reflecting a tendency to interpret the world in terms of Western and especially European or Anglo-American values and experiences" [6]. Others elaborate on the term and indicate that a Eurocentric approach assumes European or Anglo-American values and experiences as absolute truth, which would make understanding the concerns of people from different cultural backgrounds almost impossible [7]. A Eurocentric approach in primary care means that physicians interpret their patients' concerns, verbal communication, nonverbal communication, and cultural background from only a European or Anglo-American perspective.

Contrary to a cross-cultural or multicultural approach to assessment and management, the Eurocentric approach virtually ignores the unique cultural variables necessary for the most effective treatment and outcomes. What is interesting about a Eurocentric approach is that most physicians are unaware they are ignoring important cultural aspects of their patients. Generally, a Eurocentric approach is not intentionally used with culturally diverse patients; rather, it is used because of a lack of awareness of the importance of addressing cultural variables in treatment.

Culture

Culture is broadly defined as referring to a group's shared set of beliefs, norms, values, and practices. A cultural group may have overlapping characteristics with other groups but differ from those other groups in specific ways, because common social groups (eg, people who share a religion, youth who participate in the same sport, or adults trained in the same profession) have their own cultures [8].

Understanding the role of culture is important, because cultural factors influence many aspects of illness, such as manifestation of symptoms, coping styles, family and community support, and willingness to seek and adhere to treatment as well as diagnosis, treatment, and service delivery. Culture is important because it has a bearing on what all people bring to the clinical setting. It can account for minor variations in how people communicate their symptoms and which ones they report. Where cultural influences end and larger societal influences begin, culture and social contexts are not only determinants but shape the mental health of minorities and alter the types of mental health services they use. Cultural misunderstandings between the patient and clinician, clinician bias, and the fragmentation of health services deter minorities from accessing and using care and prevent them from receiving appropriate care. These possibilities intensify with the demographic trends [8].

Physicians must remember that (1) culture provides the system of information that dictates beliefs and patterns of behavior within any given environment and (2) behavior and behavioral practices are learned and displayed within a cultural context. Therefore, effective assessment and intervention require attention to the cultural context in which the patient and his or her parents are immersed. Some fundamental differences that influence health values, communication, and interaction styles between American/Western and non-Western cultures are summarized in Table 1 [9].

Culture of the patient

Culture bears on (1) whether parents even seek help for their children in the first place, (2) what types of help they seek, (2) what types of coping styles they have and which ones they teach their children, (4) what type of social supports they have, (5) how much stigma they attach to physical and mental illnesses (Box 2), and (6) the meanings that people impart to their illness. The identified culture of a patient also varies between and within groups, making it essential that health care providers attempt to understand these differences when assessing, diagnosing, and treating all patients [8].

Culture of the physician

Physicians must also increase their awareness of the influence of culture on them personally. Health care in the United States is embedded in Western science and medicine, which emphasize scientific inquiry and objective evidence [9]. As physicians coming from diverse backgrounds (ie, ethnicities, cultures, religions, sexual orientations), and from other countries, enter the health care professions, they also bring with them different cultural views of the practice of medicine. Their cultures may or may not reflect Western or American science and medicine.

A group of professionals can be said to have a "culture" in the sense that they have a shared set of beliefs, norms, and values. This culture is reflected

Table 1
Cultural dynamics influencing the clinical encounter

American/Western cultures	Concepts	Non-Western cultures
Health is the absence of disease	Core health beliefs and practices	Health is a state of harmony within body, mind, and spirit
Seeks medical system to prevent disease and treat illness		
Seeks specialty practitioners (eg, physicians, nurses, psychiatrists, surgeons)		Seeks herbalists, midwives, *santiguadoras, curanderos*, priests, shamans, *espiritistas*, or voodoo priests, for example
Prevention is practiced to avoid disease in the future		Prevention of disease is not a recognized concept
Foods are used to affect biologic functioning		Foods are used to restore imbalances (eg, hot/cold, ying/yang)
Values individualism: focus on self-reliance and autonomy	Cultural values, norms, customs	Values collectivism: reliance on other and group acceptance
Values independence and freedom		Values interdependence with family and community
Values youth over elderly status		Values respect for authority and elderly status
Personal control over environment and destiny		Fate controls environment and destiny
Future oriented		Present oriented: here and now
Efficiency: time is important, tardiness is viewed as impolite		Efficiency: time is flexible, viewed as impolite or insulting
Greeting on first-name basis denotes informality to build rapport	Communication styles	Greeting on first-name basis denotes disrespect
Being direct avoids miscommunication		Being direct denotes conflict
Eye contact signifies respect and attentiveness		Eye contact is considered disrespectful
Personal distance denotes professionalism and objectivity		Close personal space is valued to build rapport
Gestures have universal meaning		Gestures have taboo meanings depending on cultural subgroups
Individual interests are valued and encouraged	Family dynamics	Individual interests are subordinate to family needs
Individual is the focus of health care decision making		Family is the focus of health care decision making
Reliance on nuclear family bonds		Reliance on nuclear and extended family networks

Adapted from University of Massachusetts Medical School, Office of Community Programs. Physician toolkit and curriculum: resources to implement cross-cultural clinical practice guidelines for Medicaid practitioners. Washington (DC): US Department of Health and Human Services, Office of Minority Health; 2004.

> **Box 2. Factors that influence care-seeking behavior**
>
> 1. Mistrust of the medical and mental health system
>   a. Minorities and poor people have historically experienced a lower quality of care.
>   b. Current medical treatments are guided by tenets of Western science and medicine, and if those treatments do not match the patient's or parents' beliefs of what is most effective for treating specific problems, they do not trust the provider and reject treatment recommendations.
> 2. Perceived negative attitudes of health care professionals
>   a. Patients and their parents may interpret the attitudes of the treating clinician as indicative of a lack of respect for them personally.
> 3. Perceptions of being discriminated against
>   a. Minorities, especially those who are poor, may believe they are being discriminated against in terms of quality of care.
> 4. Financial limitations
> 5. Lack of transportation
> 6. Language barriers
> 7. Fear of deportation
>   a. Patients and their parents who are in this country illegally may be afraid that if they seek care, they are going to be reported to immigration and deported.

in the jargon that members of a group use, in the orientation and emphasis in their textbooks, and in their mindset or way of looking at the world. Health professionals in the United States, and the institutions in which they train and practice, are rooted in Western medicine. The culture of Western medicine, launched in ancient Greece, emphasizes the primacy of the human body in disease. Further, Western medicine emphasizes the acquisition of knowledge through scientific and empiric methods, which hold objectivity paramount (Table 2) [9]. Through these methods, Western medicine strives to uncover universal truths about disease and its causation, diagnosis, and treatment.

The impact of the combination of biologic phenomena, income, lifestyle, diet, employment, and family structure was not a part of disease conceptualization until around 1900; this way of thinking gave rise to the broader field of public health. Physicians bring their personal and professional cultures into patient care [9]. Thus, when the physician and patient do not come from the same ethnic or cultural background, there is greater potential for cultural differences to emerge. Clinicians may be more likely to ignore symptoms that the patient deems important or less likely to understand the patient's fears, concerns, and needs. The physician and patient also may harbor different assumptions about what a clinician is supposed to do, how a patient should act, what causes the illness, and what treatments are available.

Role of physician bias and stereotype. Cultural backgrounds, personal biases, and stereotypes all combine to influence the attitudes and beliefs that physicians hold regarding various groups of people. These attitudes and beliefs also influence how physicians see their patients' (who are members of those groups) needs and influence what type of care the physician delivers. Clinicians often reflect the attitudes and discriminatory practices of their society. These factors can affect patient care in many ways; for example, misdiagnosis can arise from clinician bias and stereotyping of ethnic and racial minorities. It is all too easy to lose sight of the importance of culture—until one leaves the country. Travelers from the United States, while visiting some distant frontier, may find themselves stranded in miscommunications and seemingly unorthodox treatments if they seek care for a sudden deterioration in their health status [9].

Multicultural

The term *multicultural* is not consistently defined in the literature [3,10]. In this article, the authors define "multicultural" as involving the physician becoming aware of and understanding broad characteristics of a variety of ethnic groups with different cultural backgrounds. Additionally, the physician is also aware of his or her personal cultural issues [11]. Defining such terms as *cross-cultural* and *multicultural* is often difficult, because the political and social climate in the United States often dictates what word is considered appropriate and at what time in our history such terms are appropriate.

Cross-cultural

The term *cross-cultural* is also not consistently defined in the literature, and most definitions are broad in scope [12–16]. The cross-cultural relationship requires doing more than just learning about the general and specific characteristic of various ethnic groups. The physician must actively elicit specific individualized information from the patient.

Cross-cultural assessment

The process of conducting cross-cultural services is not linear. More often than not, the processes of cross-cultural assessment and management occur simultaneously. Therefore, cross-cultural assessment and management in primary care must take into account the unique cultural variables of the provider and patient that could ultimately affect the quality and outcome of

Table 2
Differences between biomedical and nonbiomedical techniques

		Nonbiomedical techniques	
Basic concepts	Biomedical techniques	Naturalistic (physical)	Personalistic (spiritual/ mental)
Views on origin of disease	Disease is caused by pathogens, biochemical, or hematologic changes attributable to environmental factors (eg, stress, poor nutrition, injury, aging process)	Illness is caused by impersonal forces (eg, cold, heat, wind, dampness) or conditions creating imbalances in bodily humors or disruption of physical function Bodily imbalances originate from foods, medicines, or changes in physical conditions (eg, pregnancy, menses, childbirth), emotions, (anger) or environment	Illness is caused by an external agent that may be supernatural (eg, God, deity), nonhuman (eg, evil spirit, ancestor), or another human being (eg, witch, sorcerer) External agent causes disease by means of theft of soul or invoking spells that affect mental or physical function
Focus of diagnosis	To identify pathogen or biochemical process responsible for abnormality Diagnostic procedure relies on physical examination and laboratory tests	To identify forces contributing to bodily imbalances Diagnostic procedure may use taking of pulse, examining tongue or eyes to determine state of internal organs, or hot-cold or ying-yang imbalances	To identify agent behind the act and render it harmless Diagnosis of physical symptoms is of secondary concern, because condition does not improve without addressing primary belief for cause of disease
Focus of treatment	Destroy or remove entity causing disease or modify or control affected body functions	Restore equilibrium of physiologic function Treatment may include herbs, food combinations, dietary restrictions, enemas, massage, poultices, acupuncture, cupping, coining, and stopping Western medication treatments Prevention includes avoiding mental, environmental, and emotional factors that affect equilibrium and balance	Primary treatment involves a curing ritual to remove object of intrusion (eg, lifting spell, reversing technique) Secondary treatment to address physical symptoms and implement cure done by herbalist Prevention of illness involves making sure social networks with people, deity, or ancestors are in good working order

(*continued on next page*)

Table 2 (*continued*)

Basic concepts	Biomedical techniques	Nonbiomedical techniques	
		Naturalistic (physical)	Personalistic (spiritual/mental)
Practitioner types used	Physicians, nurses, psychiatrists, chemists, surgeons, and specialists	Herbalists, body workers, midwives, *santiguadora*, or *curanderos*, for example	Priests, shamans, *espiritistas*, sorcerers, or voodoo priests, for example
Practicing countries	US and European societies	China (traditional), India (Ayurveda) Greece, Latin America, Caribbean, Philippines, Pakistan, or Malaysia, for example	Indigenous groups of Americas, African tribes, Asian tribes, Latin American or Caribbean groups (eg, Cuban, Puerto Rican, Haitian)

Adapted from University of Massachusetts Medical School, Office of Community Programs. Physician toolkit and curriculum: resources to implement cross-cultural clinical practice guidelines for Medicaid practitioners. Washington (DC): US Department of Health and Human Services, Office of Minority Health; 2004.

treatment. The literature offers many suggestions of how one can become more culturally competent and, ultimately, conduct a cross-cultural assessment.

Regardless of whether one is developing multicultural or cross-cultural competence, a general theme emerges suggesting that physicians focus their learning efforts on four areas: awareness, knowledge, skills, and techniques [3,17–22].

A cross-cultural approach assumes that some techniques are universal but that others are culturally unique. The cross-cultural approach expands on the multicultural approach. Whereas the multicultural approach focuses on understanding various cultures, the cross-cultural approach also takes into account how the cross-cultural relationship is experienced by the patient and the physician (see Table 1) [11]. Therefore, it is imperative to understand the purpose of universal and culturally unique factors. Cross-cultural service delivery emphasizes that providing care respectful of, and responsive to, individual patient values and preferences, which does not vary in quality based on ethnicity, socioeconomic status, or geographic location, is essential.

Awareness

The first step of cross-cultural assessment in primary care is to develop awareness of the cross-cultural variables affecting the physician-patient relationship (see Table 2). Diversity in the United States is often viewed as a dichotomous variable between black and white interactions, such that a more holistic definition of diversity is lost. The diversity is far more inclusive (eg, ethnicity, religion, social class, age, country of origin, citizenship, language, disability, language, socioeconomic status), however, and must be expanded to include many more characteristics of individuals and groups. A narrow-sighted focus excludes many other aspects of diversity and culture. To function effectively in cross-cultural interactions, physicians must develop an awareness of attitudes, beliefs, and stereotypes about race, ethnicity, country of origin, sexuality, and religion, for example [19]. A cross-culturally competent physician must be aware of the many variables in cross-cultural interactions (see Box 2; see Table 2) that shape values, beliefs, and biases toward culturally different groups [3,18].

The next part in developing awareness is understanding how one's cultural background (age, gender, race, ethnicity, national origin, religion, sexual orientation, disability, language, and socioeconomic status) shapes the physician's values, beliefs, and biases toward culturally different groups [3,18] and how these factors function in the lives of their patients [17].

The physician must also become aware of his or her personal communication style and its impact on his or her patients. This is another key component of becoming culturally competent. Verbal communication is an important aspect of data collection and decision making in medicine. Diagnosis and treatment rely on what patients and their parents tell the physician about symptoms and their nature, intensity, and impact on functioning. This can lead to a greater potential for miscommunication when physicians and patients or their parents come from different cultural backgrounds, even if they speak the same language. Overt and subtle forms of miscommunication and misunderstanding can lead to (1) misdiagnosis, (2) conflicts over treatment, and (3) poor adherence to a treatment plan. When the patient and clinician do not speak the same language, these problems intensify (see Table 2).

Conflicts between the cultural values of ethnic minorities and the more mainstream values often used in conventional medical treatment may arise if physicians do not understand the cultural values of these groups. For example, conventional treatment approaches tend to promote individualistic value systems (ie, differentiation, individuation) rather than the interdependent value systems (ie, familialism) within which minority communities are often socialized (see Table 1). The role of spirituality in healing processes, which is being increasingly acknowledged in the realm of mental health care, has not traditionally been part of formal treatment approaches, and this, too, may have an important intra- and interpersonal role among ethnic minorities [18]. Each of the factors presented in this section represents examples of what must be considered when embarking on conducting a cross-cultural assessment.

Knowledge

The next step in conducting a cross-cultural assessment in primary care is to ensure that the physician has knowledge of how these cross-cultural variables influence the interaction with his or her patient and, ultimately, the effectiveness of treatment. It is important that the physician be able to understand how professional practices are often culturally determined sociopolitical influences of various cultures, patient beliefs about illness and help-seeking behavior, interactional styles of various cultures, and knowledge of the family structure of various cultures [3].

Similar to developing awareness of one's own cultural background, the physician now needs to have knowledge of how his or her own cultural background affects his or her definition of what constitutes normal or abnormal behavior. Many behaviors, such as hallucinations, are a sign of a severe pathologic condition to many European Americans but are a normal part of some religious practices and ceremonies of some Native Americans. Physicians also need knowledge about how racism, oppression, and discrimination affect cross-cultural interactions with their patients and the appropriateness of various forms of treatment [18]. In addition, physicians need knowledge of their patients' racial identity, ethnicity, acculturation, world views, and value differences [17] as well as the ability to acquire a working knowledge of their patients' cultural practices, daily experiences, norms, and family and social structures [22].

Cross-cultural management

In this article, cross-cultural management refers to how physicians use their awareness and knowledge of cultural variables to maximize the benefit of the cross-cultural interaction. Without paying proper attention to skills and techniques, understanding, awareness, and knowledge are not sufficient for cross-cultural management [11,23].

Skills

The term *skills* refers to a combination of one's awareness and knowledge of cultural variables as well as general guidance with how to apply that awareness and knowledge in patient-specific situations. Culturally competent physicians should have the ability to recognize appropriate use of universal and cultural-specific factors and then to design and provide effective nonbiased treatment to diverse groups [3].

As part of practicing evidenced-based medicine, physicians should be aware of the exclusion of minorities in most studies of effective treatments in medical and mental health. They must work to stay abreast of new and innovative treatments and techniques that are culturally specific and relevant to diverse individual patients [18]. More specifically, physicians must be comfortable in exploring cultural differences with their patients and not view cultural differences as pathologic or negative. Of critical importance is the ability to distinguish between what is normal versus impaired functioning within specific cultures [22] and to match interventions to the expectation of the client [17].

Techniques

The current literature supports a universalistic view of cross-cultural interactions and focuses on techniques that have been proven to be effective across most cultures (universal techniques) [24]. Universal techniques remain an important component of any physician-patient interaction and should not be ignored. These techniques include (1) establishment of a positive therapeutic relationship, (2) actively eliciting and understanding patient expectations for physician-patient interactions and care, and (3) actively involving patients and their parents in clinical care and decision making [24].

Culturally specific techniques

Although a person may belong to a cultural or ethnic group, there are significant within-group differences between individual members of the group; these differences may seem minor to the physicians but are usually viewed as significant to group members. For example, the four most frequently recognized racial and ethnic minority groups in the United States are themselves quite diverse. For instance, Asian Americans and Pacific Islanders include at least 43 separate subgroups who speak more than 100 languages. Hispanics are of Mexican, Puerto Rican, Cuban, Central and South American, or other Hispanic heritage [6]. American Indian/Alaskan Natives consist of more than 500 tribes with different cultural traditions and languages. Even among African Americans, diversity has recently increased as immigrants of mixed African ancestry arrive from the Caribbean and South America. Immigrants from Africa may share ancestors with African Americans but share little else. Some members of these subgroups have largely acculturated or assimilated into mainstream US culture, whereas others speak English with difficulty and interact almost exclusively with members of their own ethnic group [6]. This means that physicians cannot simply look at a patient and his or her parents and then assume cultural characteristics. Questions about demographics generally asked during a psychosocial history interview need to be expanded (Box 3).

For example, use of personal space varies across cultures. In the United States, social space ranges from approximately 4 to 12 ft. This likely explains why many people are uncomfortable when seeing a physician, even when the physician and patient are both from the United States. The nature of the physician-patient relationship often requires that the two persons stand much closer that a minimum of 4 ft. Because of this, physicians should be aware

Box 3. Factors to address in cross-cultural assessment in primary care

Country of origin
Social class
Religion
Citizenship status
First or primary language
Parent demographics
Gender identity
Marital status of parents
Language spoken in the home
Literacy of parents
Family resources (eg, financial, social)
Family composition (parents and children and their ages and living status)

Ethnicity
Self- or parent-identified racial group
Self- or parent-identified ancestry
Psychologic resources
Sexual orientation
Academic functioning
Social functioning (eg, home, school)
Trauma history (eg, physical, emotional)
Other violence exposure
Mental health history of the youth
Mental health history of family
View of health and wellness (physical and mental health for child, adolescent, and parents)

that many of their patients feel uncomfortable at a clinic visit simply because societal norms of distance cannot always be maintained. Latin-American, Africans, African-American, and French patients are generally more comfortable with much closer social space than are many Europeans. Also part of communication style is body movement, such as eye contact and facial expressions. In many Native American cultures, direct eye contact is perceived as hostile and should not be perceived as indicative of disrespect, a lack of assertiveness, or a pathologic finding [25].

Another example of how different groups like to interact with their physician involves the communication styles of being directive and nondirective [25]. Many patients from culturally diverse backgrounds, such as Native Americans, African Americans, Latin Americans, and Asian Americans, tend to value directive forms of helping rather than nondirective forms. A directive communication style helps many culturally diverse patients, as previously mentioned, to believe that their physician is more approachable.

Summary

The increasing number of culturally diverse patients in primary care and the demands to provide culturally sensitive health care make it essential that physicians provide care that is responsive to a culturally diverse population. Physicians must use cross-cultural techniques in their assessment and management practices [6]. A cross-cultural approach in primary care has the ability to affect the quality of patient care by potentially (1) increasing effective communication between patients, their parents, and clinicians; (2) reducing misdiagnosis of patient illness; (3) increasing parental understanding of treatment recommendations; (4) increasing patient and parental trust of the treating physician and related health care professionals; and (5) increasing patient and parent (who must administer treatments) compliance with the prescribed treatment regimen [9]. The cross-culturally competent physician has the potential to increase his or her ability to provide effective and culturally responsive treatment to a wider spectrum of patients, resulting in more positive treatment outcomes [26,27].

Physicians can also benefit from using a cross-cultural approach. If physicians understand cross-cultural variables, such as (1) the patient's perception of the illness (see Table 2) and compliance, (2) the physician-patient relationship, and (3) the patient's perception of illness, they are less likely to underdiagnose or inaccurately diagnose a patient [28]. In addition, by expanding knowledge of various cultures, physicians can recognize effective trends of treatment across cultures that are not always visible when treating a homogeneous group [12].

Summary

Cross-cultural assessment and management in primary care are essential to (1) productive physician-patient relationships, (2) effective treatment, (3) increased patient compliance, and (4) improved treatment outcomes. To provide effective cross-cultural assessment and management, physicians should focus on increasing their awareness and knowledge about their own personal cultural heritage as well as that of their patients. It is also essential that physicians consistently seek out learning experiences, such as multicultural or cross-cultural classes, workshops, and seminars, to maintain current awareness and knowledge as well as effective skills and techniques. More research is needed to strengthen and refine the terms *cross-cultural* and *multicultural* as well as to develop guidelines that provide specific and detailed explanations of effective skills and techniques. This article provides a brief description of cross-cultural assessment and management in primary care; the task is now for active participation from the medical community.

References

[1] Valdez JN. Psychotherapy with bicultural Hispanic clients. In: Psychotherapy: theory, research, practice, training, 37(3): Division of Psychotherapy (29), American Psychological Association; 2000; 37(3): 240–6.
[2] Bernal G, Saez-Santiago E. Culturally centered psychosocial interventions. J Community Psychol 2006;34(2):121–32.
[3] Hansen ND, Pepitone-Arreola-Rockwell F, Greene AF. Multicultural competence: criteria and case examples. Prof Psychol Res Pr 2000;31(6):652–60.
[4] Pettigrew TF. Ethnic group. In: Nault WH, editor. World book encyclopedia, vol. 6. Chicago: World Book; 1983. p. 297.
[5] Vander Zanden JW. Ethnocentrism. In: Nault WH, editor. World book encyclopedia, vol. 6. Chicago: World Book Author; 1983. p. 297.
[6] Merriam-Webster online dictionary. Eurocentric [Web page]. Available at: http://www.m-w.com/cgibin/dictionary?book=Dictionary&;va=Eurocentric. Accessed date, 2006.
[7] Hall RE. Eurocentric bias in women's psychology journals: resistance to issues significant to people of color. European Psychologist 2003;8(2):117–22.
[8] US Department of Health and Human Services. Mental health: culture, race, and ethnicity—a supplement to mental health: a report of the surgeon general. Rockville (MD): U.S. Department of Health and Human Services, Substance Abuse and Mental Health Services Administration, Center for Mental Health Services; 2001. SMA-01–3613. Available at:. http://www.mentalhealth.org/cre/toc.asp.
[9] University of Massachusetts Medical School, Office of Community Programs. Physician toolkit and curriculum: resources to implement cross-cultural clinical practice guidelines for Medicaid practitioners. Washington, DC: U.S. Department of Health and Human Services, Office of Minority Health; 2004.
[10] Pope-Davis DB, Reynolds AL, Dings JG, Nielson D. Examining multicultural counseling competencies of graduate students in psychology. Prof Psychol Res Pr 1995;26(3):322–9.
[11] Pope-Davis DB, Liu WM, Toporek RL, Brittan-Powell CS. What's missing from multicultural competency research: review, introspection, and recommendations. Cultur Divers Ethnic Minor Psychol 2001;7(2):121–38.
[12] Zern D. Relationships among selected child-rearing variables in a cross-cultural sample of 110 societies. Dev Psychol 1984;20(4):683–90.
[13] Power M, Bullinger M, Harper A. The World Health Organization WHOQOL-100: tests of the universality of quality of life in 15 different cultural groups worldwide. Health Psychol 1999;18(5):495–505.
[14] Butcher JN, Braswell L, Raney D. A cross-cultural comparison of American Indian, Black, and White inpatients on the MMPI and presenting symptoms. J Consult Clin Psychol 1983;51(4):587–94.
[15] Leung K. Cross-cultural differences: individual-level vs. cultural-level analysis. Int J Psychol 1989;24:703–19.
[16] Triandis HC, Brislin RW. Cross-cultural psychology. Am Psychol 1984;39(9):1006–16.
[17] Sodowsky GR, Taffe RC, Gutkin TB, Wise SL. Development of the multicultural counseling inventory: a self-report measure of multicultural competencies. J Couns Psychol 1994;41(2):137–48.
[18] Fraga ED, Atkinson DR, Wampold BE. Ethnic group preferences for multicultural counseling competencies. Cultur Divers Ethnic Minor Psychol 2004;10(1):53–65.
[19] Suzuki LA, McRae MB, Short EL. The facets of cultural competence: searching outside the box. Couns Psychol 2001;29(6):842–9.

[20] Neville HA, Heppner MJ, Louie CE, Thompson CE, Brooks L, Baker CE. The impact of multicultural training on white racial identity attitudes and therapy competencies. Prof Psychol Res Pr 1996;27(1):83–9.
[21] Roberts MC, Borden KA, Christiansen MD, Lopez SJ. Fostering a cultural shift: assessment of competence in the education and careers of professional psychologists. Prof Psychol Res Pr 2005;36(4):355–61.
[22] White TM, Gibbons MBC, Schamberger M. Cultural sensitivity and supportive expressive psychotherapy: an integrative approach to treatment. Am J Psychother 2006;60(3):299–316.
[23] Maxie AC, Arnold DH, Stephenson M. Do therapists address ethnic and racial differences in cross-cultural psychotherapy? In: Psychotherapy: theory, research, practice, training. US: Division of Psychotherapy (29), American Psychological Association; 2006; 43(1): 85–98.
[24] Fischer AR, Jome LM, Frank DR, Frank JD. Reconceptualizing multicultural counseling: universal healing conditions in a culturally specific context. Couns Psychol 1998;26(4): 525–91.
[25] Sue DW. Culture-specific strategies in counseling: a conceptual framework. Prof Psychol Res Pr 1990;21(6):424–33.
[26] Chen SX, Hui NH, Bond MH, Sit AF, Wong S, Chow VY, et al. Reexamining personal, social, and cultural influences on compliance behavior in the United States, Poland, and Hong Kong. J Soc Psychol 2006;146(2):223–44.
[27] Kaul V, Khurana S, Munoz S. Management of medication noncompliance in solid-organ transplant recipients. BioDrugs 2000;13(5):313–26.
[28] Yeung A, Yu S, Fung F, Vorono S, Fava M. Recognizing and engaging depressed Chinese Americans in treatment in a primary care setting. Int J Geriatr Psychiatry 2006;21:819–23.

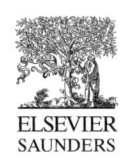

Depression in Children and Adolescents
Joseph L. Calles Jr, MD[a,b,*]

[a]College of Human Medicine, Michigan State University, Department of Psychiatry, A236 East Fee Hall, East Lansing, MI 48824, USA
[b]Psychiatry Residency Training Program, Michigan State University/Kalamazoo Center for Medical Studies, 1722 Shaffer Road, Suite 3, Kalamazoo, MI 49048, USA

Sadness is one of the basic human emotions [1] and can be triggered by any number of disturbing events—most commonly, a loss, such as the death of a loved one. The syndrome of depression may be present when sadness has no apparent triggers, is sustained beyond a time that is considered a "normal" response to identified triggers, causes a significant amount of mental suffering, or interferes with normal functioning. This article discusses the antecedents, clinical features, treatments, and course of depression in children and adolescents, focusing on major depression disorder (MDD) and dysthymic disorder (DT).

Epidemiology

An oft-quoted review of depression in childhood and adolescence [2] reports the prevalence of depression in community settings as 0.4% to 2.5% in children and 0.4% to 8.3% in adolescents. In a more recent community study of children without depression who were initially assessed between the ages of 9 and 13 years, more than 7% of boys and almost 12% of girls developed a depressive disorder by the age of 16 years [3]. From a preventative mental health perspective, it may be important to ask at what ages depression can be identified.

Infants

The exact prevalence of depression in infants is unknown. The use of a specific diagnostic system for children up to the age of 3 years was able to identify depression in 0.5% to 3% of the infants evaluated [4]. A

---

* Psychiatry Residency Training Program, Michigan State University/Kalamazoo Center for Medical Studies, 1722 Shaffer Road, Suite 3, Kalamazoo, MI 49048.
E-mail address: calles@kcms.msu.edu

researcher at New York University's Child Study Center reported to the media that "maybe one in 40 or so" of infants (or 2.5%) is depressed [5].

Preschool age

In the American Preschool Age Psychiatric Assessment Test-Retest Study (PTRTS), reported rates of depressive disorders in preschoolers (nonclinical samples) were 1.4% for MDD and 0.6% for DD [6]. Not surprisingly, MDD was more common in older preschoolers (3%) than in toddlers (0.3%). A German study [7] found that of 1887 preschoolers, 12.4% had symptoms in the clinical range of mental health problems, with the highest scale scores (for boys and girls) in the anxious/depressed category (prevalence not reported).

Children

An earlier review of the epidemiology of childhood depression [8] noted that the accurate assessment of rates of depression in children (aged 6–11 years) was hampered by inconsistent sampling and measurement techniques. Nonetheless, the authors thought that the prevalence of MDD in children was likely less than 3%, regardless the type of informant (child, parent, or teacher).

Adolescents

The rates of depression increase during childhood and into adolescence and young adulthood. At the age of 13 years, the annual incidence is 1% to 2%, and at 15 years of age, the annual incidence is 3% to 7%. Estimates are that approximately 28% of adolescents are likely to have had an episode of MDD by the age of 19 years [9].

Diagnostic features

The diagnosis of MDD and DD in younger patients follows, in general, the criteria set forth in the *Diagnostic and Statistical Manual of Mental Disorders*, 4th edition [text revision] (DSM-IV-TR) [10]. A convenient way to remember the symptoms of MDD is the use of the mnemonic "SIGECAPS" (Box 1).

Modifications in the diagnostic criteria for MDD or DD, which are established for adults, depend on the age of the patient. For example, younger patients with MDD or DD can have a mood that is irritable rather than sad. Children with MDD may not experience weight loss but may fail to gain weight as normally expected. For the diagnosis of DD in adults, the duration of illness must be at least 2 years; for children and adolescents, the diagnosis requires symptoms for only 1 year.

> **Box 1. Criteria (SIGECAPS) for the diagnosis of major depressive disorder**
>
> Two weeks of sad/irritable mood[a] and at least four of the following:
> Sleep disturbance: insomnia or hypersomnia
> Interest in activities is diminished or absent[a]
> Guilt or other thoughts of self-blame or low self-worth
> Energy is low, and the person fatigues easily
> Concentration is poor, and thinking and decision making are impaired[a]
> Appetite is poor or weight is lost (or not gained appropriately)
> Psychomotor retardation or agitation[b]
> Suicidal thoughts, plans, or attempts
>
> ---
> [a] Self-reported or observed by others.
> [b] Must be observed by others.

Infants

Sixty years ago, the psychiatrist René Spitz observed that infants separated from their mothers for extended periods (≥3 months) exhibited several pathologic signs that were indistinguishable from those of depression, including poor appetite and sleep, psychomotor retardation, emotional withdrawal, and physical illnesses [11]. In the most extreme cases, the babies died from malnutrition, even though food had been provided. What had not been provided was adequate emotional support, and he termed this unfortunate phenomenon *anaclitic* (not being able to "lean upon") depression. In the current care of infants, a failure-to-thrive picture should thus include depression as part of the differential diagnosis [12].

Preschool age

It was previously thought that younger children would express their depression indirectly through "masked" (ie, nonaffective) symptoms, such as somatic complaints and behavioral disturbances. More recent research [13] has shown that depressed preschoolers show the "typical" symptoms that are seen in older children and adolescents, however. When evaluating children in this age group, it is important to be aware that a sad or irritable mood is a sensitivity symptom for MDD but that anhedonia (loss of pleasure in usually enjoyed activities) seems to show specificity.

Children

The older school-aged child with depression tends to manifest symptoms similar to those seen in depressed adolescents and adults. Younger children who look sad may have difficulty in articulating that they feel sad, however. In prepubertal children, there may be loss of interest in social activities, but they are "unlikely to experience decreased libido" [14].

Adolescents

Depression in adolescents is diagnosed using the same criteria as used with adults. Farmer [15] approached the characterization of adolescent depression in a rather unique manner. She evaluated five depressed adolescents in great detail, which generated eight theme categories (and their associated symptom clusters). The themes can be summarized as feelings of (1) mental and physical weariness; (2) aloneness and disconnectedness, (3) uncertainty and vulnerability, (4) anger and irritability, (5) parental/familial disintegration, (6) self-punishment and escape, (7) ambivalence toward friends (relied on but also mistrusted), and (8) wanting things to be better and willing to engage in therapy.

Comorbid conditions

Anxiety disorders

There is a high degree of co-occurrence of depression and anxiety in younger people; having one of the disorders predicts the presence of the other in anywhere from around 16% to 62% of clinically identified samples [16]. Considering youth with depression, approximately 20% to 75% also have an anxiety disorder [17]. As a group, the anxiety disorders tend to develop before the depressive disorders in children who are comorbid for both [18], but there is debate as to whether the anxiety actually causes the depression [19].

Attention-deficit/hyperactivity disorder

Citing his previous work, Gillberg and colleagues [20] reported that 16% to 26% of school-aged children with attention-deficit/hyperactivity disorder (ADHD) in the community met criteria for a "depressive syndrome." Well-designed prevalence studies have shown rates of depression in the ADHD population of between 9% and 38% [21].

Oppositional defiant disorder

There is a bidirectional relation between oppositional defiant disorder (ODD) and MDD. In clinically referred youth (mean age of 10.7 years) with "severe" MDD (ie, with marked impairment), approximately 45% also met criteria for ODD; conversely, in those patients with ODD (but without conduct disorder [CD]), approximately 30% met criteria for the MDD [22].

Conduct disorder

The combination of CD and ODD increases the rate of severe MDD to almost 55% of those patients [22]. For patients with MDD, CD and ODD were present at the same time in only approximately 33% of the patients. In a detailed review of comorbidity in child and adolescent psychiatric disorders [23], the median odds ratio for the association of depression with conduct disorder was 6.6.

Substance use disorders

In one study, compared with adolescents (by the age of 16 years) without psychiatric disorders, girls with depression started using alcohol significantly earlier and boys with depression started using and abusing any drug (especially cannabis) significantly earlier [24]. In the same study, also in comparison to the nonpsychiatric group, a significant number of girls with depression (88.6%) had used any sort of drug by the age of 16 years; 86.5% of depressed boys had used any substance but also had significantly greater use of individual substances, which was different than for the girls. Although there is not a one-to-one correlation between level of depression and degree of substance use, it has been noted that, generally, a decrease in the severity of substance use is associated with a decrease in depression [25].

Developmental disorders

There are several developmental disorders in which the rate of depression is higher than that seen in the general population. In Down syndrome, depression increases with age and may confound diagnostic efforts to rule out dementia, which also occurs at higher rates in this population [26].

In a sample of 23 children (range: 5–13 years of age) with heavy prenatal exposure to alcohol and with IQs of 70 or greater, 13% were diagnosed with MDD [27]. Of those with MDD, none were diagnosed with fetal alcohol syndrome (FAS) or partial FAS and all were diagnosed with alcohol-related neurodevelopmental deficits (ARNDs), which occur three times more often than FAS.

Depression seems to be quite common in girls with fragile X syndrome, especially those with the full mutation; however, the exact prevalence is unknown, because there is a lot of overlap with other mood problems and with anxiety [28].

The various mood states and mood-driven behaviors (eg, aggression, self-injury) seen in patients with Prader-Willi syndrome can obscure an underlying depressive disorder, delaying diagnosis and treatment [29].

A study of 84 children (mean age of 11.9 years) with velocardiofacial syndrome (VCFS) showed that when compared with controls, a significant number (12%) met criteria for MDD [30].

The parents of children and adolescents with neurofibromatosis type 1 (NF-1) completed standardized behavioral checklists in two different studies [31,32]. Results show that when compared with their unaffected siblings, the children with NF-1 have increased rates of a variety of psychologic symptoms, including depression.

Medical disorders

Although many medical conditions could be discussed in relation to depression, only two, diabetes mellitus and asthma, are mentioned here.

A study conducted at an inpatient specialty unit for diabetic children reported on 92 patients who were initially enrolled with new-onset insulin-dependent diabetes mellitus (IDDM) between the ages of 8 and 13 years [33]. The median follow-up time was 9.1 years from first assessment to last visit. At entry, none of the children had a history of a depressive disorder. During follow-up, 24 patients (26.1%) had MDD or DD, and each of 4 patients with DD also had MDD.

It is well known to clinicians who care for asthmatic youth that anxiety is quite common in that patient population. Richardson and colleagues [34] looked at how anxiety and depressive symptoms (which were combined) might affect symptoms of asthma in 767 patients aged 11 to 17 years. They found that in the 2 weeks before the survey, patients with an anxiety or depressive disorder reported more symptom days, and more symptoms, than did the patients without the psychiatric disorders.

Risk factors

Risk factors for depression in childhood and adolescence can be divided into four major categories: genetics, environmental factors, negative life events, and child characteristics [35].

Genetic factors

The presence of depression in parents greatly increases the risk of their offspring developing depression, and the risk is essentially the same whether one or both parents have been depressed [36]. In addition, the onset of depression occurs earlier in those children, and the prognosis is poorer, with recurrence, severity, and associated impairment being greater than in those children without depressed parents. In multigenerational depression studies [37,38], children who had at least one grandparent and one parent with depression were at greater risk for developing an early-onset anxiety disorder. As alluded to in the section on comorbid conditions, anxiety disorders in children increase the risk for developing a depressive disorder.

Environmental factors

Interactions between a child and his or her environments (home, school, and community) affect the child's development in a cumulative fashion. The nature of environmental stressors contributes to the direction (health or illness) and degree of the developmental outcome. In the home, for example, the risk for depression in children increases when parents are negative in their outlooks, are emotionally unavailable or uninvolved, lack warmth in their interactions, are overcontrolling, or use harsh physical discipline [39]. Another variable is the use by parents (especially mothers) of a critical communication style, which is significantly higher in families with depressed children [40].

The school environment plays an important part in the lives of children and adolescents because they essentially spend half of their waking days in that setting. In addition to academic demands, there are increasing social demands, especially as children transition into adolescence. A 3-year follow-up study, beginning when the subjects were in the sixth grade, showed that peer rejection increased the risk for the development of depression, possibly by means of the element of low self-esteem [41]. There was no evidence that depression led to the rejection. On the opposite pole from rejection is victimization, including bullying. A meta-analysis of 20 years' worth of research in this area determined that of all the possible negative psychologic outcomes, depression was the most strongly correlated to peer victimization [42].

In the community, exposure to violence increases the risk for depression in younger people. The risk is especially high if they are directly victimized, if they witness someone known to them being hurt, or if they are in the early-adolescent age group [43].

Negative life events

In addition to the more chronic and pervasive effects of negative home and school environments, specific events that are out of the ordinary can lead to depression. In nonclinical protective service caseloads, the rates of MDD were found to be 18% in preadolescents and 40% in adolescents who had been abused, or approximately eight to nine times the rate seen in the general population [44].

Parental divorce adversely affects the severity and time course of child and adolescent depression. In an 11-year longitudinal study, Ge and colleagues [45] found that when compared with youth from families without divorce, boys and girls from divorced families had higher rates of depression. Girls had an earlier onset of depression, and boys had a more sustained duration of depression. Divorce also seemed to make the children and adolescents more vulnerable to concurrent stressors.

A variety of severe life events (eg, loss of parental job, death of a friend) were found to be significantly greater in the year preceding the onset of symptoms in depressed adolescents versus adolescents without depression [46]. In fact, one half of the depressed youth had experienced two or more events during that period.

Child (individual) characteristics

The findings of greater rates of depression in girls, compared with boys, after puberty have been fairly consistent [47]. The clinical phenomenology also differs in that adolescent girls develop comorbid anxiety and eating disorders, whereas adolescent boys tend to develop disruptive behavioral problems. Although the gonadotropins may play a part in the postpubertal increase in female depression, other hormonal changes (eg, dehydroepiandrosterone [DHEA], cortisol) may increase the risk for depression in both genders [48,49].

Emotional unavailability on the part of parents has been previously mentioned as a risk factor for depression. One mechanism by which this may come about is by means of a failure of the child to develop a secure attachment to caregivers [50]. More specifically, the combination of insecure attachment and a need for excessive reassurance seems to place a child at great risk for the development of severe depression [51].

If a young person lacks external support, he or she may still be able to do well relying on internal psychologic strengths. What of the child or adolescent with a negative view of the self (low self-esteem) and a pessimistic view of the world, however? That particular, fatalistic outlook increases the chances of an adolescent developing depression to twice as often as an adolescent without fatalism [52].

Protective factors

In addition to preventing, minimizing, or eliminating the previously noted risk factors, the development of depression in children and adolescents may be prevented or reduced by certain protective factors.

Social support

Beginning by the time of early elementary school, the popularity of a child increases his or her opportunities for friendships. Having friends of sufficient quantity and quality reduces loneliness and the likelihood of a child developing depression (whereas few or absent friendships lead to loneliness, which, in turn, increases the risk for becoming depressed) [53]. There is evidence that establishing dependable peer relationships in kindergarten has protective effects against depression three and four grades later [54]. In adolescents, the impact of anticipated peer support interacts with parental support; when both are high, levels of depression are low at 2-year follow-up, but when parental support is low and anticipated peer support is high, levels of depression at follow-up are actually high. This latter finding likely represents the adolescent seeking support from a deviant peer group, an obvious poor replacement for the absent support at home [55].

Personal competence

The ability to set reasonable goals and achieve them, despite intervening obstacles, leads to a sense of self-efficacy and a lowered risk of developing depression [56]. Feeling good about one's own competence, about being good at something (eg, academics or sports), is so important that it protects adolescents from becoming depressed, even in the face of maternal criticism or absence of positive feedback [57]. Involvement in sports seems to reduce the risk of depressive symptoms for boys and girls; possible mechanisms include increased social acceptance and body image satisfaction [58].

Religion and spirituality

Participation in religious activities may reduce depressive symptomatology in adolescents [59], although it is unclear if the connection is directly related to religious beliefs or indirectly related through family cohesiveness and social support. The importance of religion in reducing depressive symptoms in adolescents does not seem to be as significant as a sense of religious well-being (ie, a personal relationship with God), which is less significant than a sense of existential well-being (ie, feeling that life has purpose, joy, and a future) [60].

Treatment modalities

Psychotherapy

Although psychotherapy has been shown to be efficacious in the treatment of depression in younger people, most of the research has been conducted using cognitive-behavioral therapy (CBT) for acute-phase treatment of adolescents [61,62]. There is less research involving interpersonal therapy (IPT), family therapy, and group therapy; less research in younger children; and less research on the use of these therapies as maintenance treatments or as relapse preventatives. Nevertheless, evolving practice guidelines (American Academy of Child and Adolescent Psychiatry, Practice parameter for the assessment and treatment of children and adolescents with depressive disorders, draft 2006) suggest the use of supportive therapy for mild or uncomplicated depression and CBT or IPT, with or without medications, for more complicated depressive disorders.

Pharmacotherapy

The use of antidepressant medications in children and adolescents has grown over time. It has been estimated that 1.4 million Americans aged 18 years or younger received antidepressants in 2002 [63], with much of the increase attributed to more prescriptions for adolescents. The initial surge in use of antidepressant medications was largely attributable to the relative ease and safety of using the selective serotonin reuptake inhibitors (SSRIs) as compared with the older tricyclic antidepressants (TCAs). In addition to the safety issue, the TCAs were never much better than placebo in terms of efficacy, especially for the treatment of depression in prepubertal children [64,65].

More recently, there have emerged questions about the efficacy of the SSRIs [66] and concerns about their safety [67]. There is also much debate in this area, with some authors questioning the trustworthiness of current academic research and publishing [68], whereas others question the reliability of governmental postmarketing surveillance [69]. From a clinical standpoint, suicidal thoughts and behaviors in children and adolescents do emerge during antidepressant use; however, those symptoms tend to be mild and transient [70] and are outweighed by what seems to be an overall decrease in suicide and suicidal behaviors with the use of antidepressants [71].

Once the clinician decides to use an antidepressant in a younger person, selection of the agent should be based on the best evidence of efficacy and safety available as well as on what would be the "best fit" for that particular patient. A logical first choice is fluoxetine, given its efficacy and safety [72,73] as well as its approval for use in children 8 years of age and older. Although not approved for persons younger than the age of 18 years, the next choice of agent would be sertraline [74] or citalopram [75]. Table 1 lists the antidepressants currently available for use, their typical dosage ranges, and ages for which they are approved.

Even though it was previously stated that the TCAs are not that effective in treating depression in younger people, some treatment algorithms still include the TCAs and other older antidepressants further down the treatment sequence. The Children's Medication Algorithm Project (CMAP) proposes one such algorithm [76], although a revision is due sometime in 2007. The author uses a fairly similar approach in his own practice (Fig. 1).

Electroconvulsive therapy

Electroconvulsive therapy (ECT) is rarely used in children and adolescents, but it does remain a treatment choice for severely depressed and medication-refractory patients. Guidelines have been established [77] and should be referred to in cases in which ECT may be a legitimate option for treatment.

Transcranial magnetic stimulation

In the search for a safer alternative to ECT for severe and refractory cases of child and adolescent depression, some researchers are looking at transcranial magnetic stimulation (TMS). This particular modality has not received

Table 1
Medications used for the treatment of depressive disorders

Class (antidepressants)	Agent	Dose (daily)	Age[a] (years)
Tricyclics	Imipramine	1–2.5 mg/kg	≥18
	Nortriptyline	1–2 mg/kg	≥18
	Amitriptyline	1–2.5 mg/kg	≥12
	Doxepin	1–2.5 mg/kg	≥12
Monoamine oxidase inhibitors	Isocarboxazid	5–40 mg	≥16
	Phenelzine	7.5–45 mg	≥16
	Tranylcypromine	5–30 mg	≥18
	Selegiline (transdermal)	6, 9, or 12 mg[b]	≥18
Selective serotonin reuptake inhibitors	Fluoxetine	5–60 mg (0.25–1 mg/kg)	≥8
	Paroxetine	5–40 mg (0.25–1 mg/kg)	≥18
	Sertraline	12.5–200 mg (1.5–3 mg/kg)	≥18
	Citalopram	5–40 mg	≥18
	Escitalopram	5–20 mg	≥18
Serotonin-Norepinephrine Reuptake Inhibitors	Venlafaxine	37.5–225 mg (1–3 mg/kg)	≥18
	Duloxetine	20–40 mg	≥18
Other	Trazodone	25–300 mg (2–5 mg/kg)	≥6
	Nefazodone	25–300 mg	≥18
	Bupropion	75–300 mg (3–6 mg/kg)	≥18
	Mirtazapine	7.5–45 mg	≥18

[a] US Food and Drug Administration–approved ages for the treatment of major depressive disorder.
[b] Each patch is effective for 24 hours.

approval for use in younger people, but ongoing studies may provide us with another tool to use in difficult-to-treat patients [78].

Complementary and alternative medicine

It is not uncommon for the parents and guardians of our patients to inquire about the use of nonpharmaceutic treatments for depression. Although the author cannot recommend complementary and alternative medicine (CAM) treatments at this time, it is interesting that the ω-3 fatty acids have shown efficacy in at least one depression treatment study [79]. Further study is indicated.

Clinical course

Diligence in identifying cases of child and adolescent depression and aggressive treatment and follow-up are crucial, because these young people simply do not "grow out of it." A study from the United Kingdom [80] re-evaluated a cohort of young adults who had been diagnosed with depression a mean of 7.8 years earlier. At that later assessment, 40% had experienced recurrent depression at some time and 18% had essentially remained

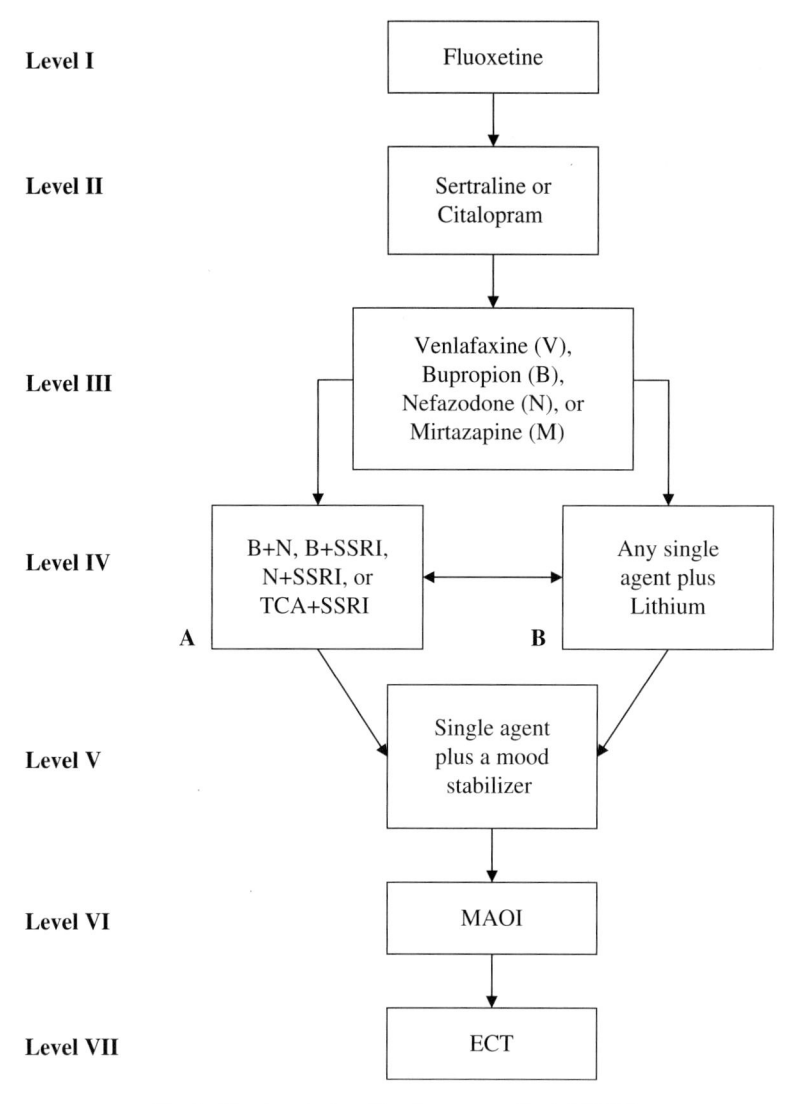

```
Level I         Fluoxetine
                   ↓
Level II        Sertraline or
                Citalopram
                   ↓
Level III       Venlafaxine (V),
                Bupropion (B),
                Nefazodone (N), or
                Mirtazapine (M)
                ↙            ↘
Level IV    B+N, B+SSRI,    Any single
            N+SSRI, or  ↔   agent plus
            TCA+SSRI         Lithium
              A                B
                ↘            ↙
Level V         Single agent
                plus a mood
                stabilizer
                   ↓
Level VI        MAOI
                   ↓
Level VII       ECT
```

Fig. 1. Treatment algorithm for uncomplicated MDD.

depressed since childhood. The greatest concern related to missed or inadequately treated depression is, of course, the increased risk of suicide (see the article by Greydanus and Calles elsewhere in this issue).

Consultation and referral

Primary care physicians usually have the first contact with a depressed child or adolescent and, in most cases, are able to provide effective treatment. Questions that may arise when treatment is not going well include the following. When should I ask for a psychiatric consult? When should I refer to a child and adolescent psychiatrist? Richardson and Katzenellenbogen [35] have recommended considering a mental health evaluation of the child when there is severity, comorbidity, suicidality, or family unreliability.

Summary

The development of depression in children and adolescents is complex and multifactorial. Similarly, the effective resolution of a depressive episode requires a multidisciplinary approach. Primary care physicians are in a unique position to provide early assessment and treatment to their depressed and vulnerable younger patients.

References

[1] Ekman P. Are there basic emotions? Psychol Rev 1992;99:550–3.
[2] Birmaher B, Ryan ND, Williamson DE, et al. Childhood and adolescent depression: a review of the past 10 years. Part I. J Am Acad Child Adolesc Psychiatry 1996;35(11):1427–39.
[3] Costello EJ, Mustillo S, Erkanli A, et al. Prevalence and development of psychiatric disorders in childhood and adolescence. Arch Gen Psychiatry 2003;60(8):837–44.
[4] Keren M, Tyano S. Depression in infancy. Child Adolesc Psychiatr Clin N Am 2006;15:883–97.
[5] ABC News- Health Online. One in 40 infants experience baby blues, doctors say. Mental health of parents can have an effect on child. 2006. Available at: http://abcnews.go.com/Health/OnCall/story?id=2640591&;page=1. Accessed December 3, 2006.
[6] Egger HL, Angold A. Common emotional and behavioral disorders in preschool children: presentation, nosology, and epidemiology. J Child Psychol Psychiatry 2006;47(3–4):313–37.
[7] Furniss T, Beyer T, Guggenmos J. Prevalence of behavioural and emotional problems among six-years-old preschool children: baseline results of a prospective longitudinal study. Soc Psychiatry Psychiatr Epidemiol 2006;41:394–9.
[8] Fleming JE, Offord DR. Epidemiology of childhood depressive disorders: a critical review. J Am Acad Child Adolesc Psychiatry 1990;29(4):571–80.
[9] Lewinsohn PM, Rohde P, Seeley JR. Major depressive disorder in older adolescents: prevalence, risk factors, and clinical implications. Clin Psychol Rev 1998;18(7):765–94.
[10] American Psychiatric Association. Diagnostic and statistical manual of mental disorders. 4th edition [text revision]. Washington, DC: American Psychiatric Association; 2000.
[11] Spitz R, Wolf KM. Anaclitic depression: an inquiry into the genesis of psychiatric conditions in early childhood. Psychoanal Study Child 1946;2:313–42.
[12] Guedeney A. From early withdrawal reaction to infant depression: a baby alone does exist. Infant Ment Health J 1997;18(4):339–49.
[13] Luby JL, Heffelfinger AK, Mrakotsky C, et al. The clinical picture of depression in preschool children. J Am Acad Child Adolesc Psychiatry 2003;42(3):340–8.
[14] Klein DN, Dougherty LR, Olino TM. Toward guidelines for evidence-based assessment of depression in children and adolescents. J Clin Child Adolesc Psychol 2005;34(3): 412–32.
[15] Farmer TJ. The experience of major depression: adolescents' perspectives. Issues Ment Health Nurs 2002;23:567–85.
[16] Brady EU, Kendall PC. Comorbidity of anxiety and depression in children and adolescents. Psychol Bull 1992;111(2):244–55.

[17] Avenevoli S, Stolar M, Li J, et al. Comorbidity of depression in children and adolescents: models and evidence from a prospective high-risk family study. Biol Psychiatry 2001; 49(12):1071–81.
[18] Kovacs M, Devlin B. Internalizing disorders in childhood. J Child Psychol Psychiatry 1998; 39:47–63.
[19] Seligman LD, Ollendick TH. Comorbidity of anxiety and depression in children and adolescents: an integrative review. Clin Child Fam Psychol Rev 1998;1(2):125–44.
[20] Gillberg C, Gillberg IC, Rasmussen P, et al. Co-existing disorders in ADHD—implications for diagnosis and intervention. Eur Child Adolesc Psychiatry 2004;13(Suppl 1):I80–92.
[21] Pliszka S. Comorbidity of attention-deficit/hyperactivity disorder with psychiatric disorder: an overview. J Clin Psychiatry 1998;59(Suppl 7):50–8.
[22] Greene RW, Biederman J, Zerwas S, et al. Psychiatric comorbidity, family dysfunction, and social impairment in referred youth with Oppositional Defiant Disorder. Am J Psychiatry 2002;159(7):1214–24.
[23] Angold A, Costello EJ, Erkanli A. Comorbidity. J Child Psychol Psychiatry 1999;40:57–87.
[24] Costello EJ, Erkanli A, Federman E, et al. Development of psychiatric comorbidity with substance abuse in adolescents: effects of timing and sex. J Clin Child Psychol 1999;28: 298–311.
[25] Chinet L, Plancherel B, Bolognini M, et al. Substance use and depression. Comparative course in adolescents. Eur Child Adolesc Psychiatry 2006;15:149–55.
[26] Chapman RS, Hesketh LJ. Behavioral phenotype of individuals with Down syndrome. Ment Retard Dev Disabil Res Rev 2000;6:84–95.
[27] O'Connor MJ, Shah B, Whaley S, et al. Psychiatric illness in a clinical sample of children with prenatal alcohol exposure. Am J Drug Alcohol Abuse 2002;28(4):743–54.
[28] Reiss AL, Dant CC. The behavioral neurogenetics of fragile X syndrome: analyzing gene-brain-behavior relationships in child developmental psychopathologies. Dev Psychopathol 2003;15:927–68.
[29] Verhoeven WMA, Tuinier S, Curfs LMG. Prader-Willi syndrome: the psychopathological phenotype in uniparental disomy. J Med Genet 2003;40:e112.
[30] Antshel KM, Fremont W, Roizen NJ, et al. ADHD, major depressive disorder, and simple phobias are prevalent psychiatric conditions in youth with velocardiofacial syndrome. J Am Acad Child Adolesc Psychiatry 2006;45(5):596–603.
[31] Kayl AE, Moore BD. Behavioral phenotype of Neurofibromatosis, Type 1. Ment Retard Dev Disabil Res Rev 2000;6:117–24.
[32] Prinzie P, Descheemaeker MJ, Vogels A, et al. Personality profiles of children and adolescents with neurofibromatosis type 1. Am J Med Genet 2003;118A:1–7.
[33] Kovacs M. Psychiatric disorders in youths with IDDM: rates and risk factors. Diabetes Care 1997;20(1):36–44.
[34] Richardson LP, Lozano P, Russo J, et al. Asthma symptom burden: relationship to asthma severity and anxiety and depression symptoms. Pediatrics 2006;118:1042–51.
[35] Richardson LP, Katzenellenbogen R. Childhood and adolescent depression: the role of primary care providers in diagnosis and treatment. Curr Probl Pediatr Adolesc Health Care 2005;35(1):6–24.
[36] Lieb R, Isensee B, Hofler M, et al. Parental major depression and the risk of depression and other mental disorders in offspring: a prospective-longitudinal community study. Arch Gen Psychiatry 2002;59:365–74.
[37] Warner V, Weissman MM, Mufson L, et al. Grandparents, parents, and grandchildren at high risk for depression: a three-generation study. J Am Acad Child Adolesc Psychiatry 1999;38:289–96.
[38] Weissman MM, Wickramaratne P, Nomura Y, et al. Families at high and low risk for depression: a 3-generation study. Arch Gen Psychiatry 2005;62:29–36.
[39] Sander JB, McCarty CA. Youth depression in the family context: familial risk factors and models of treatment. Clin Child Fam Psychol Rev 2005;8(3):203–19.

[40] Asarnow JR, Tompson M, Woo S, et al. Is expressed emotion a specific risk factor for depression or a nonspecific correlate of psychopathology? J Abnorm Child Psychol 2001; 29(6):573–83.
[41] Nolan SA, Flynn C, Garber J. Prospective relations between rejection and depression in young adolescents. J Pers Soc Psychol 2003;85(4):745–55.
[42] Hawker DSJ, Boulton MJ. Twenty years research on peer victimization and psychosocial maladjustment: a meta-analytic review of cross-sectional studies. J Child Psychol Psychiatry 2000;41(4):441–55.
[43] Lynch M. Consequences of children's exposure to community violence. Clin Child Fam Psychol Rev 2003;6(4):265–74.
[44] Kaufman J, Charney D. Effects of early stress on brain structure and function: implications for understanding the relationship between child maltreatment and depression. Dev Psychopathol 2001;13:451–71.
[45] Ge X, Natsuaki MN, Conger RD. Trajectories of depressive symptoms and stressful life events among male and female adolescents in divorced and nondivorced families. Dev Psychopathol 2006;18:253–73.
[46] Williamson DE, Birmaher B, Frank E, et al. Nature of life events and difficulties in depressed adolescents. J Am Acad Child Adolesc Psychiatry 1998;37(10):1049–57.
[47] Weller EB, Kloos A, Kang J, et al. Depression in children and adolescents: does gender make a difference? Curr Psychiatry Rep 2006;8(2):108–14.
[48] Goodyer IM, Herbert J, Tamplin A, et al. First-episode major depression in adolescents. Affective, cognitive and endocrine characteristics of risk status and predictors of onset. Br J Psychiatry 2000;176:142–9.
[49] Goodyer IM, Herbert J, Tamplin A, et al. Recent life events, cortisol, dehydroepiandrosterone and the onset of major depression in high-risk adolescents. Br J Psychiatry 2000;177: 499–504.
[50] Sund AM, Wichstrom L. Insecure attachment as a risk factor for future depressive symptoms in early adolescence. J Am Acad Child Adolesc Psychiatry 2002;41(12):1478–85.
[51] Abela JRZ, Hankin BL, Haigh EAP, et al. Interpersonal vulnerability to depression in high-risk children: the role of insecure attachment and reassurance seeking. J Clin Child Adolesc Psychol 2005;34(1):182–92.
[52] Roberts RE, Roberts CR, Chen IG. Fatalism and risk of adolescent depression. Psychiatry 2000;63(3):239–52.
[53] Nangle DW, Erdley CA, Newman JE, et al. Popularity, friendship quantity, and friendship quality: interactive influences on children's loneliness and depression. J Clin Child Adolesc Psychol 2003;32(4):546–55.
[54] Schrepferman LM, Eby J, Snyder J, et al. Early affiliation and social engagement with peers: prospective risk and protective factors for childhood depressive behaviors. Journal of Emotional and Behavioral Disorders 2006;14(1):50–61.
[55] Young JF, Berenson K, Cohen P, et al. The role of parent and peer support in predicting adolescent depression: a longitudinal community study. J Res Adolesc 2005;15(4):407–23.
[56] Bandura A, Pastorelli C, Barbaranelli C, et al. Self-efficacy pathways to childhood depression. J Pers Soc Psychol 1999;76(2):258–69.
[57] Jacquez F, Cole DA, Searle B. Self-perceived competence as a mediator between maternal feedback and depressive symptoms in adolescents. J Abnorm Child Psychol 2004;32(4): 355–67.
[58] Boone EM, Leadbeater BJ. Game on: diminishing risks for depressive symptoms in early adolescence through positive involvement in team sports. J Res Adolesc 2006;16(1): 79–90.
[59] Schapman AM, Inderbitzen-Nolan HM. The role of religious behaviour in adolescent depressive and anxious symptomatology. J Adolesc 2002;25:631–43.
[60] Cotton S, Larkin E, Hoopes A, et al. The impact of adolescent spirituality on depressive symptoms and health risk behaviors. J Adolesc Health 2005;36:529.e7–529.e14.

[61] Asarnow JR, Jaycox LH, Tompson MC. Depression in youth: psychosocial interventions. J Clin Child Psychol 2001;30(1):33–47.
[62] Curry JF. Specific psychotherapies for childhood and adolescent depression. Biol Psychiatry 2001;49:1091–100.
[63] Vitiello B, Zuvekas SH, Norquist GS. National estimates of antidepressant medication use among U.S. children, 1997–2002. J Am Acad Child Adolesc Psychiatry 2006;45(3):271–9.
[64] Geller B, Reising D, Leonard HL, et al. Critical review of tricyclic antidepressant use in children and adolescents. J Am Acad Child Adolesc Psychiatry 1999;38:513–6.
[65] Hazell P, O'Connell D, Heathcote D, et al. Tricyclic drugs for depression in children and adolescents. Cochrane Database of Systematic Reviews 2002;2:CD002317. doi: 10.1002/14651858.
[66] Safer DJ. Should selective serotonin reuptake inhibitors be prescribed for children with major depressive and anxiety disorders? Pediatrics 2006;118(3):1248–51.
[67] Wohlfarth TD, van Zwieten BJ, Lekkerkerker FJ, et al. Antidepressants use in children and adolescents and the risk of suicide. Eur Neuropsychopharmacol 2006;16(2):79–83 [Epub 2005 Nov 18].
[68] Leo J. The SSRI trials in children: disturbing implications for academic medicine. Ethical Hum Psychol Psychiatry 2006;8(1):29–41.
[69] Klein DF. The flawed basis for FDA post-marketing safety decisions: the example of antidepressants and children. Neuropsychopharmacology 2006;31(4):689–99.
[70] Gualtieri CT, Johnson LG. Antidepressant side effects in children and adolescents. J Child Adolesc Psychopharmacol 2006;16(1–2):147–57.
[71] Bostwick JM. Do SSRIs cause suicide in children? The evidence is underwhelming. J Clin Psychol 2006;62(2):235–41.
[72] Emslie GJ, Rush J, Weinberg WA, et al. A double blind, randomized, placebo-controlled trial of fluoxetine in children and adolescents with depression. Arch Gen Psychiatry 1997;54:1031–7.
[73] Emslie GJ, Heiligenstein JH, Wagner KD, et al. Fluoxetine for acute treatment of depression in children and adolescents: a placebo-controlled, randomized clinical trial. J Am Acad Child Adolesc Psychiatry 2002;41:1205–15.
[74] Wagner KD, Ambrosini P, Rynn M, et al. Efficacy of sertraline in the treatment of children and adolescents with major depressive disorder: two randomized controlled trials. JAMA 2003;290(8):1033–41.
[75] Wagner KD, Robb AS, Findling RL, et al. A randomized, placebo-controlled trial of citalopram for the treatment of major depression in children and adolescents. Am J Psychiatry 2004;161:1079–83.
[76] Hughes CW, Emslie GJ, Crismon ML, et al. The Texas Children's Medication Algorithm Project: report of the Texas Consensus Conference Panel on medication treatment of childhood Major Depressive Disorder. J Am Acad Child Adolesc Psychiatry 1999;38(11):1442–54.
[77] American Academy of Child and Adolescent Psychiatry. Practice parameter for use of electroconvulsive therapy with adolescents. J Am Acad Child Adolesc Psychiatry 2004;43(12):1521–39.
[78] Morales OG, Henry ME, Nobler MS, et al. Electroconvulsive therapy and repetitive transcranial magnetic stimulation in children and adolescents: a review and report of two cases of epilepsia partialis continua. Child Adolesc Psychiatr Clin N Am 2005;14(1):193–210, viii–ix.
[79] Nemets H, Nemets B, Apter A, et al. Omega-3 treatment of childhood depression: a controlled, double-blind pilot study. Am J Psychiatry 2006;163(6):1098–100.
[80] Dunn V, Goodyer IM. Longitudinal investigation into childhood- and adolescence-onset depression: psychiatric outcome in early adulthood. Br J Psychiatry 2006;188:216–22.

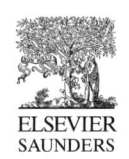

Suicide in Children and Adolescents
Donald E. Greydanus, MD[a],*, Joseph Calles, Jr., MD[b]

[a] *Pediatrics and Human Development, Michigan State University College of Human Medicine, Michigan State University/Kalamazoo Center for Medical Studies, 1000 Oakland Drive, Kalamazoo, MI 49008–1284, USA*
[b] *Department of Psychiatry, Michigan State University College of Human Medicine, Psychiatry Residency Training Program, Michigan State University/Kalamazoo Center for Medical Studies, 1722 Shaffer Road, Suite 3, Kalamazoo, MI 49048, USA*

Suicide in children and adolescents has long been of concern to society. In 1910, the Vienna Psychoanalytic Society held a conference dealing with what was perceived to be a growing epidemic of youth suicide. Experts who attended included Sigmund Freud, who believed that major reasons for adolescent suicide included conflicts over love and academic pressure from schools. One of the publications blamed for the increase in youth suicide was Goethe's *The Sorrows of Young Werner*, which centered on a youth who committed suicide by shooting himself after the loss of his love interest; although this work was published in the early nineteenth century, it was believed to be a factor at the 1910 Vienna conference. The conclusion of this meeting was that more research into adolescent suicide was needed, similar to the conclusion of the US Surgeon General's report published several decades later [1].

Childhood suicide

There are limited data on the subject of childhood suicide, because there is limited research on this subject, and because of the conclusion of some researchers that children are not capable of suicide per se [2,3]. Such data are often hidden in data that look at ages 10 to 14 or 5 to 14 years, whereas other information only looks at adolescent suicide. Because the start of puberty can vary widely, it may be difficult to separate out "childhood" from "adolescent" suicide. Despite this ambiguity, experts conclude that rates of suicide in the 5 to 14 year old has increased over the past 30 years in the

---

* Corresponding author.
E-mail address: greydanus@kcms.msu.edu (D.E. Greydanus).

United States, going from 0.4 per 100,000 in 1979 to 0.8 per 100,000 in the 1990s [2,3]. There were approximately 324 suicides among 5 to 14 year olds in 1998; worldwide, there are 0.5 per 1000 in girls and 0.9 per 1000 in boys in this same age cohort [2,3]. The male to female ratio for 5 to 14 year olds is 3:1 versus a 1:1 for 10 to 14 year olds and 6:1 for 15 to 24 year olds [2,3].

Reasons for childhood suicides are listed in Box 1. The concept of "death" is a complex and emotional issue; only very slowly does the child learn what it actually means from an adult perspective [4]. Preschool children usually identify death with sleeping, although most 6 or 7 year olds state they know that everyone dies. Death is often a concept that is observed by children as they see their relatives die and as they see animals die. Children do not typically appreciate the finality of death before puberty is reached, and even then, those in early puberty do not understand that healthy individuals also can die.

The concept that children can really attempt suicide is a controversial one, although one study of 1528 parents noted that these parents stated 4% of their children had attempted suicide [4]. Most parents are reluctant to discuss the topic of suicide with their children, who often learn about this topic from the media. School officials also typically do not discuss the concept of suicide with the children in their schools. The media teaches children that suicide is what cartoon characters or movie humans do after the loss of a romantic love or when one becomes very angry or frustrated; depression is typically not a motive for suicide in the media's portrayal of ending one's own life. Other reasons for movie characters to end their life are when one does get one's way or because there is a need for revenge after being seriously wronged in some way.

Adolescent suicide

Worldwide

An estimated 2 million people die each year as a result of homicide or suicide [5–7]; in 2002, there were an estimated 877,000 suicides in the world [8].

Box 1. Reasons for childhood suicide

1. Depression
2. Family and environmental dysfunction
3. Disruptive behavior (males)
4. Substance abuse (males)
5. Schizophrenia
6. Suicide behavior as a child predicts suicide behavior as a teenager or adult

---

Suicides are among the three leading causes of death for adolescents in the world and rates are rising faster in teenagers than in other age groups; at least 90,000 adolescents (up to age 19) commit suicide each year in the world (one every 5 minutes) in the context of 4 million suicide attempts each year [9,10]. Research suggests that 100,000 to 200,000 young people (15–24 years) commit suicide each year [8,11–18].

Suicide rates vary around the world, as noted in Table 1. The lowest rates are reported in Latin America and Middle East Arabic countries, with rates under 6.5 per 100,000 [8]. Countries with suicide rates over 30 per 100,000 are Finland, Latvia, Lithuania, New Zealand, Russian Federation, and Slovenia. Suicide rates globally are underreported because they may be

Table 1
1996 Global suicide rates (per 100,000) 15 to 24 year olds

Country	Males	Females
Greece	3.8	0.8
Portugal	4.3	2
Italy	5.7	1.6
Spain	7.1	2.2
Netherlands	9.1	3.8
Sweden	10	6.7
Japan	10.1	4.4
Israel	11.7	2.5
United Kingdom	12.2	2.3
Germany	12.7	3.4
Denmark	13.4	2.3
France	14	4.3
Bulgaria	15.4	5.6
Czech Republic	16.4	4.3
Poland	16.6	2.5
Ukraine	17.2	5.3
Hungary	19.1	5.5
Austria	21.1	6.5
Ireland	21.5	2
United States	21.9	3.8
Belarus	24.2	5.2
Canada	24.7	6
Switzerland	25	4.8
Australia	27.3	5.6
Norway	28.2	5.2
Estonia	29.7	10.6
Finland	33	3.2
Latvia	35	9.3
Slovenia	37	8.4
New Zealand	39.9	6.2
Russian Federation	41.7	7.9
Lithuania	44.9	6.7

Data from World Health Organization. Available at: http://www.unicef.org/pon96/insuicid.htm.

classified as accidents or not classified at all. In industrialized countries, four times as many males commit suicide as females. The exact place that suicide has in the deaths of adolescents and young people depends on what other factors are operational in that country, as noted in Box 2 [9,11,12].

Suicide was more common in adolescent boys of European descent in Australia, United States, and New Zealand. It is now equal or more prevalent in minority and indigenous populations: African Americans and Native Americans in the United States, Aboriginal and Torres Straight Islanders in Australia, and Pacific Islanders in New Zealand. Increased suicide rates over the last part of the twentieth century were reported in Spain, China, and other parts of Asia, the Caribbean, and Africa [9,19].

United States

Suicides in the 15 to 24 year old have changed historically in the United States in response to various factors. These rates were high in the 1930s, dropped in the 1940s to 1950s, increased in the late 1950s to 1980s, and then stabilized or dropped somewhat from the 1990s to the middle of the twenty-first century's first decade [20,21]. In the United States, suicide rates for 15 to 19 year olds doubled from 1960 to 2001, peaking in the early 1990s; there was a 250% increase from the 1960s to the 1980s. Epidemiologists call the increase in suicides in the 15- to 24-year-old group after World War II the "baby boomer cohort." The estimated suicide rate for those 15 to 19 years of age in 2000 was 10 per 100,000 (14.6 in boys and 2.9 in girls) [18]. Suicide represents about 12% of annual deaths in the 15 to 19 year old (Table 2). In 1998, there were 4135 suicides for those 15 to 24 years of age and in 2001, the rates were 12.9 in males and 2.7 in females. Ethnic distribution of suicides in 15 to 24 year olds in 1998 are listed in Table 3;

Box 2. Causes of death in adolescents and young adults in different countries (decreasing order of frequency)

Africa: AIDS, other IFs, homicide or war, UIs, suicide
South East Asia: UIs, other IFs, AIDS, suicide, homicide or war
South America and Caribbean: Homicide or war, UIs, suicide, other IFs, AIDS
Western Pacific: UIs, suicide, other IFs, homicide or war, AIDS
Europe: UIs, suicide, homicide or war, other IFs, AIDS
Eastern Mediterranean: UIs, other IFs, homicide or war, AIDS, suicide
North America: UIs, suicide, homicide, cancer, other IFs, AIDS

IFs, infections; UIs, unintended injuries.

Table 2
Causes of death in 15 to 24 year olds in 2000

Unintentional injuries	14,113
Homicide	4939
Suicide	3994
Malignant neoplasms	1713
Cardiac causes	1031
All causes	31,307

Data from references [8], [15], and [17].

annual rates for African American males increased from 2.9 per 100.000 in 1981 to 6.1 per 100,000 in 1998 [17].

In the United States, there were 31,655 deaths from all causes in 2002 in the 15- to 24-year age group; this included about 2000 suicides in the 15- to 19-year age group and 2000 in those 20 to 24 years of age with an overall prevalence of 11 per 100,000 [8]. More adolescents and young people die from suicide than from deaths of these combined disorders: heart disease, cancer, cerebrovascular accidents, HIV-AIDS, chronic lung disease, pneumonia, influenza, and birth defects [1].

Twenty percent to 25% of American adolescents have seriously considered suicide and 9% have tried it at least once [22]. The 2001 Centers for Disease Control and Prevention Youth Risk Behavioral Survey noted that 19% had a suicidal ideation, 14.8% with a suicide plan; 8.8% of these youth had attempted suicide and medical attention was provided in 2.6% [17,23].

Completed suicides in the United States increased 250% in teenagers from the 1960s to the 1980s, leveling off in the late 1990s [18]. There has been a decrease in suicide rates in 10 to 19 year olds from 1992 to 2001 (6.2 per 100,000 to 4.6). Suicide is the third leading cause of death in older teenagers and fifth in those 5 to 14 years of age. The ratio of suicide attempts to actual suicide varies widely and is difficult to study because there is no national registry on suicide attempts. One study noted 6200 attempts that produced 13 deaths in boys with a ratio of 1:470; in girls there were 3 deaths in 11,200 attempts for a ratio of 1:3700 [24]. The ratio of suicide attempts to completed suicides is 3 to 1 (female to male), whereas three to five times as many boys versus girls completed suicide in 15 to 19 year olds [25,26]. Completed suicide rates are higher in girls versus boys in China and India [9].

Table 3
Ethnic distribution of suicides in 15 to 24 year olds in 1998

Group	Males	Females
White	19.3	3.5
African American	15	2.2
Hispanic	13.4	2.8

Table 4 lists methods of death in 10 to 19 year olds. In 10 to 14 year olds, hanging has become more popular than firearms; there was a drop in firearm suicides of 0.9 in 1992 to 0.4 in 2001 versus an increase in suffocation suicide of 0.5 in 1992 to 0.8 in 2001 [15,17]. In 15 to 19 year olds, there was a drop of firearm suicides of 7.3 in 1992 to 4.1 in 2001 versus an increase of suffocation suicide of 1.9 in 1992 to 2.7 in 2001. The suicide methods of choice for boys are the gun, hanging, or a motor vehicle accident, whereas girls tend to choose pill overdose or wrist cutting [26,27]. There has been a tendency for girls to use more deadly methods of suicide attempt since the mid-1990s [27].

Etiology

Although there is no biologic test for suicide or suicide risk, a number of biologic factors have been noted (Box 3) [3,28]. A major cause or precipitant to suicide in adolescents and young adults is depression. Studies note that 35% to 50% of depressed adolescents make a suicide attempt and that 5% to 10% of adolescents with severe depression (major depressive disorder) complete a suicide within 15 years of their diagnosis [29]. Table 5 lists psychiatric diagnoses noted in 121 adolescents who had attempted suicide and were then evaluated [30]. Andrews and Lewinsohn [30] reviewed six studies that contained 1265 depressed youth, noting that 60% had a history of suicidal ideation and 30% had attempted suicide; in this review, three studies looked at 466 youth after treatment and noted that 24% had attempted suicide.

One fifth to one third of disability in adolescents (10–19 years) is caused by mental disorders (psychosocial, behavioral, developmental, or psychiatric) [31]. Major depression is a major cause of such disability, and increases with age and is noted in 9 of every 1000 preschool children and 20 per 1000 of school-aged children; it is nearly 50 per 1000 in adolescents, a rate similar to that found in adults [22,32,33]. In childhood depression, there is a 1:1 male/female ratio; in adolescents and adults, there is a 1:2 male/female ratio. Depression can lead to a number of adverse events, as reflected in Box 4, and can be found with a number of comorbidities, including anxiety disorders, substance abuse disorders, and disruptive behavior disorders [33].

Table 4
Methods of suicide in 10 to 19 year olds

Firearms	49%
Suffocation (mainly hanging)	38%
Poisoning	7%
Miscellaneous[a]	6%

[a] Running into traffic, motor vehicle accidents, burning, and others.
Data from Centers for Disease Control and Prevention. Methods of suicide among persons age 10–19 years—United States, 1992–2001. MMWR Morb Mortal Wkly Rep 2004;53:471–4.

> **Box 3. Biologic factors of suicide**
>
> Low cerebrospinal fluid levels of 5-hydroxy-indolacetic acid
> Low platelet imipramine binding sites
> Nonsuppressed plasma cortisol after the Dexamethasone Challenge Test
> Abnormal hypothalamic-pituitary-adrenal axis
> Abnormal sleep electroencephalogram with decreased rapid eye movement

Mental health of the world's children and adolescents is worsening with increase in overall stress, psychosomatic symptoms, school dropouts, substance abuse, and violence [34–36].

In a study of 112 adolescent suicides, at least one previous suicide attempt was known in 28% of the boys and 50% of the girls [37]. Suicide completion is five times more common in 15- to 19-year-old boys than similar age girls [26]. In a review of 14 studies looking at 2012 adolescent boys who were hospitalized for a suicide attempt, 1.3% had committed suicide at an average of 3.6 years follow-up; 0.2% of 5189 of the girls in this study had committed suicide at an average of 3.6 years follow-up [38].

Box 5 lists suicide precipitants or risks in youth [26–28,39–43]. The New York Psychological Autopsy Study looked at 173 adolescent suicides and noted that the most important factor in boys was a previous suicide attempt; other factors that were also important were a history of major depression disorder and substance abuse disorder in these boys [44,45]. This same study noted that the most important factor for suicide in girls was major depression disorder; substance abuse disorder was also an important risk factor [44,45]. In this study by Shaffer and coworkers [44,45], a family history of suicide results in a 5 times increased risk for suicide in boys and a 3 times increased risk in girls.

Table 5
Diagnoses in 31 adolescent boys and 90 girls with suicide attempt

Disorder	Boys (%)	Girls (%)
Major depression or dysthymia	71	64.5
Disruptive behavior disorder	32.3	12.2
Drug abuse or dependence	29	13.3
Alcohol abuse or dependence	19.4	14.4
Anxiety disorder	9.7	18.9
Adjustment disorder	6.5	10
Eating disorder	0	3.3
Some type of psychiatric disorder	87.1	77.8

Data from Andrews JA, Lewinsohn PM. Suicidal attempts among older adolescents: prevalence and co-occurrence with psychiatric disorders. J Am Acad Child Adolesc Psychiatry 1992;31:655–62.

Box 4. Potential consequences of depression

Suicide
Failing grades or reduced academic success
Substance abuse disorders
Social isolation
Intimate relationship disruption
Abuse
Sexual dysfunction
Sexual promiscuity (with unwanted pregnancy and sexually transmitted diseases)
Others

Suicide may occur in a youth without a specific psychiatric diagnosis when one's life is complicated by such factors as legal difficulties, homosexuality, intense personality conflicts, widespread availability of firearms, narcissistic traits, and factors leading to a withdrawal from one's environment shortly before the attempt [46]. Bisexual and homosexual youth constitutes

Box 5. Risk factors for suicide and suicide attempts

Depression
Severe irritability or agitation
Schizophrenia
Violent behavior (including aggressive conduct disorder)
Schizophrenia
Previous attempts
Substance abuse disorder
Widespread availability of firearms and suffocation methods
Personal acceptability of suicide
Being bullied
Homosexual male
Community chaos or dysfunction
Personality disorder (borderline, antisocial)
School failure
Family history of completed suicide
Noncompliance with mental health treatment
History of abuse (sexual or physical)
Chronic illness
Life on the street (throwaway or runaway adolescents)
Involvement in war

a high risk for suicide; 20% to 42% of homosexual youth attempt suicide, often between 15 and 17 years of age [11,47]. Chronic illness can lead to an increase in suicide attempts; this includes factors that lead to central nervous system damage from epilepsy, infection, chemotherapy, or trauma. Alcohol use contributes to 25% to 50% of the deaths in adolescents (caused by motor vehicle accidents, suicide, and so forth) [48–50].

Millions of youth are victims of physical and sexual abuse and sexual coercion; although most abuse goes unreported, the consequences remain [11,51,52]. There are approximately 3 million reported annual cases of abuse in those under age 18 years in the United States; reported abuse cases are subdivided into neglect in 53%, physical abuse in 26%, sexual abuse in 14%, and emotional abuse in 5% [53–56].

Millions of children and adolescents are incarcerated in the world, as a result of their conduct disorder or other negative behavior [57]. There are over 800,000 youth in jail-like facilities in the United States, such as jails, detention centers, or lock-ups [58–60]. They have various health care needs and often are not eligible for health care coverage [60]. They represent a very vulnerable and high-risk group of youth in America and the world.

It is noted that 100 to 140 million adolescents in the world are vulnerable to the adverse effects of war as solders, civilians, or refugees [9]. Estimates suggest there are 300,000 child soldiers around the world, some as young as 10 years of age [34]. Their duties are varied, from being overt soldiers to providing sexual services for the older solders [51].

Estimates of the number of children and adolescents who live on the world's streets range from 30 to 170 million [9]. This includes over 40 million in Latin America, 30 million in Asia, over 10 million in Africa, and several hundred thousand in the United States; there are over 450,000 runaways and 127,000 throwaways (ie, thrown out by their guardians) in the United States [61–67]. There are 10,000 children on the streets in South Africa, and 100,000 in three cities of India (Calcutta, Delhi, and Mumbai). There are an estimated 1 million children abducted or coerced into the global sex trade industry each year. About 40% of sex workers in India are under 18 years of age (some as young as 8 or 9). The average age for girls to enter prostitution in Moscow (Russian Federation) is age 16. Asia and Africa account for over 90% of the total world child labor force. Many street children enter a world of prostitution. Children and adolescents living on the streets of the world are the product of war; poverty; domestic violence; and abuse (physical, sexual, or mental). Homeless youth are subject to many dangers of the street: physical or sexual abuse, substance abuse, sexually transmitted diseases, various medical disorders, and others [67–70]. Their main medical treatment is usually through the hospital emergency room, if they receive any care at all. Suicide and homicide become predictable results of life on the streets.

Repeat suicide

In one survey study of adolescents, 5% reported over one suicide attempt per year; factors leading to repeated attempts included depression (13 times increase); sexual assault (seven times increase); substance abuse disorder; violent behavior in boys; and increased weight problems in girls [71]. In a 2001 Centers for Disease Control and Prevention Youth Risk Behavioral Survey of 13,601 adolescents in school (9th grade to 12th grade), 53% of those who had attempted suicide did so only once per year [27]. One attempt increased the risk for further attempts by 15-fold, however, and 30% had two or three attempts per year; 17% had four or more attempts in a year [27].

Selective serotonin reuptake inhibitors and the risk of suicide

Recent research in England and the United States has indicated that most selective serotonin reuptake inhibitors (SSRIs) are not proved to be of benefit to children and adolescents with depression; some research also suggests that the use of SSRIs may increase suicidal ideation in a small number of children and adolescents. On March 22, 2004, the US Food and Drug Administration issued a statement that pediatric and adult patients who are placed on these medications receive close observation for the potential worsening of depression and development of suicidality. One manufacturer (GlaxoSmithKline) provided the Food and Drug Administration with their results of a study of 1385 patients aged 7 to 18 years of age who were placed on paroxetine; 3.4% developed emotional liability that included crying, mood fluctuations, suicidal ideation, or attempted suicide [72]. This was in contrast to the findings in 1.2% of placebo controls, and no completed suicide was reported in those on paroxetine.

A potential link between the use of SSRIs and suicide remains controversial. Simon [73] reported from a study of health plan data in Washington and Idaho that included 82,285 treatment episodes with SSRIs; 5107 were age 17 or less. The highest risk for suicidal attempt was the month before SSRI treatment and there was no evidence from these data that the use of SSRIs increased suicidal behaviors [73]. Olfson and coworkers [29] reports a drop of 0.23 suicides per 100,000 per year in the United States from 1990 to 2000 at the same time there was an increase in use of SSRI. In the United Kingdom, Gunnell and Ashby [74] concluded that an increase in antidepressants (SSRIs) from 1991 to 1998 led to a stabilization of suicide rates in males aged 12 to 29. Historically, there was a 3- to 10-fold increase in SSRI use in children and adolescents from 1987 to 1996, a 50% increase from 1998 to 2002, and a 9% increase in 2003; however, there was also a 10% to 20% decrease in use in 2004 that is attributed to the concern over a potential link between SSRIs and suicidality.

Concepts of management

Adolescents who are considering suicide are often relieved to tell someone and receive help to overcome these disturbing thoughts. There is no research evidence that hospitalization per se prevents eventual completed suicide [44,45]. Box 6 lists some reasons to hospitalize a youth voicing suicidal thoughts. It should be remembered that suicide ideation or attempt reflects symptoms of underlying issues and is not a psychiatric diagnosis in itself. Nearly one third of multiple suicide attempts have signed a previous safely contract, and such a contract is not a guarantee against future attempts. Research notes that asking a youth about potential suicidal thoughts can prevent a suicide and not cause a suicide [75]. Box 7 provides advice to give to an adolescent who tells the clinician he or she has a friend who is "suicidal."

Medication itself is not useful in preventing the acute suicide and antidepressant medication is not the treatment of choice for the suicidal youth. Flupenthixol has been used for multiple suicide attempters and lithium has been tried with adults who have bipolar disorder and suicidal ideations. Clozapine has been attempted for adults with schizophrenia and acute suicidal ideations.

When talking to a suicidal youth, ask about the availability of firearms and drugs in his or her home; clinicians often fail to ask about such risk factors that can contribute to a completed suicide [76]. The parents or guardians should be asked to drug-proof and gun-proof the youth's home. Some research notes that 17% of caregivers buy a firearm after a youth in the home attempts suicide [3]. Caregivers are three times more likely to improve home factors, however, if given education about this by the clinician [45]. A youth placed on antidepressants should receive close monitoring for

---

Box 6. Reasons to hospitalize a youth with suicidal ideation

Agitated behavior
Mania
Intoxication state
Unmanageable as an outpatient
Active psychosis
Medical-legal considerations
Positive family history for suicide completion (doubles the risk)
Male gender (10 times the risk)
Prior attempts (15 times the risk)
History of aggressive outbursts
Substance abuse disorder
Support for the family to provide education
Inadequate home care or supervision

> **Box 7. Advising an adolescent with a suicidal friend or peer**
>
> 1. Note that you (the friend) are concerned
> 2. Advise the suicidal person to get professional help by contacting
>   Suicide prevention hotline
>   Hospital emergency department
>   Local crisis center
> 3. Make a contract that no suicide will occur now and that he or she will get help
> 4. Do not allow the teenager to swear you to secrecy about the suicide
> 5. Do not leave the suicidal youth alone
> 6. Do not assume it will be resolved by no action
> 7. Do not be shocked by what the suicidal youth says
> 8. Do not argue moral, religious, or ethical issues
> 9. Do not challenge, dare, or use verbal "treatments" on the youth
> 10. Seek information on any suicide plan and its specifics to relay to others

increased suicidal ideations [77]. Follow-up care is very important for youth with a suicide attempt, although research notes 16% to 59% do not receive such care [45]. Prevention of suicide among adolescents and young adults should be a major priority of health providers and society at large [1,45,78–84].

References

[1] Satcher W. National strategy for suicide prevention: goals and objectives for action. Washington, DC: SAMHSA, CDC, NIH, HRSA; 2001.
[2] Pfeffer CR. The suicidal child. New York: Guilford Press; 1986.
[3] Pfeffer CR. Suicide. In: Wiener JM, editor. Textbook of child and adolescent psychiatry. 2nd edition. Washington, DC: American Psychiatric Press; 1997. p. 727–38.
[4] Mishara BL. How the media influences children's conceptions of suicide. Crisis 2003;24(3): 128–30.
[5] Romer C. Global health problems of violence. In: Romer C, editor. Violence and health: proceedings of a WHO global symposium. Kobe (Japan): WHO Center for Health Development; 2000. p. 25–33.
[6] Miller M, Hemenway D. Firearm prevalence and the risk of suicide: a review. Harvard Health Policy Journal 2001;2:1–3.
[7] United Nations Childrens Fund (UNICEF). The progress of nations, 1996. Available at: www.unicef.org/pon96/insuicid.htm. Accessed November 23, 2006.
[8] Mann JJ, Apter A, Bertolote J, et al. Suicide prevention strategies: a systematic review. JAMA 2005;294(16):2064–74.
[9] World Health Organization. The second decade: improving adolescent health and development. Geneva (Switzerland): World Health Organization; 2001.

[10] Centers for Disease Control and Prevention. Programs for the prevention of suicide among adolescents and young adults; and suicide contagion and the reporting of suicide: recommendations from a national workshop. MMWR 1994;43(No. RR-6):13–8.
[11] Barker G. What about boys: a literature review in the health and development of adolescent boys. Geneva (Switzerland): WHO Department of Child and Adolescent Health and Development; 2000.
[12] Brown P. Choosing to die: a growing epidemic among the young. Bull World Health Organ 2001;79(12):1175–7.
[13] Diekstra R. Suicide and the attempted suicide: an international perspective. Acta Psychiatr Scand 1989;80(Suppl 354):1–24.
[14] Ryland D, Kruesi M. Suicide among adolescents. Int Rev Psychiatry 1992;4:185–95.
[15] Keith CR. Adolescent suicide: perspectives on a clinical quandary. JAMA 2001;286:3126–7.
[16] Anderson RN, Minino AM, Fingerhut LA, et al. Deaths: injuries 2001. Natl Vital Stat Rep 2004;52(21):1–86.
[17] Centers for Disease Control and Prevention. Suicide and attempted suicide. MMWR 2004; 53:471.
[18] Pfeffer CR. Suicide in mood disordered children and adolescents. Child Adolesc Psychiatr Clin N Am 2002;11:639–48.
[19] Eddleston M, Sheriff MHR, Hawton K. Deliberate self harm in Sri Lanka: an overlooked tragedy in the developing world. Br Med J 1998;317:133–5.
[20] Holinger PC. Epidemiologic issues in youth suicide. In: Pfeffer CR, editor. Suicide among youth: perspectives on risk and prevention. Washington, DC: American Psychiatric Press; 1989. p. 41–2.
[21] Kessler RC, Bergland P, Borges G, et al. Trends in suicide ideation, plans, gestures, and attempts in the United States, 1990-1992 to 2001-2003. JAMA 2005;293(20):2487–95.
[22] Zamekin A, Alter MR, Yemini T. Suicide in teenagers: assessment, management, and prevention. JAMA 2001;286:3120–5.
[23] Goldsmith SK, Pellmar TC, Kleinman AM, et al, editors. Reducing suicide: a national imperative. Washington, DC: National Academies Press; 2002.
[24] Anderson RN, Smith BL. Deaths: leading causes for 2001. Natl Vital Stat Rep 2003;52(9): 1–85.
[25] Pfeffer CR. Suicidal behavior in prepubertal children: from the 1980s to the new millennium. In: Maris RW, Canetto SS, McIntosh JL, et al, editors. Review of suicidology. New York: Guilford; 2000. p. 159–69.
[26] Maris RW. Suicide. Lancet 2002;360:319–26.
[27] Centers for Disease Control and Prevention. Methods of suicide among persons age 10-19 years- United States, 1992-2001. MMWR 2004;53:471–4.
[28] Pfeffer CR. Suicidal behavior in children and adolescents: causes and management. In: Lewis M, editor. Child and adolescent psychiatry: a comprehensive textbook. 3rd edition. Philadelphia: Lippincott Williams & Wilkins; 2002. p. 796–805.
[29] Olfson M, Shaffer D, Marcus SC, et al. Relationship between antidepressant medication treatment and suicide in adolescents. Arch Gen Psychiatry 2003;60(10):978–82.
[30] Andrews JA, Lewinsohn PM. Suicidal attempts among older adolescents: prevalence and co-occurrence with psychiatric disorders. J Am Acad Child Adolesc Psychiatry 1992;31(4):655–62.
[31] Demyttenaere K, Bruffaerts R, Posada-Villa J, et al. Prevalence, severity, and unmeet need for treatment of mental disorders in the World Health Organization World Mental Health Surveys. JAMA 2004;291(21):2581–90.
[32] Besseghini VH. Depression and suicide in children and adolescents. Ann N Y Acad Sci 1997; 816:94–8.
[33] Elliott GR, Smiga S. Depression in the child and adolescent. Pediatr Clin North Am 2003;50: 1093–106.
[34] Greydanus DE, Patel DR, Pratt HD, editors. Behavioral pediatrics, Part II. Pediatr Clin North Am 2003; vol. 50. p. 963–1231.

[35] World Health Organization. A Healthy Start in Life. Report on the Global Consultation on Child and Adolescent Health and Development. March 12–13, 2002. Stockholm (Sweden): World Health Organization; 2002.
[36] Satcher D. Global mental health: its time has come. JAMA 2001;285(13):1697–8.
[37] Shaffer D, Gould MS, Fisher P, et al. Psychiatric diagnosis in child and adolescent suicide. Arch Gen Psychiatry 1996;53(4):339–48.
[38] Safer DJ. Adolescent/adult differences in suicidal behavior and outcome. Ann Clin Psychiatry 1997;9(1):61–6.
[39] Jenkins RR. Adolescent health. In: Behrman RE, Kliegman RM, Jenson HB, editors. Nelson textbook of pediatrics. 16th edition. Philadelphia: WB Saunders; 2004. p. 641–80.
[40] Dube SR, Anda RF, Felitti VJ, et al. Childhood abuse, household dysfunction and the risk of attempted suicide throughout the life span: findings from the Adverse Childhood Experiences Study. JAMA 2001;286:3089–96.
[41] Beautrais AL. Risk factors for suicide and suicide attempt among young people. Aust N Z J Psychiatry 2000;34:420–36.
[42] Stewart L, Sebastiani A, Delgado G, et al. Consequences of sexual abuse of adolescents. Reprod Health Matters 1996;1(7):129–34.
[43] Edelsohn GA, Gomez JP. Psychiatric emergencies in adolescents. Adolesc Med 2006;17:183–204.
[44] Shaffer D. The epidemiology of teen suicide: an examination of risk factors. J Clin Psychiatry 1988;49:36–41.
[45] Shaffer D, Garland A, Gould M, et al. Preventing teenage suicide: a critical review. J Am Acad Child Adolesc Psychiatry 1988;27(6):675–87.
[46] Marttunen MJ, Aro HM, Henriksson MM, et al. Adolescent suicide with adjustment disorder or no psychiatric diagnosis. Eur J Child Adolesc Psychiatry 1994;3:101–10.
[47] Greydanus DE, Sison AC. Homosexual attraction and sexual behavior in adolescents. In: Greydanus DE, Patel DR, Pratt HD, editors. Behavioral pediatrics. 2nd edition. New York: iUniverse Publishers; 2006. p. 331–52.
[48] Greydanus DE. Substance abuse in adolescents. Int Pediatr 2002;17:1–3.
[49] Greydanus DE, Patel DR. Substance abuse in adolescents: a complex conundrum for the clinician. Pediatr Clin North Am 2003;59:1179–223.
[50] Greydanus DE, Patel DR. Substance abuse in the adolescent. Curr Probl Pediatr 2005;35(3):73–104.
[51] Young People and HIV/AIDS. Opportunity in crisis. Geneva (Switzerland): United Nations Children's Fund, Joint United Nations Programme on HIV/AIDS, and World Health Organization; 2002.
[52] Gushurst CA. Child abuse: behavioral aspects and other associated problems. Pediatr Clin North Am 2003;50:919–38.
[53] United States Department of Health and Human Services, National Center on Child Abuse and Neglect. Child maltreatment, 1994. Report from States to the National Center for Child Abuse and Neglect. Washington, DC: U.S. Government Printing Office; 1996.
[54] Kaplan DW, Feinstein RA, Fisher MM, et al. Care of the adolescent sexual assault victim. Pediatrics 2001;107(6):1476–9.
[55] Kellogg ND, Hoffman TJ. Unwanted and illegal sexual experiences in childhood and adolescence. Child Abuse Negl 1995;19(12):1457–68.
[56] Mitchell KJ, Finkelhor D, Wolak J. Risk factors for and impact of online sexual solicitation of youth. JAMA 2001;285:3011–4.
[57] Goldhagen J. Child health in the developing world. In: Behrman RE, Kliegman RM, Jenson HB, editors. Nelson textbook of pediatrics. 16th edition. Philadelphia: WB Saunders; 2000. p. 11–4.
[58] World Health Organization. Health care for incarcerated youth. Position paper of the Society for Adolescent Medicine. J Adolesc Health 2000;27:73–5.
[59] World Health Organization. US Congress, Office of Technology Assessment. Adolescent health, vol. 2. Background and effectiveness of selected prevention and treatment services. Washington, DC: U.S. Government Printing Office; 1991.

[60] American Academy of Pediatrics. Committee on Adolescence. Health care for children and adolescents in the juvenile correctional care system. Pediatrics 2001;107:799–803.
[61] Patel DR, Greydanus DE. Homeless adolescents in the United States. Int Pediatr 2002;17: 71–5.
[62] US General Accounting Office. Children and youths: about 68,000 homeless and 186,000 in shared housing at any given time (Report to congressional committees No. PEMD-89–14). Washington, DC: U.S. General Accounting Office; 1989.
[63] Finkelhor D, Hotaling G, Sedlak A. Missing, abducted, runaway, and throwaway children in America. First report: numbers and characteristics, national incidence studies. executive summary. Washington, D.C.: U.S. Department of Justice, Office of Juvenile Justice and Delinquency Prevention; 1990.
[64] Farrow JA, Deisher W, Brown R, et al. Health and health needs of homeless and runaway youth: a position paper of the Society for Adolescent Medicine. J Adolesc Health 1992;13:717–26.
[65] American Academy of Pediatrics. Committee on Community Health Services. Health needs of homeless children and families. Pediatrics 1996;98:351–3.
[66] Le Roux J. Street children in South Africa: findings from interviews on the background of street children in Pretoria, South Africa. Adolescence 1996;31:423–31.
[67] Abdalian SE. Street youth mortality: leaning with intent to fall. JAMA 2004;292:624–6.
[68] Pratt HD, Patel DR, Greydanus DE, et al. Adolescent sexual offenders: issues for pediatricians. Int Pediatr 2001;16:1–12.
[69] Pratt HD. Homeless adolescents in the United States. International Pediatrics 2002;17:70–1.
[70] Boris NW, Heller SS, Sheperd T, et al. Partner violence among homeless young adults: measurement issues and associations. J Adolesc Health 2002;30:355–63.
[71] Rosenberg HJ, Jankowski MK, Senguptga A, et al. Single and multiple suicide attempts and associated health risk factors in New Hampshire adolescents. Suicide Life Threat Behav 2005;35(5):545–57.
[72] World Health Organization. Are SSRIs safe for children? Med Lett Drugs Ther 2003; 45(1160):53–4.
[73] Simon GE. Suicide risk during antidepressant treatment. Am J Psychiatry 2006;163:41–7.
[74] Gunnell D, Ashby D. Antidepressants and suicide: what is the balance of benefit and harm. BMJ 2004;329(7456):34–8.
[75] Elliott GR, Smiga SM. Mood disorders in children and adolescents. In: Greydanus DE, Patel DR, Pratt HD, editors. Behavioral pediatrics. 2nd edition. New York: iUniverse Publishers; 2006. p. 589–617.
[76] Greenhill LL, Waslick B. Management of suicidal behavior in children and adolescents. Psychiatr Clin North Am 1997;20:641–66.
[77] Simon GE. The antidepressant quandary: considering suicide risk when treating adolescent depression. N Engl J Med 2006;355:2722–3.
[78] Fergusson DM, Horwood LJ, Ridder EM, et al. Suicidal behaviour in adolescence and subsequent mental health outcomes in young adulthood. Psychol Med 2005;35:983–93.
[79] Gould MS, Greenberg T, Velting DM, et al. Youth suicide risk and preventive interventions: a review of the past 10 years. J Am Acad Child Adolesc Psychiatry 2003;42:386–405.
[80] Knox KL, Caine ED. Establishing priorities for reducing suicides and its antecedents in the United States. Am J Public Health 2005;95:1898–903.
[81] Lewis G, Hawton K, Jones P. Strategies for preventing suicide. Br J Psychiatry 1997;171: 351–4.
[82] Teplin LA, McClelland GM, Abram KM, et al. Early violent death among delinquent youth. Pediatrics 2005;115:1586–93.
[83] Friedman RA. Uncovering an epidemic: screening for mental illness in teens. N Engl J Med 2006;355:2717–9.
[84] Brent DA, Mann JJ. Familial pathways to suicidal behavior: understanding and preventing suicide among adolescents. N Engl J Med 2006;355:2719–21.

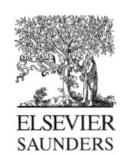

Sexuality in the Child, Teen, and Young Adult: Concepts for the Clinician

Helena Fonseca, MD[a], Donald E. Greydanus, MD[b,c],*

[a]Faculty of Medicine, University of Lisbon, Lisbon, Portugal
[b]Pediatrics & Human Development, Michigan State University College of Human Medicine
[c]Michigan State University/Kalamazoo Center for Medical Studies, 1000 Oakland Drive, Kalamazoo, MI 49008-1284 USA

Sexuality begins at birth or even at conception. Freud described five psychosexual stages of development (Box 1) [1,2]. According to Freud's psychoanalytic theory, the Oedipus and Electra complex is described as boys and girls having competitive feelings toward their fathers and the mothers, respectively. Children view the same-gender parent as a rival for the attention of the other parent. This complex is resolved when boys and girls develop normal identification with fathers and mothers, respectively. The complex is typical during the phallic stage and the genital stage. Moreover, according to this theory, the development of normal sexual health dictates successful resolution of this complex.

Normal development of sexuality

Infancy

During the first year of life (infancy), exploration is through mouthing and sucking. Trust in a caretaker (usually the mother) is critical for healthy development of infants. Babies start building their sexuality by touching and being touched. The quality of this first relationship has an impact on their emerging sexuality and is a determinant for their future sexual life.

Toddler period

During the toddler period (ages 2 to 3 years), children develop new mobility and language skills. They learn what boys and girls are expected to do

---

* Corresponding author. Michigan State University/Kalamazoo Center for Medical Studies, 1000 Oakland Drive, Kalamazoo, MI 49008-1284.
  E-mail address: greydanus@kcms.msu.edu (D.E. Greydanus).

> **Box 1. Psychosexual stages of Freud**
>
> 1. Oral (birth through 1 year of age)
> 2. Anal (1 year through 3 years of age)
> 3. Phallic (3 years through 6 years of age)
> 4. Latency (6 years through 9 years of age)
> 5. Genital (9 years through adolescence)

and the names of body parts. Self-genital manipulation for pleasure is common. During this time, health professionals should begin providing sexual education and guidance for families. Children's normal curiosity about their body and the differences between boys and girls should be anticipated. It is important to use correct terms for all body parts, including genitals. Questions, for example, "where babies come from," always need to be answered by parents or guardians in a developmentally adequate way.

Preschool period

During the preschool period (ages 3 to 5 years), children develop further curiosity about the differences between boys and girls and continue to have an interest in masturbation. The manner in which parents deal with their children's increasing sexual curiosity influences the incorporation of sexuality into children's self-value. At this stage, health care professionals should provide guidance to parents that children's sexual curiosity and exploration are normal. Parents should begin to teach children about sexuality through the use of age-appropriate sex education picture books. Children need to understand that certain parts of the body are private and should not be touched without their permission. Questions asked by children should be answered at a level appropriate to their understanding. Children should be encouraged to feel comfortable asking additional questions in the important arena of sexuality.

Latency

During the latency period (age 5 to the beginning of puberty), school-age children are expected to establish their gender identity. This latency stage, as Freud defined it, is characterized mainly by having same-gender friends, and sexuality often is expressed by a major interest in sexual jokes, stories, or songs. They are curious about the anatomy of the opposite gender. Nevertheless, usually, masturbation recedes during this period.

Parents should have age-appropriate sex education books at home that help answer some questions and encourage children to ask further questions. If children are receiving sex education at school or in the community, parents should discuss this information with them to be sure the children understand the parents' views. Parents of girls should start to prepare their daughters for menstruation. The transition into adolescence is characterized by a reinforced interest regarding sexuality.

Adolescence

Adolescence is a critical period of psychologic and physical growth and pubertal development. A key component to the healthy development of adolescents is how they proceed with the stages of adolescent sexuality. The progression through puberty is predictable, but there is considerable variation in its onset, timing, and magnitude of changes. Peer relationships play a major role in adolescents' emotional separation from parents and emerging individuality. Peer and social influences may expose adolescents to values that differ significantly from their family's values. There is a need to balance peer pressure and family expectations, and sometimes conflicts may arise. Adolescents' struggle to gain autonomy often is a source of family tension. Parents may describe this period as a critical and challenging one for the family. A family physician can be a key person in this process, offering guidance and support for adolescents and families as they adapt to these changes [3].

The sequential changes of puberty are classified in five stages, the Tanner stages (also called the sexual maturity stages) (Tables 1 and 2) [4]. Breast buds (thelarche) are the first clinical event of puberty in females and represent a sexual maturity rating (SMR) of 2. Menarche (onset of menstruation) happens in SRM 4, between 12 and 13 years of age in the average pubertal female; menarche may occur in a late SMR 3 stage. In males, the first clinical event of puberty is enlarged testicles (over 4 mL in volume). Ejaculation is noted at SMR 3.

Female adolescents may be concerned about vaginal discharge (physiologic leukorrhea). Male adolescents may be concerned about spontaneous erections or nocturnal emissions. Transient development of breasts (gynecomastia), which happens in approximately two thirds of male adolescents by Tanner stage of SMR 2 to 3, also can be a source of confusion and anxiety for males. Female and male adolescents may be concerned about homosexual interests, sexual experimentation, and pressure from peers and society to become sexually active. In both genders, acne, body odor, and seborrheic dermatitis may have a negative impact on body image and decrease self-esteem.

For adolescents who mature early (ie, precocious puberty) or late (ie, delayed puberty), there can be considerable psychosocial consequences. An association between early maturation and earlier onset of sexual intercourse is documented [4]. Moreover, it is shown that young women who mature early have higher rates of psychopathology and, thus, are at unique risk for persistent difficulty during adolescence; they should be targeted for preventive efforts [5]. It also is noted that bulimic-type eating pathology among girls is

Table 1
Sexual maturity rating or Tanner staging in females

Stage	Breasts	Pubic hair	Range
I	None	None	Birth to 15 years
II[a]	Breast bud (thelarche): areolar hyperplasia with small amount of breast tissue	Long downy pubic hair near the labia; may occur with breast budding or several weeks to months later (pubarche)	8.5 to 15 years (some use 8 years)
III[b]	Further enlargement of breast tissue and areola	Increase in amount of hair with more pigmentation	10 to 15 years
IV[c]	Double contour form: areola and nipple form secondary mound on top of breast tissue	Adult type but not distribution	10 to 17 years
V[d]	Larger breast with single contour form	Adult distribution	12.5 to 18 years

[a] Peak height velocity often occurs soon after stage II.
[b] 25% develop menarche in late III.
[c] Most develop menarche in stage IV 1 to 3 years after thelarche.
[d] 10% develop menarche in stage V.

Reproduced with permission from Greydanus DE, Fonseca F, Pratt HD. Childhood and adolescent sexuality. In: Behavioral pediatrics. 2nd edition. Lincoln (NE): iUniverse Publishers; 2006. p. 308–10.

associated with early menarche and early sexual experiences [6]. Alternatively, girls who mature late may be teased more frequently by their peers than other youth and be an object of bullying at school [7].

Psychosocial development

Adolescent psychosocial development typically is divided into three periods: early (ages 10 to 14), middle (ages 15 to 17), and late adolescence (ages 18 to 21+) (Table 3). Early adolescence is characterized mainly by feelings of confusion because of the rapid physical changes, exploration of one's own body, and need for comparison with peers of the same gender due to concerns about normality. Much energy is spent acquiring social skills and interacting with individuals of the same gender. In this interaction, however, adolescents' interests come first and concerns of others become secondary.

Early adolescents behave as if they are the only actor on the stage of life. According to the psychoanalytic theories, this period typically is the time for re-emergence of the Oedipus complex [2]. Many young adolescents do not have accurate information about sexual development and the consequences of early and unprotected sexual activity. Anticipatory guidance by clinicians

Table 2
Sexual maturity rating or Tanner staging in males

Stage	Testes	Penis	Pubic hair	Range
I	No change, testes 2.5 cm or less	Prepubertal	None	Birth to 15 years
II	Enlargement of testes, increased stippling, and pigmentation of scrotal sac	Minimal or no enlargement	Long downy hair often occurring several months after testicular growth; variable pattern noted with pubarche	10 to 15 years
III[a]	Further enlargement	Significant penile enlargement, especially in length	Increase in amount, now curling	10.5 to 16.5 years
IV[b]	Further enlargement	Further enlargement, especially in diameter	Adult type but not distribution	Variable; 12 to 17 years
V[c]	Adult size	Adult size	Adult distribution (medial aspects of thighs, linea alba)	13 to 18 years

[a] Peak height spurt usually between III and IV.
[b] Axillary hair develops and some facial hair.
[c] 20% have peak height velocity now. Body hair, increase in musculature, and so forth continue for several months to years.

Reproduced with permission from Greydanus DE, Fonseca F, Pratt HD. Childhood and adolescent sexuality. In: Behavioral pediatrics. 2nd edition. Lincoln (NE): iUniverse Publishers; 2006. p. 308–10.

must include a talk with the adolescents about body changes during puberty, including individual variations in the rate of growth and development [1,4].

Middle adolescence is characterized by the acquisition of diverse experiences, typically short and intensive, with the opposite gender. At an early stage, it begins with interest in the opposite gender, then group dating, individual dating, and, finally, eventual sexual intimacy in many adolescents. These relationships mainly are narcissistic, generated from self-interest. Anticipatory guidance by clinicians should address adolescents' concerns while also providing information on sexual development, contraception, and prevention of sexually transmitted diseases (STDs) [1,4]. Moreover, parents and health professionals should discuss with adolescents ways to resist sexual pressures. According to the resilience theories, the identification of a supportive adult who can give adolescents accurate information about sexuality is important [1]. Health supervision must address sexual experimentation, its risks, and prevention of negative results.

Late adolescence is characterized by building relationships that are more adult-like. The ability to integrate emotional and physical intimacy in a love relationship is an important developmental task for older adolescents and young adults. Anticipatory guidance by clinicians should include a talk about sexual maturity and sexual feelings (for the same or opposite gender), contraceptive methods, and sexually transmitted disease prevention [1,4].

Table 3
Adolescent psychosocial development

	Early adolescence (11–14 years)	Middle adolescence (15–17 years)	Late adolescence (18–25 years)
Cognitive thinking	Concrete thinking: here and now. Appreciate immediate reactions to behavior but no sense of later consequences	Early abstract thinking: inductive/deductive reasoning. Able to connect separate events, understand later consequences. Self-absorbed, introspective, lots of daydreaming and rich fantasies	Abstract thinking: adult ability to think abstractly. Philosophic. Intense idealism about love, religion, social problems
Task areas			
1. Family—independence	• Transition from obedient to rebellious • Rejection of parental guidelines • Ambivalence about wishes (dependence/independence) • Underlying need to please adults • Hero worship ("crushes")	• Insistence on independence, privacy • May have overt rebellion or sulky withdrawal • Much testing of limits • Roleplaying of adult roles (but not felt to be "real"—easily abandoned)	• Emancipation (leave home) • Re-establishment of family ties • Assume true adult roles with commitment
2. Peers—social/sexual	• Same-gender "best friend" • "Am I normal?" concerns • Giggling boy-girl fantasies • Sexual experimentation not normal at this age: done to counteract fears of worthlessness • Obtain "friends" • Humiliate parents	• Dating, intense interest in "boys" • Sexual experimentation begins • Risk-taking actions • Unrealistic concept of partner's role • Need to please significant peers (of either sex)	• Partner selection • Realistic concept of partner's role • Mature friendships • True intimacy possible only after own identity is established • Need to please self too ("enlightened self-interest")

(*continued on next page*)

Table 3 (*continued*)

	Early adolescence (11–14 years)	Middle adolescence (15–17 years)	Late adolescence (18–25 years)
3. School—vocation	• Still in a structured school setting • Goals unrealistic, changing • Want to copy favorite role models	• More class choices in school setting • Beginning to identify skills, interests • Start part-time jobs • Begin to react to system's expectations: may decide to beat the establishment at its own game (super achievers) or to reject the game (dropouts)	• Full-time work or college • Identify realistic career goals • Watch for apathy (no future plans) or alienation, because lack of goal-orientation is correlated with unplanned pregnancy, juvenile crime, and so forth
4. Self-perception	• Incapable of self-awareness while still concrete thinkers	• Confusion about self-image	• Realistic, positive self-image
Identity	• Losing child role but do not have adult role; hence, low self-esteem	• Seek group identity • Very narcissistic	• Able to consider others' needs, less narcissistic
Social responsibility	• Tend to use denial (it can't happen to me)	• Impulsive, impatient	• Able to reject group pressure if not in self-interest
Values	• Stage II values (back-scratching) (good behavior in exchange for rewards)	• Stage III values (conformity) (behavior that peer group values)	• Stage IV values (social responsibility) (behavior consistent with laws and duty)
Chief health issues (other than acute illness)	• Psychosomatic symptoms • Fatigue and "growing pains" • Concerns about normalcy • Screening for growth and development problems	• Outcomes of sexual experimentation • Prevention of pregnancy, STDs, AIDS • Health-risk behaviors (drugs, alcohol, and driving) • Crisis counseling (runaways, acting-out, family, and so forth)	• Health promotion/healthy lifestyles • Contraception and STD/AIDS prevention • Self-responsibility for health and health care

(*continued on next page*)

Table 3 (*continued*)

	Early adolescence (11–14 years)	Middle adolescence (15–17 years)	Late adolescence (18–25 years)
Professional approach. To retain sanity, you and your staff should: • Like teenagers • Understand development • Be flexible • Be patient	• Firm, direct support • Convey limits—simple, concrete choices • Do *not* align with parents, but do be an objective caring adult • Encourage transference (hero worship) • Sexual decisions—directly encourage to wait, to say "NO" • Encourage parental presence in clinic, but interview teens alone	• Be an objective sounding board (but let them solve own problems) • Negotiate choices • Be a role model • Don't get too much history ("grandiose stories") • Confront (gently) about consequences, responsibilities • Consider: what will give them status in eyes of peers? • Use peer-group sessions • Adapt system to crises, walk-ins, impulsiveness, "testing" • Ensure confidentiality • Allow teens to seek care independently	• Allow mature participation in decisions • Act as a resource • Idealistic stage, so convey "professional" image • Can expect patients to examine underlying wishes, motives (eg, pregnancy wish if poor compliance with contraception) • Older adolescents able to adapt to policies/needs of clinic system

From Greydanus DE, Fonseca F, Pratt HD. Childhood and adolescent sexuality. In: Behavioral pediatrics. 2nd edition. Lincoln (NE): iUniverse Publishers; 2006. p. 308–10; with permission. *Courtesy of* Roberta K. Beach, MD, Denver, CO.

Researchers have shown considerable differences between genders concerning the way they view sexuality [8]. Western society conditions men at an early stage of their development that dominance, aggressiveness, and achievement are synonymous with masculinity. Alternatively, contraceptive responsibility remains a female responsibility instead of a shared one for heterosexual couples. Lack of role models, the influence of the media, and exposition to limited or inadequate sexual education may explain some conflict and confusion regarding sexuality and gender roles in men.

The media are believed to play a significant role in encouraging early sexual activity among adolescents [1,7]. Adolescents rank the media second only to school sex education programs as a leading source of information about sex [9]. The dramatic changes that have occurred in contemporary families are partially responsible for that [7]. Most parents have a decreased amount of time to spend with their adolescents, leading to decreased communication and support. At the crucial period in development, when adolescents are likely to experiment with behaviors that can have serious health consequences, parental involvement and supervision are needed more than ever. Primary care physicians can play an important role in helping families adapt to relationship changes between parents and changing adolescents while maintaining a balance that provides parental supervision and promotes adolescents' normal autonomy [1,7].

Adolescent sexual behavior

Oral sex

As adolescents experiment with their sexuality, oral sex becomes a common practice, often without understanding that several STDs may result (Box 2) [10–12]. A survey of 212 adolescents in the tenth grade identified 42% of the female adolescents and nearly 38% of the male adolescents reporting oral sex behavior in contrast to 35% of these female adolescents and 22% of these male adolescents involved in coital behavior [10]. In a survey of 580 ninth graders, nearly 20% had been involved in oral sex in contrast to 13.5% with coital sex [11]. Youth involved in oral sex often feel it is safer than coital sex.

Coital sex

The Centers for Disease Control and Prevention's 2005 Youth Risk Behavior Surveillance notes that 46.8% of all high school students have had sexual (coital) experience, with a range of 43% for whites, 51% for Hispanics, and 67.6% for African American youth [13]. In addition, 33.9% currently are sexually active (ie, have had sexual intercourse during the 3 months preceding the survey). This report notes that nationwide, 6.2% are coitally active before age 13 (8.8% of males and 3.7% of females), and 14.3% of youth have four or more partners (16.5% of males and 12% of females) [1,13]. Youth who have experience with more than one partner usually

---

Box 2. Sexually transmitted microbes spread by oral sexual behavior

Herpes simplex virus
HIV/AIDS
Human papillomavirus
Neisseria gonorrhoeae
Treponema pallidum

practice serial monogamy—having one partner and then moving on to another, usually one at a particular time [14]. There is an increased coital rate with increased drug or alcohol use and those engaged in survival sex. In the United States, millions of coitally active youth produce approximately 900,000 pregnancies and more than 6 million cases of STDs each year [1,7,15].

Adolescent pregnancy

Approximately 900,000 adolescent pregnancies are reported annually in the United States [16,17]. A decrease in adolescent pregnancies was noted from 1973 (the date of legalized abortion in the United States) until 1986; there was an increase from 1986 until 1991, and then a decrease until the present. However, 40% of female adolescents still become pregnant at least once. Female adolescents present 13% of all United States births (4,158,212 in 1992) and 26% of all abortions (approximately 400,000) [18].

The 2005 birth rate of 40.4 per 1000 female adolescents ages 15 to 19 years in the United States is the highest among all developed nations and is in stark contrast to a birth rate of 4 per 1000 in Japan; rates lower than the United States are noted in Canada, Great Britain, France, Sweden, and other countries [19–21].

In the United States, 14% of adolescent pregnancies end in miscarriages, 51% in live births, and 35% in abortions. In 2005, approximately 20% of births to adolescents were not first births, representing a 7.5% increase in repeat childbearing during adolescence since 1985. The 2005 data reveal a birth rate of 60.9 per 1000 female adolescents, ages 15 to 19, in the African American population versus 26 for 15- to 19-year-old white, 81.5 for Hispanic, 52.7 for American Indian, and 16.9 for Asian American, or Pacific Islander mothers 15 to 19 years old [20,22].

Summary

Limited sexuality education can be invoked as a partial explanation for the tragic statistics of American adolescent sexuality (ie, high rates of STD, sexual assault, and unwanted pregnancy) noted throughout the United States [14,15,17,18,23–30]. Simply discouraging or banning sexuality education on cultural and religious bases does not resolve these issues fully, if these youth are sexually active. Limited knowledge of sexuality can be dangerous for the youth of America and of the world [27–31]. Concepts of sex education are presented in Appendix 1. Adolescents should be taught that abstinence is an important goal while they are preparing to become adults [29]. They also can be taught several strategies to prevent negative consequences of sexual behavior:

1. How to avoid sexual abuse
2. How to resist unwanted sexual advances (including "date rape")

3. How to negotiate peer pressure
4. How to avoid media messages for sexual behavior without responsibility.

Teenagers who are mothers or fathers should receive parental, school, and societal support to become the best possible parents and to reduce potential negative consequences of teenage pregnancy [1,15,18]. Pregnancy prevention programs should be tailored to the needs of each region, involving multidimensional solutions. Cultural and religious beliefs of each person must be respected [29].

Adolescents who become sexually active must be taught how to use contraceptives effectively ("safe sex") and receive access to contraception, including emergency contraceptives [28–35]. Clinicians should encourage immunization with the human papillomavirus vaccine and ensure that the hepatitis B vaccine is provided. Adolescents also can be taught about the dangers from sexual abusers found on the Internet and the problems that bullying present to many youth [36–38]. Many dangers await children, adolescents, and young adults as they traverse the normal stages of human sexuality. Family physicians can be a helpful guide in this regard, with positive lifelong results for these important patients.

Appendix 1

Anticipatory guidance: sex education

Age	Children's needs or interests	Anticipatory guidance
Newborn	• Cuddling, sucking, loving touch (foundations for security, trust and later ability to give physical affection are established now)	• Teach parents the importance of touch, of warm, loving cuddling • Encourage breastfeeding, front packs, rocking chairs • "You can't spoil a baby at this age—it's okay to pick her up when she cries" • Observe parents' interactions with newborn—demonstrate behaviors if parents seem uncomfortable • Comment on role expectations—by choosing "pink or blue" we are already sending gender role messages to infants
6 months	• Infant discovers body • Self-stimulation and touching of genitals	• Tell parents to expect this behavior and that it's normal • Ask parents about their own attitudes toward infant self-stimulation

(*continued on next page*)

Appendix 1 (*continued*)

Age	Children's needs or interests	Anticipatory guidance
		• Remind them, "Don't slap his hands," as this sets up negative messages (ie, that part of your body is "bad")
		• Show the parents the parts of genitalia—teach them the vocabulary to use
		• Encourage questions—let them know sexually related topics are appropriate to discuss during health care visits
1 year	• Curiosity as to what daddy and mommy look like without clothes on	• Guidelines for household nudity. Explore parents' own attitudes—what's best is what they are comfortable with
		• Children begin to establish gender identity by observing differences in male and female bodies
		• Use picture books if nudity is uncomfortable
		• Parents should avoid messages that convey nudity as "dirty" or "pornographic"
1.5–3 years	• Self-respect and self-esteem develop.	• Teach parents how self-esteem is developed. Need for lots of positive feedback ("catch them being good"). Give praise and positive messages about being either a girl or a boy. Let children seek own preferences for gender role behavior (okay for boys to play with dolls or girls to play with trucks)
	• Feelings form about being a boy or a girl	
	• Effectiveness of toddler discipline at this age determines later ability to handle frustration and have self-control	
	• Exploration of body parts is common	• Discuss plans for discipline. Teach parents methods (eg, time out). Emphasize how to give positive reinforcement ("I like it when you__")
	• Bathroom activities are of great interest (toilet training)	
	• Sense of privacy develops	• Encourage parents to help children learn correct words for genitals and body functions (penis, vulva, bowel movement)
		• Discuss toilet training—using rewards and reinforcing positive attitudes about genitals
3–5 years	• Children need answers to "sexual questions" appropriate to cognitive level of development	• Tell parents to expect sexual questions ("where do babies come from") and give examples of how to answer them

(*continued on next page*)

Appendix 1 (*continued*)

Age	Children's needs or interests	Anticipatory guidance
	• Grasping genitals clearly is pleasurable, may occur when children are upset • Children become very seductive toward opposite-gender parent • Role-modeling (assimilation of characteristics of same-gender role model) takes place • Children begin learning what is socially acceptable, what behaviors are public or private, and how to show respect for others	• Give techniques for determining level of understanding ("where do you *think* they come from") • Children need to learn it's okay to talk about sex • Give booklets or suggest additional educational materials • Prepare parents for children's seductive behavior • Encourage parents to support each other and put their needs as a couple first (bad time to get divorced) • Remind them to role model the kind of male-female relationship they want their children to imitate (because the kids will) • This is the time to begin demonstrating that women have rights and men are equally responsible for outcomes
5–7 years	• "Playing doctor" is universal • Kids have learned parents' discomforts, starting "keeping secrets" about sex • Peer discussions provide many ideas about sex—dirty jokes among playmates common • Four-letter words (for exhibitionist behavior) used for shock value • Starting school—so stranger awareness is important	• Let parents know that childhood genital exploration is typical—it satisfies curiosity about opposite gender • Ask parents about their own childhood experiences "playing doctor" • Discuss ways to handle the situation ("It's normal to be curious—we consider other people's bodies private— I'd like you to get dressed and play other games") • Same with four-letter words ("be cool") • Encourage parents to bring up sexual questions, rather than waiting to be asked, use "teachable moments" to reinforce that it's okay to talk about sex. Need ample family discussion to balance what is learned from playmates • Discuss sexual molestation as a risk—discuss prevention techniques to teach children
7–9 years	• Children need answers to more advanced sexual questions (often scientific) (eg, "How does the baby get into the womb")	• Ask if parents have been getting any sexual questions (if not, children may feel it's not okay to ask). Dispel myth that information leads to sexual experimentation or

(*continued on next page*)

Appendix 1 (continued)

Age	Children's needs or interests	Anticipatory guidance
	• Need preview of changes in sexual development that will be associated with puberty • Values are instilled now that will last a lifetime (eg, self-responsibility, kindness)	that children are "too innocent" to hear about sex • Encourage them to use experiences, such as TV shows, mating animals, new babies in neighborhood, as opportunities to bring up questions • Assure parents it's okay not to know all the answers. Guide them to resources (books) for information • Give parents an understanding of wide range of pubertal development (eg, breast budding at age 8–9 is normal) • Encourage parents to teach difference between facts and opinions (eg, that nearly all young men masturbate is a fact; that masturbation is bad [or good] is an opinion, with which others may not agree) • Important to teach children the family values and beliefs, as well as facts
10–12 years	• Pubertal changes are of great importance—hormone levels rise • Both genders need to know about body changes, menarche, wet dreams, and sexual fantasies • Gender behavior "rehearsal" is common (looking through *Playboy*, spin-the-bottle games) • Questions about homosexuality arise • Need for privacy intensifies • Self-esteem is fragile	• By now, caregivers should start giving anticipatory guidance directly to young teens and to parents • Parents need to understand the normalcy of preadolescent sexual concerns and be willing to discuss them in a nonjudgmental way (last chance to be an important source of information—later it will be peers) • Empathize with parental discomfort ("sometimes we feel uneasy talking about sex, but—") • Model nonjudgmental ways of asking questions ("some parents don't mind their children looking at *Playboy*, and some parents disapprove. What are your feelings about that?") • Parents must set aside time to talk with children about puberty and sexual changes • School and community groups (scouts, church) should be encouraged to provide sex education for young adolescents

(continued on next page)

Appendix 1 (*continued*)

Age	Children's needs or interests	Anticipatory guidance
11–15 years (early adolescence)	• Obsessive concern with body and appearances (breast size, penile erections, acne, and so forth) • Pubertal changes are completed—need for a solid understanding of reproductive physiology • Sexual behaviors emerge (masturbation, homosexual encounters, sex dreams) • "First dates" start—questions about "what is love" • Peer pressure become significant • Need for assertiveness skills, right to say "NO" • Boys need to know they are equally responsible for consequences of sexual activity • Both genders need to be prepared to use contraception when the time comes • Educations about STDs, AIDS prevention is a priority • Self-esteem still low	• Build self-esteem—preteens need lots of positive feedback • At puberty, parents will reap the results of their past efforts • Parents need to learn how to "let go with love" and let teens take responsibility for choices • Reflective listening is far more important than talking • Affirm wholesomeness of sexual feelings ("it's natural to want to have sex") while conveying own opinions ("it would be wiser to wait until you're sure") • Parents should be sure teens have access to educational resources (eg, books) that will answer questions in detail • Many heterosexual young teens have some experimental homosexual encounters before dating. They may need reassurance and information • Parents need to prepare teens to use contraception—discuss realities, give permission, explain about resources. Dispel parental myths (eg, that access to family planning promotes promiscuity) • Message should be "wait until you're sure you're ready, then use reliable birth control each and every time" • Do not give messages that "good girls" don't have sex—guilt induction leads to denial and inability to accept responsibilities for choices (eg, unprotected sex) • Risks for STDs and AIDS should be discussed openly. Help teens plan realistically for self-protection (abstinence, monogamy, and condoms) • Continue to discuss personal values (continue to separate facts from opinions) • Continue to reinforce positive self-esteem

(*continued on next page*)

Appendix 1 (*continued*)

Age	Children's needs or interests	Anticipatory guidance
15–17 years (middle adolescence)	• Sexual activity begins • Services for sexual issues (family planning, STD, pregnancy tests) are essential • Meaning of relationships is explored ("Does he really love me") • Life planning becomes serious (high-risk, low-income teens need to see options beyond pregnancy) • Increased independence can lead to risks (date-rape, sexual assault) • Sexual preference becomes apparent to self—homosexual teens may feel much confusion and self-doubt	• Caregivers: the same anticipatory guidance should be given directly to teens in the office setting. • Ask parents, "What have you done to prepare your teen to use contraception when the time comes?" "How much have you discussed STD or AIDS with your teen?" • Encourage parents to give teens permission to obtain contraception and acquaint them with resources and means • Allow confidentiality and independence for teens seeking health care • Parents can continue to raise questions ("What did you think of that TV scene that showed __?") and give teens a chance to look at choices and consequences. But be prepared for either unwillingness to talk or challenges to parental viewpoints • Most teens do not want to discuss their personal sexual activities with their parents • Suggest to parents that they discuss teens' plans for the future, and then ask how plans would be affected by pregnancy, or marriage, and so forth • Teens need to know family, society expect them to prevent unplanned pregnancy, STDs if they choose to have sex • Discuss prevention techniques for sexual assault • Sexual orientation should be asked about (rather than presumed) • Referral to support resources may be helpful to gay teens or their parents if emotional or societal stress is present

From Greydanus DE, Fonseca F, Pratt HD. Childhood and adolescent sexuality. In: Behavioral pediatrics. 2nd edition. Lincoln (NE): iUniverse Publishers; 2006. p. 326–30; with permission. *Courtesy of* Roberta K. Beach, MD, Denver, CO.

References

[1] Greydanus D, Fonseca H, Pratt H. Childhood and adolescent sexuality [Chapter 12]. In: Greydanus D, Patel D, Pratt H, editors. Behavioral pediatrics. 2nd edition. New York: iUniverse, Inc; 2006. p. 295–330.
[2] Freud S. Three essays on the theory of sexuality. vol. 7. London: Hogarth Press; 1953. p. 125–43.
[3] Green M, Palfrey JS, editors. Bright futures: guidelines for health supervision of infants, children, and adolescents. 2nd edition. Arlington (VA): National Center for Education in Maternal and Child Health; 2000.
[4] Sigel EJ. Adolescent growth and development [chapter 1]. In: Greydanus DE, Patel DR, Pratt HD, editors. Essential adolescent medicine. New York: McGraw-Hill Medical Publishers; 2006. p. 3–15.
[5] Graber JA, Seeley JR, Brooks-Gunn J, et al. Is pubertal timing associated with psychopathology in young adulthood? J Am Acad Child Adolesc Psychiatry 2004;43:718–26.
[6] Kaltiala-Heino R, Rimpela M, Rissanen A, et al. Early puberty and early sexual activity are associated with bulimic-type eating pathology in middle adolescence. J Adolesc Health 2001; 28:346–52.
[7] Greydanus DE, Bashe P. Caring for your teenager. American Academy of Pediatrics. New York: Bantam Books; 2003. p. 600.
[8] Bell DL, Ginsburg KR. Connecting the adolescent male with health care. Adolesc Med 2003; 14:555–64.
[9] American Academy of Pediatrics. Sexuality, contraception and the media. Committee on public education. Pediatrics 2001;07:191–4.
[10] Prinstein MJ, Meade CS, Cohen GL. Adolescent oral sex, peer popularity, and perceptions of best friends' sexual behaviour. J Pediatr Psychol 2003;28:243–9.
[11] Halpern-Fisher BL, Cornell JL, Kropp RY, et al. Oral versus vaginal sex among adolescents: perceptions, attitudes, and behaviour. Pediatrics 2005;115:845–51.
[12] Brady SS, Halpern-Felsher BL. Adolescents' reported consequences of having oral sex versus vaginal sex. Pediatrics 2007;119:229–36.
[13] Eaton DK, Kann L, Kinchen S, et al. Youth risk behavior surveillance–United States, 2005. Centers for Disease Control and Prevention. MMWR Surveillance Summaries 2006;55.
[14] Adolescent pregnancy—current trends and issues: 1998. American Academy of Pediatrics. Committee on adolescence. Pediatrics 1999;103(2):516–20.
[15] Alan Guttmacher Institute. Into a new world: young women's sexual and reproductive lives. New York: The Alan Guttmacher Institute, (120 Wall Street, NY,NY USA 10005); 1998. p. 1–56 (www.agi-usa.org)
[16] Kirby D. Emerging answers: research findings on programs to reduce teen pregnancy [Summary]. . Washington, DC: National Campaign to PreventTeen Pregnancy; 2001.
[17] Klein JD, the Committee on Adolescence. Adolescent pregnancy: current trends and issues. Pediatrics 2005;116:281–6.
[18] Jenkins RR. Adolescent pregnancy and abortion [Chapter 26]. In: Greydanus DE, Patel DR, Pratt HD, editors. Essential adolescent medicine. New York: McGraw-Hill Medical Publishers; 2006. p. 559–68.
[19] Darroch JE, et al. Differences in teenage pregnancy rates among five developed countries: the roles of sexual activity and contraceptive use. Fam Plann Perspect 2001;33(6):244–50 281.
[20] Hamilton BE, Miniño AM, Martin JA, et al. Annual summary of vital statistics: 2005. Pediatrics 2007;119:345–60.
[21] Martin JA, Hamilton BE, Sutton PD, et al. Births: final data for 2004. MMWR 2007;55(51): 1383.
[22] Births: preliminary data for 2005, Centers for Disease and Controls, National Vital Statistics Survey 2005.

[23] Centers for Disease Control and Prevention. 2006 Guidelines for treatment of sexually transmitted diseases. MMWR 2006;55(RR-11):1–94.
[24] Weinstock H. STDs among American youth: incidence and prevalence estimates, 2000. Perspect Sex Reprod Health 2004;36(1):6–10.
[25] Johnson J. Sexually transmitted diseases in adolescents [chapter 24]. In: Greydanus DE, Patel DR, Pratt HD, editors. Essentials of adolescent medicine. New York: McGraw-Hill Medical Publishers; 2006. p. 511–42.
[26] Greydanus DE, Patel DR. Sexually transmitted diseases in adolescents [Section 6]. In: Burg FD, Ingelfinger JR, Polin RA, et al, editors. Current pediatric therapy. 18th edition. Philadelphia: Elsevier; 2006. p. 326–9.
[27] Greydanus DE, Senanayake P, Gaines MJ. Reproductive health: an international perspective. Indian J Pediatr 1999;66:339–48.
[28] Greydanus DE, Pratt HD, Dannison LL. Sexuality education programs for youth: current state of affairs and strategies for the future. J Sex Educ Ther 1995;21:238–54.
[29] Greydanus DE, Rimsza ME, Matytsina L. Contraception. Pediatr Clin North Am 2005;52: 135–61.
[30] Kahn JA. Maximizing the potential public health impact of HPV vaccines. J Adolesc Health 2007;40:101–3.
[31] Sionean C, DiClemente RJ, Wingood GM, et al. Psychosocial and behavioral correlates of refusing unwanted sex among African-American adolescent females. J Adolesc Health 2002; 30:55–63.
[32] Trenholm C, Devaney B, Fortson K, et al. Impacts of Four Title V, Section 510 Abstinence Education Programs. Final Report. Mathematica Policy Research, Inc. HHS-98–0010; MPR Reference No: 8549-110, 1–164, 2007 (April). Available at: http://mathematica-mpr.com/publications/PFDs/impactabstinence.pdf. Accessed on April 18, 2007.
[33] Greydanus DE, Rimsza ME, Newhouse PN. Sexuality and disability in adolescence. Adolesc Med 2002;13:500–14.
[34] Santelli JS, Lindberg LD, Finer LB, et al. Explaining recent declines in adolescent pregnancy in the United States: the contribution of abstinence and improved contraceptive use. Am J Public Health 2007;97:150–6.
[35] Kaunitz AM. Long-acting hormonal contraceptives—indispensable in preventing teen pregnancy. J Adolesc Health 2007;40:1–3.
[36] Wolak J, Mitchell K, Finkelhor D. Unwanted and wanted exposure to online pornography in a national sample of youth internet users. Pediatrics 2007;119:247–57.
[37] Ybarra ML, Mitchell KJ, Finkelhor D, et al. Internet prevention messages: targeting the right messages. Arch Pediatr Adolesc Med 2007;161:138–45.
[38] Vreeman RC, Carroll AE. A systemic review of school-based interventions to prevent bullying. Arch Pediatr Adolesc Med 2007;161:78–88.

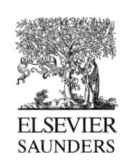

Deconstructing Adolescent Same-Sex Attraction and Sexual Behavior in the Twenty-First Century: Perspectives for the Clinician

Antonio C. Sison, MD[a], Donald E. Greydanus, MD[b]

[a]*Department of Psychiatry, University of the Philippines, Philippine General Hospital, 1906 Taft Avenue, Malate, Manila 1004, Philippines*
[b]*Michigan State University College of Human Medicine, Michigan State University/ Kalamazoo Center for Medical Studies, 1000 Oakland Drive, Kalamazoo, MI 49008-1284, USA*

Homosexuality or same-sex attraction is a highly controversial aspect of human sexuality that has caused conflict for thousands of years [1,2]. Although condemned by many religions since the dawn of theologic thought, it has persisted throughout human existence. The American Psychiatric Association, the American Psychological Association, and other organizations have officially declared that homosexuality in the male and lesbianism in the female are normal aspects of human sexuality [3–6].

Research notes that 2% to 4% of male adults are homosexual and 3% are bisexual and that 3% to 7% of female adults are lesbians [7–12]. Societal condemnation of nonheterosexual orientation extends to other groups as well, now summarized with the term *gay, lesbian, bisexual, transgender, and questioning* (GLBTQ) youth. This controversy regarding homosexuality has continued into the twenty-first century. The potential consequences of homosexuality in youth are noted in Table 1 [1,2,13–26], and this highlights the importance of the clinician acquiring a better perspective of the psychosocial issues confronting the adolescent with same-sex attraction.

Sexual side of technologic advancements in the twenty-first century

Because of the rapid technologic advances in the twenty-first century, the generation divide has been reframed into a technologic divide. The Internet

E-mail address: greydanus@kcms.msu.edu (D.E. Greydanus).

Table 1
Potential biopsychosocial consequences of homosexuality in youth

Medical	Reproductive tract infections (sexually transmitted diseases)
Psychologic	Depression
	Suicidal ideations, attempts, and completions
	Substance abuse disorders
	Eating disorders
Social	Family rejection (parents and siblings)
	Peer rejection
High-risk situations	Trauma from beatings, murder, rape, murder
	Victims of hate crimes
	Runaway behavior or rejected by family ("throwaway")
	Street life with prostitution and sex survival

is a whole universe that includes the whole range of human interest at the click of the mouse [27,28]. To the curious adolescent, cyberspace offers the whole range of sex sites that cater to all possible ranges of sexual interest. Some sites offer dating services and chat rooms. The adolescent who is attracted to the same sex is able to access gay and lesbian sites that may provide information, and possibly misinformation, on sexual practices, especially in terms of safe sex practices.

Chat rooms have opened a new arena for communication with other people who share the same interests, especially with regard to sexual encounters. For the trusting adolescent, the chat room is a potentially harmful area because of the sexual predators and opportunists who prey in this twenty-first century medium. The phenomenon of the blog has created a whole new arena for individuals to share personal interests, pictures, and videotapes with the rest of the millions who access the site, often all for free. It is not surprising that adolescents have taken up blogging as an activity to connect with friends and other people who may find them interesting. There are blogs mainly featuring content that is of interest to gays and lesbians as well.

Cellular telephone technology has expanded its abilities to include taking pictures and recording short videotapes in technology that is further refined on a frequent basis. The cellular telephone is also used to meet new friends and possible sex partners. This is another area that the adolescent may explore, and it may lead to risky sexual encounters.

The twenty-first century is defined by rapid technologic advances, although, paradoxically, with continued ambivalent attitudes regarding homosexuality. Some regions of the world retain a negative view of same-sex attraction. Some countries still prosecute any adolescent or adult who engages in homosexual activity, leading to a death sentence in some cases, all within the framework of the local legal and religious systems. Gay, lesbian, bisexual, and transgender (GLBT) adolescents living in such conditions continue to live under the sword of persecution.

In contrast, in recent years, some countries have legally acknowledged same-sex marriages that afford similar rights of male and female married couples, including immigration, inheritance, and adoption rights. The GLBT adolescent living in a more tolerant society is not necessarily safe either. GLBT adolescents may be subjected to various degrees of harassment, and some suffer serious injury, including loss of life (see Table 1).

Discrimination based on sexual orientation is considered illegal in most cases. A special category of hate crimes reflects the unique focus of illegal activities against a selected population—gays and lesbians. Immigration of families from various parts of the world to industrialized countries presents unique challenges to the adolescent, who must balance traditional values and perceptions with the current values of his or her adoptive country.

Some pioneering companies have started to develop marketing strategies targeting the GLBT market. Adolescents are exposed to various images of vague homoeroticism in advertisements. Gay-themed movies have started to be viewed as economically viable projects, as evidenced by the commercial success of "Brokeback Mountain," which features the strained relationship of two cowboys across the years and societal prejudice. Television now has sitcoms that feature prominently gay characters, such as "Will and Grace," and even openly gay talk show hosts, such as the "The Ellen Degeneris Show." Although there is more visibility of gay characters in media, homophobia in various levels is still pervasive and damaging.

How can the clinician integrate these influences in the context of adolescent sexuality—specifically gay, lesbian, bisexual, and transgender adolescents?

There are negative and positive influences that have an impact on the adolescent in the twenty-first century, some of which may affect the physical and mental health of the adolescent. Is the clinician aware of these developments? How can the clinician help the GLBTQ adolescent in the twenty-first century? In attempting to address this issue, it is necessary to deconstruct the GLBT gestalt into smaller frameworks. The Clinician's Framework Guide Questions for the GLBT Adolescent (Appendix) allow the clinician to appreciate the different aspects that may be overlooked in routine health care evaluation of this adolescent and show each framework in terms of possible questions that may tap the thoughts and feelings of the adolescent. This gives the clinician a sense of possible issues that may be easily overlooked in routine health consultation; these include a general framework with various aspects: physical, gender-specific, sexual orientation, psychologic mood-anxiety, drug use, impulsive behavior, sexual, family, financial, living conditions, school, social support, cultural-religious, and legal issues.

How can the clinician be more sensitive to and understanding of the gay, lesbian, bisexual, and transgender adolescent patient?

The past adolescent experience of the clinician is the starting framework that he or she can use to understand the difficult and sometimes confusing issues, experiences, and choices of the GLBT adolescent [2]. The first process toward understanding the new world of the twenty-first century adolescent is recognizing the role of technology in the current adolescent gestalt. The adolescent has a different world view today because of the push of technology that influences world views, values, language, platonic relationships, sexual relationships, and sex-seeking behaviors.

The second process is for the clinician is to be aware of his or her own thoughts, feelings, and reactions regarding GLBT issues [2]. The Clinician Reaction to GLBT Issues Checklist is a tool that the clinician can use to obtain an overview of his or her personal thoughts, feelings, and interactions, which have positive or negative ratings (Table 2). Should the clinician have more negative than positive personal reactions to GLBT issues, it is important to be aware of these personal issues and to seek to prevent their negative influence on the assessment of the GLBT adolescent. The role of the clinician is to be of help to patients and not to reject them.

Table 2
Clinician reaction to gay, lesbian, bisexual, or transgender issues checklist

Clinician	Positive reaction to GLBT issues	Neutral reaction to GLBT issues	Negative reaction to GLBT issues
Personal thoughts			
Religious values			
Cultural values			
Friends' values			
Family's values			
Personal values			
Personal feelings			
Emotions			
Social interaction			
Strangers			
Colleagues			
Friends			
Patients			

Abbreviation: GLBT, gay, lesbian, bisexual, or transgender.

How can the clinician integrate this broader knowledge of adolescent gay, lesbian, bisexual, and transgender high-risk factors in the doctor-patient process?

Issues of confidentiality, respect, and referral are integral for the clinician to articulate to GLBT youth at the initial phase of the consultation.

> Confidentiality. The clinician respects the right to privacy of the adolescent patient; however, the safety and security of the patient are the priority [29]. Should the clinician believe that the adolescent is at risk, confidentiality can be breeched. Should there be any issues that should be disclosed to the parents, the clinician may encourage the patient to open this topic with his or her parents. The clinician may facilitate a family session or refer to another professional to facilitate this adolescent-family discussion.
>
> Respect. The clinician should be nonjudgmental and not make comments regarding the patient's opinions and sexual activity. Should there be any episode that makes the clinician feel uncomfortable, the clinician may shift the topic or shorten the session. The reason for the discomfort is an area the clinician should understand, and it may be an area of needed personal growth.
>
> Referral. If the clinician cannot help the GLBT adolescent because of personal issues, referral to an unbiased clinician who may be of help is recommended.

After establishing rapport in the initial phase, the clinician may use a checklist that can help to identify areas that may require prevention, treatment, or referral. The Global GLBT Checklist for Biopsychosocial Risk Factors by Greydanus and Sison [2] is a guide that helps the clinician to obtain an evaluation of the biopsychosocial dimension of the adolescent's same-sex attraction and sexual behavior (Table 3). After the using the checklist, the clinician can discuss areas for prevention, treatment, and referral with the adolescent. Hopefully, the GLBT adolescent of today not only has medically competent clinicians but clinicians who are nonjudgmental and comfortable in discussing nuances of sex-seeking behavior in the twenty-first century [30].

Summary

Although the twenty-first century is defined by rapid technologic advances, this is not the case with regard to ambivalent attitudes regarding the GLBT individual. Many regions of the world retain negative views of same-sex attraction. There are negative and positive influences that have an impact on the physical and mental health of the GLBT adolescent. For the clinician to develop a global perspective, it is necessary to deconstruct the GLBT gestalt into smaller frameworks. The Clinician's Framework Guide Questions for the

Table 3
Global gay, lesbian, bisexual, or transgender checklist for biopsychosocial risk factors

Biopsychosocial framework	Clinical focus prevention	Clinical focus treatment	Clinical focus referral
Biologic			
Physical			
Psychologic			
Gender			
Sexual orientation			
Psychological			
Mood, anxiety, and thinking			
Drug			
Impulsive behavior			
Sexual behavior			
Social			
Family			
Living condition			
School			
Social support			
Culture and religious			
Legal			

GLBT Adolescent (see Appendix) show the different frameworks of possible questions that may tap the thoughts and feelings of the adolescent.

The Clinician Reaction to GLBT Issues Checklist (see Table 2) is a tool that the clinician can use to obtain an overview of his or her positive, neutral, or negative personal thoughts, feelings, and interactions on GLBT issues, which may potentially compromise the benefit of the clinical evaluation. The Global GLBT Checklist for Biopsychosocial Risk Factors by Greydanus and Sisson [2] (see Table 3) is a guide that clinicians can use to help them obtain a beneficial systematic evaluation of the biopsychosocial dimensions of adolescent same-sex attraction and sexual behavior. This guide may allow the clinician to appreciate the different aspects that may be missed in the routine evaluation of the GLBT adolescent who needs a health care professional to reach out and help this teen's journey through adolescent and adult life. These three checklists may aid the clinician to appreciate the global dynamics between the adolescent with same-sex attraction, the clinician's sensitivity, and the impact of social realities.

References

[1] Greydanus DE, Bhave SY. Alternative sexual orientation. In: Bhave SY, Bhalerao-Ghandi A, editors. Handbook of adolescent gynecology and ARSH (adolescent reproductive and sexual health). New Delhi (India): Jaypee Brothers Medical Publishers; 2007. p. 27–34.
[2] Greydanus DE, Sisson A. Homosexual attraction. In: Greydanus DE, Patel DR, Pratt HD, editors. Behavioral pediatrics. 2nd edition. Lincoln (Nebraska): iUniverse Publishers; 2006. p. 344–76.
[3] American Psychiatric Association. Diagnostic and statistical manual of mental disorders (DSM-IV). 4th edition. Washington, DC: American Psychiatric Association; 2000.
[4] International classification of diseases and related health problems (ICD-10). 10th edition. Los Angeles (CA): Professional Medical Information Corporation; 2004.
[5] American Medical Association. Council on Scientific Affairs. Health needs of gay men and lesbians in the United States. JAMA 1996;275:1354–9.
[6] American Academy of Pediatrics. Homosexuality and adolescence. Committee on Adolescence. Pediatrics 1993;92:631–4.
[7] Kinsey A, Pomeroy W, Martin C. Sexual behavior in the human male. Philadelphia: WB Saunders; 1948.
[8] Kinsey A, Pomeroy W, Martin C. Sexual behavior in the human female. Philadelphia: WB Saunders; 1953.
[9] Diamond M. Homosexuality and bisexuality in different populations. Arch Sex Behav 1993; 22:291–310.
[10] Seidman SN, Rieder RO. A review of sexual behavior in the United States. Am J Psychiatr 1994;151:330–41.
[11] Sell RL, Wells JA, Wyrij D. The prevalence of homosexual behavior and attraction in the United States, the United Kingdom, and France: results of national population-based samples. Arch Sex Behav 1995;24:235–48.
[12] Rowlett J, Greydanus DE. Gender identity. In: Greydanus DE, Wolraich M, editors. Behavioral pediatrics. New York: Springer-Verlag; 1991. p. 40–65.
[13] Eisenberg ME, Resnick MD. Suicidality among gay, lesbian, and bisexual youth: the role of protective factors. J Adolesc Health 2006;39:662–8.
[14] Remafedi G, Farrow JA, Deisher RW. Risk factors for attempted suicide in gay and lesbian youth. Pediatrics 1991;87:869–75.
[15] Remafedi G. Sexual orientation and youth suicide. JAMA 1999;282:1291–2.
[16] Shaffer D, Fisher P, Hicks RH, et al. Sexual orientation in adolescents who commit suicide. Suicide Life Threat Behav 1995;25(Suppl):64–71.
[17] Garofalo R, Wolf RC, Kessel S, et al. The association between health risk behaviors and sexual orientation among a school-sample of adolescents. Pediatrics 1998;101:895–902.
[18] Garofalo R, Wolf C, Wissow LS, et al. Sexual orientation and risk of suicide attempts among a representative sample of youth. Arch Pediatr Adolesc Med 1999;153:487–93.
[19] Garofalo R, Harper GW. Not all adolescents are the same: addressing the unique needs of gay and bisexual male youth. Adolesc Med 2003;14:595–611.
[20] Nicholas J, Howard J. Better dead than gay: depression, suicide ideation, and attempt among a sample of gay and straight-identified males 18 to 24. Youth Stud Aust 1998;17: 28–33.
[21] Harrison AE, Silenzio VMB. Comprehensive care of lesbian and gay patients and their families. Prim Care 1996;23:31–45.
[22] Kruks G. Gay and lesbian homeless/street youth: special issues and concerns. J Adolesc Health 1991;12:515–8.
[23] Zea MC, Reisen CA, Poppen PJ. Psychological well-being among Latino lesbians and gay men. Cultur Divers Ethnic Minor Psychol 1999;5:371–9.
[24] Federal Bureau of Investigation. Hate crime statistics, 2003. Washington, DC: US Department of Justice; 2004. p. 9–12.

[25] Sadock BJ, Sadock VA. Human sexuality. In: Kaplan and Sadock's synopsis of psychiatry. 9th edition. New York: Lippincott Williams and Wilkins; 2003. p. 692–729.
[26] Sadock BJ, Sadock VA. Gender identity disorders. In: Kaplan and Sadock's synopsis of psychiatry. 9th edition. New York: Lippincott Williams and Wilkins; 2003. p. 730–8.
[27] Saini S, Bhave SY. Internet and sexual activity. In: Bhave SY, Bhalerao-Gandhi A, editors. Handbook of adolescent gynecology and ARSH (adolescent reproductive and sexual health). New Delhi (India): Jaypee Brothers Medical Publishers; 2007. p. 35–40.
[28] Ybarra ML, Mitchell KJ, Finkelhor D, et al. Internet prevention messages: targeting the right online behaviors. Arch Pediatr Adolesc Med 2007;161:138–45.
[29] Ford C, English A, Sigman G. Confidential health care for adolescents: position paper of the Society for Adolescent Medicine. J Adolesc Health 2004;35:160–7.
[30] Greydanus DE, Sison AC. Focus on adolescents with same sex attraction and sexual attraction. Asian J Padiatr Practice 2007;11:12–20.

Appendix

Clinician's framework guide questions for the gay, lesbian, bisexual, or transgender adolescent

Physical framework	GLBT adolescent issues	
1. Body image	How do you view yourself?	
	Do you consider yourself attractive?	
	How would you compare yourself with your friends?	
	Do you have any part of your body that you feel would need improvement?	
2. Chest/breasts	Male:	Female:
	Are you content with your chest?	Are you content with your breasts?
	Do you want any modification done?	Do you want any modification done?
3. Genitals	Male:	Female:
	Are you content with your penis and testes?	Are you content with your vagina?
	Do you wish to have a vagina instead of a penis?	Do you wish to have a penis instead of a vagina?
	Do you want any modification done?	Do you want any modifications done?
	Do you have any problems with your penis?	Do you have any problems with your vagina?
4. Body markings and modifications	Have you had any modifications done like tattoos, piercing, scarring, branding, or other modifications?	
	Are you planning to have any modification in the future?	
	Do your friends have any modifications?	
	What are your attitudes regarding body modifications?	
5. Use of substances	Male:	Female:
	Do you use any illegal substances?	Do you use any illegal substances?
	Do you use any hormones like estrogen to make yourself look more feminine?	Do you use any hormones like testosterone to make yourself look more masculine?
	Do you use any steroids to improve your sports performances?	Do you use any steroids to improve your sports performances?

Appendix (*continued*)

Physical framework	GLBT adolescent issues	
4. Body fat	Do you have any concerns with regard to your weight?	
	Do your friends comment about your weight?	
	Do you have a good appetite?	
	Do you exercise?	
	Do you vomit or use laxatives to lose weight?	
5. Sexually transmitted diseases	Are you sexually active?	
	Do you consistently practice safe sex?	
	Do you have multiple sex partners?	
	Have you had any sexually transmitted disease?	

Gender-specific behavior framework	Adolescent issues	
1. Gender-specific grooming	Male:	Female:
	Do you want to look like a girl instead of a boy?	Do you want to look like a boy instead of a girl?
	Do you use make-up or pluck your eyebrows?	Do you groom your hair to look like a boy?
2. Gender typical behavior	Male:	Female:
	Do you feel completely masculine, mixed masculine and feminine, or completely feminine?	Do you feel completely feminine, mixed feminine and masculine, or completely masculine?
3. Gender-specific voice projection	Male:	Female:
	Do you think your voice sounds masculine or not?	Do you think your voice sounds feminine or not?
4. Gender identification	Male:	Female:
	Do you want to change into a girl?	Do you want to change into a boy?
	Do you feel you have both male and female qualities?	Do you have both female and male qualities?

Sexual orientation framework	Adolescent issues
1. Sexual attraction	Are you sexually attracted to the opposite sex, same sex, or both?
	Are you confused about your sexual attraction?
	Do you think your attraction to the same sex is experimental?
	Is your sexual attraction a source of anxiety or distress?

Psychologic framework	Adolescent issues
1. Intelligence	Do you have problems learning?
	Do you have problems understanding lessons?
	How are your grades at school?
2. Emotional	Would you consider yourself too emotional, sensitive, or irritable?
	Do you keep a grudge for a long time?
3. General self-image	Do you like yourself?
	How would compare yourself with your friends?

(*continued on next page*)

Appendix (*continued*)

Mood, anxiety, and thinking framework	Adolescent issues
1. Depression	Do you have episodes of depression?
	Do you have episodes of feeling exhausted or having lower energy levels than usual?
2. Suicidal ideation or plans	Do you sometimes wish you were dead?
	Do you have plans to kill yourself?
3. Anxiety	Do you have episodes of feeling nervous even for no reason?
	Do you have fears of being alone?
	Do you feel scared to leave the house?
4. Psychosis	Do you hear voices that only you can hear?
	Do you see things that only you can see?
	Are you suspicious of everyone, including your family?

Drug use framework	Adolescent issues
1. Illegal drugs	Have you tried any illegal drugs?
	Do you compulsively use illegal drugs?
2. Source of drugs	Who is the source of your use of illegal drugs?
3. Amount of money for drugs	How much do you spend on illegal drugs a week?
	Where do get the money to pay for illegal drugs?
4. Friends who use drugs	How many of your friends use illegal drugs?
	Did any of your friends who use illegal drugs get into legal problems or any medical problems?

Impulsive behavior framework	Adolescent issues
1. Impulsive behavior	Do you have any problems with regard to impulsive behavior?
2. Petty theft	Do you steal sometimes?
3. Gun and knives	Do you carry guns or knives?

Sexual behavior framework	Adolescent issues
1. Knowledge of safe sex practices	Are you knowledgeable with regard to safe sex?
2. Source of knowledge of sexual practices	What are your sources of information with regard to safe sex?
3. Sexual partners	Do you have multiple sex partners?
	Do you have sex with prostitutes?
4. Sex for pay	Have you ever paid for sex?
	Have you ever been paid for sex?
5. Use of drugs	Do you use drugs when you have sex?
6. Use of pornography	How much pornography do you use?
	Does your pornography use affect your school work, social life, or recreational activities?
7. Use of cybersex	Do you use the Internet to look for sex partners?
8. Sexual asphyxiation	Do you use asphyxiation as part of you sexual activities?
9. Participation in pornography	Have you ever participated in any form of pornography?
10. Sexual behavior	Have you been coerced into sexual activity?
	Have you ever had a traumatic sexual experience?
	Do you have sex in high-risk situations?
	Have you had any legal problems because of your sexual behavior?

Appendix (*continued*)

Family and financial framework	Adolescent issues
1. Family structure	Can you describe your family situation?
	How do you feel about your family situation?
	How is discipline implemented at home?
2. Verbal abuse	Are there any episodes of shouting between family members?
3. Physical abuse	Are there any episodes when family members would hurt each other?
4. Mental illness	Do you have any family history of any form of mental illness or drug use?
5. Financial resources	Do you have adequate finances?
	Do you have other sources of income?
6. Attitudes toward homosexuality	What are your family's attitudes about GLBT?
	Do you have family friends that are GLBT?
	Do you have problems with regard to your family's attitudes about GLBT?
7. Family member with GLBT identification	Do you have a family member who has GLBT identification?
	How is this family member treated?

Living condition framework	Adolescent issues
1. Presence of responsible related adult	Is there always a parent at home?
	Do you live with your extended family, such as grandparents, uncles, aunts, and cousins?
2. Other nonrelated adults	Is there any adult who is not a relative who is at home after school?

School framework	Adolescent issues
1. Academic performance	How are your grades at school?
	Do you have any problems related to school?
	Are you able to focus on your studies?
2. Extracurricular activities	Do you engage in sports?
	Do you have any hobbies?
	Have you joined any clubs?
3. Teachers	What do you feel your teachers think of you?
	Do you have any problems with your teachers?
	What is the general attitude of your teachers with regard to GLBT issues?
4. Peers	Do you have close friends in school?
	Are you being teased, bullied, or harassed at school?
5. Stigma against same-sex attraction and sexual behavior	What are the general attitudes of students in your school with regard to GLBT issues?

(*continued on next page*)

Appendix (*continued*)

Social support framework	Adolescent issues
1. Family	Can you talk with your parents or siblings with regard to problems, including GLBT issues?
2. Extended family	Could you talk with any other relative with regard to problems, including GLBT issues?
3. Neighborhood	Could you talk with any friends in your neighborhood with regard to problems, including GLBT issues?
4. School	Can you talk with any friends in school with regard to problems, including GLBT issues?
5. Other friends	Can you talk with any friends with regard to problems, including GLBT issues?
6. Family member with GLBT identification	Do you have any friends who have GLBT identification? How are your GLBT friends treated?

Cultural and religious framework	Adolescent issues
1. Immigrant status	Have you recently immigrated to the United States? Did you grow up in the United States?
2. Language	Do you speak other languages?
3. Cultural attitudes	Do you belong to an ethnic community? What are the attitudes of your ethnic community with regard to GLBT issues?
4. Religious attitudes	Do you belong to any religious denomination or group? What are the attitudes of this religious community with regard to GLBT issues?

Legal framework	Adolescent issues
1. Laws regarding sexual behavior	Is homosexual behavior a crime in your community or state?
2. Laws regarding adolescent sex	What is the age of consent for sex in your state or community?

Abbreviation: GLBT, gay, lesbian, bisexual, or transgender.

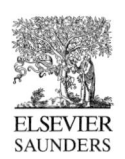

The Adolescent Sexual Offender

Helen D. Pratt, PhD*, Donald E. Greydanus, MD, Dilip R. Patel, MD

Division of Behavioral-Developmental Pediatrics, Michigan State University Kalamazoo Center for Medical Studies, 1000, Oakland Drive, Kalamazoo, MI 49008, USA

The family physician plays a vital role in recognition and management of child sexual abuse. There is a large body of literature on the various aspects of abused children; however, few data are available in the literature on adolescent sexual offenders or teenagers who are involved in sexual abuse of younger children [1–3]. In a review of the literature on adolescent sexual offending, the authors found that physicians may encounter adolescent sexual offenders in their practice under several circumstances, such as with adolescent revelation, parental report, or at the request of legal representatives. Few adolescents are caught or prosecuted, however, and those offenders who are arrested and convicted often receive minimal punishments (ie, probation, community service) [1–3]. The costs to society for the crimes of juvenile sex offenders are considerable, not only those inflicted on crime victims and society as a whole but also those imposed on offenders and their families [1,2].

Although a significant number of adolescents are referred to treatment programs, the treatment interventions remain controversial [4–13]. Many of the treatment interventions have not been scientifically evaluated on adolescents; instead, they have been adapted from experience with adult sexual offenders. Most treatment programs focus on rehabilitation of adolescent offenders in the private sector and on the prevention of re-offending [4–6,14–20]. Unfortunately, there is little empiric evidence of the long-term effects of different interventions with adolescent sexual offenders. Most treatments are controversial and result in high (50%) rates of recidivism [4,7,11,13,16,20]. Righthand and Welch (2001) contend that, as with other delinquent behaviors, early intervention can be critical [21]. This article reviews some practical aspects of this topic for family physicians; issues

* Corresponding author.

E-mail address: pratt@kcms.msu.edu (H.D. Pratt).

0095-4543/07/$ - see front matter © 2007 Elsevier Inc. All rights reserved.
doi:10.1016/j.pop.2007.04.016   *primarycare.theclinics.com*

reviewed included definitions, characteristics, comorbidity, assessments, and legal issues regarding adolescent sexual offenders.

Presentation in the office

Adolescents and their families may be reluctant to openly discuss acts of sexual offending because of the serious psychosocial and legal implications for the offender and his or her family. More often the offender is brought to the family physician by an appropriate agency in the course of a child abuse investigation. The family physician's assistance may be sought in medical and psychologic evaluation or to facilitate further expert or specialized referral and to coordinate ongoing care [2].

Occasionally, the clinician may be presented with indirect or nonspecific indicators of an adolescent being involved in the sexual abuse of younger children [2]. Presentation may involve parental concerns about their teen's sexual activities with a younger child (ie, sibling, other relative, or acquaintance); they may ask if such activities are "normal." In other circumstances the parents of the victim may report fear of the offender or incidents of sex play with an older teen to the offender's parents; again, the physician is asked for advice on how to help their offending teen [2].

Theories of etiology

Theories offered to explain the cause of deviant sexual behavior in adolescents toward younger children are primarily based on adult models. Researchers generally agree that there are multiple factors (ie, psychologic, biologic, and sociologic) that interact in complex and poorly understood ways [22]. Studies suggest some association between adolescent sexual offending and a combination of individual characteristics, family variables, and socioeconomic factors [23,24]. A history of prior physical or sexual abuse, impaired family functioning, alcohol and substance abuse, exposure to erotica, neurobiologic factors, and psychiatric comorbidity have been found to be associated with a higher prevalence of adolescent sexual offending. Unfortunately, most theories do not relate the cause of deviant sexual behavior to other factors that may impair treatment [2].

Incidence

The sexual victimization of children by adolescents has become a serious problem in our society [25,26]. Approximately one third of sexual offenses against children are committed by teenagers. Sexual offenses against young children are typically committed by boys between the ages of 12 and 15 years old [1]. The percentages of adolescents arrested for sexual offending in 2004 are as follows: 28% of adolescents were aged 12 to 14 years, 37%

aged 15 to 17 years, and 42% aged 18 to 20 years; about 6% of all statutory rapes and 12% of forcible rapes involved the arrest of a juvenile [27,28]. In 2003 law enforcement agencies reported 2.2 million arrests of people less than 18 years of age for criminal acts. Of those arrested 15% were males and 20% were females less than 18 years of age; these sexual offenses (excluding forcible rape and prostitution) included 20% that were committed by males and 22% by females [29].

Legal definition

Adolescent sex offenders are described as youth between the ages of 13 and 17 years who commit illegal sexual behavior as defined by the sex crimes statues of the legal jurisdictions in which they reside [1]. Legal meanings of sexual offenses vary from state to state [30,31]. Statutes typically define sexual offenses as: (a) penetration offenses, which include penetration of virtually any body orifice for a sexual purpose and are felonies; and (b) crimes not involving physical contact (eg, voyeurism, exhibitionism, obscene phone calls). Such offenses progress from privacy issues at the misdemeanor level to the felony level, depending on the specific circumstances of each case [2,30–32]. The addition of physical force or coercion almost always results in a felony life offense [30–32].

The offender

Biologic factors

In an earlier published review the authors found that there is little consistent empiric evidence to support biologic factors as direct causal agents of adolescent sexual offending. Adult studies of the effects of antiandrogens, the luteinizing hormone–releasing hormone (LHRH) antagonists and serotonergics, have looked at the impact these agents have had on sexual offending [19]; few studies have focused on adolescents [2,33,34]. High levels of androgens are theorized to contribute to increased libido in adult males; similar data in adolescents are not known [19,33,34].

Individual characteristics

Juveniles who have committed sex offenses are a heterogeneous mix, commit multiple offenses, usually assault more than one victim, and may not limit their offenses to one type of victim [23,35]. They differ according to victim and offense characteristics and a wide range of other variables, including types of offending behaviors, histories of child maltreatment, sexual knowledge and experiences, academic and cognitive functioning, and mental health issues [1].

A small percentage of adolescent offenders (2%–4%) are responsible for most of sexual assaults committed by adolescents [35,36]. These adolescent offenders account for the victimization of approximately one half of boys and one quarter of girls who are molested or sexually abused. Most adolescent offenders are males who victimize females. Few data are available on female sexual offenders. When adolescent molesters (male or female) violate very young children, however, they tend to select male victims [23,37–40].

Adolescent sex offenders rarely have previous convictions for sexual assault, but 63% are likely to have committed nonsexual offenses [35,41]. Most incest offenses occur in the victim's home, often when the perpetrator is providing child care services [42]. Adolescent rapists, on the other hand, tend to victimize strangers [43]. Offenses commonly include intercourse as the age of the perpetrator and victim increase [35,36,39,42].

Contrary to common assumption, most adolescent sex offenders have not been victims of childhood sexual abuse [1]. Of particular note is that children and adolescents who had been physically abused were 7.6 times more likely to rape or sodomize other children when compared with adolescents who were sexually abused or neglected [24]. Additionally, one in two adult sex offenders began sexually abusive behavior as a juvenile [1].

Family characteristics

Most offenders lived at home with both parents and at least one other juvenile at the time of their offending [43,44]. Their families more closely resemble those of youth who have severe emotional or behavioral problems [44,45]. The parents often deny sexual tensions [39] and exhibit a paucity of sexual knowledge or education [43]; one quarter of the parents have known sexual pathology [46]. Adolescent sexual offenders who had committed sexual homicides experienced exaggerated personal and family dysfunction [32].

Comorbid disorders

Concurrent diagnoses of psychopathology can exist in adolescent sexual offenders [2]. The most common psychiatric diagnoses are listed in Box 1 [39,44,47–50]. Similar to other delinquents, adolescent sexual offenders frequently engage in distorted thinking to make their offenses more socially acceptable to themselves and others [49–51]. Gender differences in comorbid diagnoses do exist. For example, male offenders are more often diagnosed with antisocial behavior and paraphilias (Box 2) [52]. On the other hand, female offenders are more likely to be diagnosed with mood disorders and engage in self-mutilation [23]. Rarely are these offenders plagued with behavioral problems; they are more likely to be shy and more comfortable with youth who are younger than they are [49].

Box 1. Psychiatric comorbidities of adolescent sexual offenders

Conduct disorder
Substance abuse disorders
Adjustment disorders
Attention deficit/hyperactivity disorder with hyperactivity
Specific phobia
Mood disorder

Data from Refs. [39,44,47–50].

Distinguishing sexual exploitation

Physicians who understand the differences between sexual exploration and exploitation are better prepared to make that distinction when faced with a report of adolescent sexual behavior. Normal or developmentally acceptable sexual play usually involves the factors listed in Box 3 [2,37].

Determination

Sexual curiosity and exploration is a normal part of the developmental process if it meets the criteria listed in Box 3; however, parents and adult caregivers need to be vigilant and give children other healthy outlets.

Action steps

If the "sex play" is determined to be experimental or exploratory, the family physician should discuss normal childhood and adolescent sexual behavior with parents and outline measures to minimize inappropriate sexual

Box 2. Paraphilias [52]

Exhibitionism
Fetishism
Frotteurism
Pedophilia
Sexual masochism
Sexual sadism
Transvestic fetishism
Voyeurism

Data from American Psychiatric Association: Diagnostic and statistical manual of mental disorders. 4th edition [DSM-IV-TR]. Washington, DC: American Psychiatric Association; 2000.

> **Box 3. Factors of normal or developmentally acceptable sexual play**
>
> 1. The two involved individuals are age and developmental peers.
> 2. Children and prepubertal adolescents may engage in exploratory behavior; the play or exploration usually involves mutual genital display, touching, and fondling only.
> 3. Curiosity about the differences and similarities in anatomy and pleasurable feelings associated with masturbation are the normal motivator to engage in sexual exploration.
> 4. Young children are motivated to exploratory behavior by curiosity about differences and similarities in anatomy and pleasurable feelings associated with masturbation. Older children and young adolescents may also be interested in sexual roles and sexual identity to the curiosity and pleasure motivations.
> 5. Exploratory sexual play is not coercive; mutual consent is typical of exploratory behaviors.
> 6. Only the two individuals discussed as above instigate and participate in the exploratory sexual play. Two children or adolescents may be involved in age-appropriate exploratory behavior, but not observers or additional participants.
> 7. Although one or both of the participants may express/demonstrate guilt feelings, they do not manifest feelings of anger, fear, sadness, or other strongly negative responses.
>
> ---
>
> *Data from* Pratt HD, Patel DR, Greydanus DE, et al. Adolescent sexual offenders: issues for family physicians. Int Pediatr 2001;16(2)1–12; and De Jong AR. Sexual interactions among siblings and cousins: experimentation or exploitation? Child Abuse Neg 1989;13:271–9.

stimulation in the home. Parents should be advised to provide closer supervision of the adolescent. Older adolescents can be instructed to stay away from compromising situations with younger children.

Exploitive sexual play

Exploitation involves the absence of the factors listed above and the inclusion of the following [2,37]:

- If one of the individuals is cognitively impaired then a peer relationship does not exist.
- Attempted intercourse is atypical among preschoolers and is rare in the young school-aged child (6–9 years).

- Abusive behavior often involves elements of pressure, misrepresentation, force, threat, secrecy, or other forms of coercion. Although some of the threat or coercion is obvious and violent, the evaluator must take care to recognize subtle emotional pressure or the use of implied authority by an older child or adolescent in some cases.
- If sexual contact has been arranged for the pleasure of another older individual, it is exploitative. One of the participants manifests feelings of anger, fear, sadness, or other strongly negative responses in this situation [1,2].

Determination

Exploitation is more often viewed in negative terms by the child; however, some abused children seem to have a neutral or positive emotional response to abuse. If the sexual behavior is determined to be exploitation, in addition to the preceding suggestions, medical examination and documentation should be performed; as required by state child abuse laws, the family should be referred to the appropriate agency for further evaluation. If the adolescent has access to other children, especially very young children, the clinician should assess the level of risk posed to those children.

Action steps

When it is determined that the child or adolescent is at high risk for sexually offending the physician should inform the family and the appropriate people. Furthermore, the family should be advised to stop all baby-sitting and childcare activities to limit the adolescent offender's opportunity to re-offend. A more definitive treatment may not be within the purview of all family physicians and generally the adolescent offender is referred to professionals and programs specializing in such treatment [1,2].

In-office assessment

The family physician is concerned mainly with medical and psychosocial assessment of the adolescent offender, and is not expected to conduct a specialized or forensic evaluation. The untrained clinician should not undertake a detailed sexual perpetration history without the assistance and guidance of highly trained professionals. Family physicians play an essential role in early recognition, medical and psychosocial evaluation, appropriate referral, and coordination and follow-up of medical services [2].

The physician should carefully document the reported information, which also includes a history of the offending incident, psychosocial history, medical history, and a general physical and neurologic examination. The extent of evaluation performed by the family physician depends on his or her experience and familiarity with such cases. It is generally neither necessary nor advisable for this clinician to go into finer details of the incident; however, enough information should be obtained to justify that an offense has occurred. Detailed investigation is best left to the authorities. In most cases the physician may elect to refer the adolescent to a colleague with more expertise in this area [23,53]. It is important that as soon as the physician realizes that the adolescent or parent is revealing information of a criminal offense, the limits of confidentiality and "Duty to Warn" must be explained before completing the examination [2].

Legal issues

The process

It is helpful for the physician to understand what happens to youth who are adjudicated for their sexual offenses.

- The age at which an adolescent can be adjudicated for criminal behavior varies. The minimum ages in those jurisdictions in which age is defined varies from 6 to 12 years of age, with most states setting 10 years as the lowest age of criminal responsibility [30,31,54].
- In most juvenile justice jurisdictions it is unimportant whether the alleged victim has consented to the act or is an involuntary participant [30]. Once there is sufficient evidence to identify an offender, a decision regarding prosecution is often made at the juvenile court level.
- Trials in the juvenile justice system are less formal and are often conducted in private without the use of a jury. Juveniles in this system are more likely to receive efforts at rehabilitation and less likely to be held fully accountable for their actions than if they were adjudicated in the adult courts. In the case of rape, sodomy, or sexual homicide, however, most states have moved to address adolescent offending in the adult criminal justice system, which can impose harsher punishments [21,26,30,31,54,55].

Physician–patient privilege

Local statutes usually govern physician–patient privileges (ie, the right to respect the confidentiality of all communications). The development of such privileges in each state is thus subject to local interpretation and state-by-state case law developments. Family physicians should explain, at the outset, to all adolescents and their families the limits of confidentiality [2,30,54,55]. As guided by local laws and standards of medical practice, certain acts that are harmful to the adolescent or others have to be reported to appropriate agencies. If the adolescent's behavior must be reported to the authorities or potential victims warned, the family physician should inform the adolescent and the family.

Reporting any crime changes the status of the act from private to criminal. Most family physicians are familiar with local child abuse reporting laws and procedures. In every state the definition of child abuse is not left to the determination of the professional; thus, professionals who deal with children have an enforceable mandate to report suspected child abuse [2,30,54–56]. All fifty states have mandated reporting laws that require professionals to report reasonable suspicions that abuse or neglect has occurred [30,54–56]. Professional obligations pertaining to confidentiality may be seriously challenged by the requirements of the law and the local community, particularly when it involves sexual conduct [30,54–56].

Serving as an expert witness in sexual offense cases

No physician should consider serving as a witness or expert witness in sexual abuse case involving adolescent offenders without specific training in this complex area [2].

Summary

Adolescent sexual offenders represent a cross section of our country's population and present a serious problem. They commit multiple offenses, usually have more than one victim, and may not limit their offenses to one type of victim. Family physicians can play a vital role in the recognition, referral, and management of their adolescent patients who sexually offend. Because most offenders are not detected, and those who are discovered are often not adjudicated, the physician can help to prevent and minimize the occurrence of sexual offending by educating parents about the importance of close supervision and seeking appropriate professional help for deviant sexual behavior in children and adolescents.

References

[1] Chaffin M, Bonner B, Pierce K. What research shows about adolescent sex offenders. National Center on Sexual Behavior of Youth at the Center on Child Abuse and Neglect Alexandria, VA American Prosecutors Research Institute 2002;5(2). Available at: http://www.ndaa.org/publications/newsletters/in_re_volume_5_number_2_2002.html. Accessed May 11, 2007.
[2] Pratt HD, Patel DR, Greydanus DE, et al. Adolescent sexual offenders: issues for family physicians. Int Pediatr 2001;16(2):1–12.
[3] Stahl AL. Person offenses in juvenile court, 1985–2002. OJJDP fact sheet. U.S. Department of Justice, Office of Justice Programs, Office of Juvenile Justice and Delinquency Prevention, 2006;6 #FS 200603. Available at: www.ojp.usdoj.gov/ojjdp. Accessed May 11, 2007.
[4] Freeman-Longo RE, Burotn D, Levins J, Fiske JA. Nationwide survey of treatment programs and models. Brandon (VT): The Safer Society Foundation, Inc.; 1998.
[5] Henggeler SW, Milton GB, Smith LA. Family preservation using multisystemic therapy: an effective alternative to incarcerating serious juvenile offenders. J Counsel Clin Psychol 1992; 60:953–61.
[6] Icenogle DL. Sentencing male sex offenders to the use of biological treatments. J Leg Med 1994;15:279–304.

[7] Lab SP, Shielf G, Schondel C. Research note: an evaluation of juvenile sexual offender treatment. Crime Delinq 1993;39:543–53.
[8] Monto M, Zgourides G, Harris R. Empathy, self-esteem, and the adolescent offender. Sexual Abuse: J Res Treat 1998;10:127–40.
[9] Prentky RA, Knight RA, Lee AFS. Child sexual molestation: research issues National Institute of Juvenile Research Report June NCJ 163390; 1997.
[10] Gijs L, Gooren L. Hormonal and psychopharmacological interventions in the treatment of paraphilias: an update. J Sex Res 1996;33:273–90.
[11] Rösler A, Witztum E. Treatment of men with paraphilia with a long-acting analogue of gonadotropin-releasing hormone. N Engl J Med 1998;338:416–22.
[12] Bradford JMW. Treatment of men with paraphilia. N Engl J Med 1998;338:464.
[13] Sipe R, Jensen EL, Everett RS. Adolescent sexual offenders grown up: recidivism in young adulthood. Crim Justice Behav 1998;25:109–24.
[14] Weinrott MR, Riggan M, Frothingham S. Reducing deviant arousal in juvenile sex offenders using vicarious sensitization. J Interperson Viol 1997;2(5):704–28.
[15] Sermabeikian P, Martinez D. Treatment of adolescent sexual offenders: theory-based practice. Child Abuse Negl 1994;18:969–76.
[16] McConaghy N. Assessment and treatment of sex offenders: the Prince of Whales programme. Aust NZ J Psychiatr 1990;24:175–81, 22.
[17] Cooper AJ. Review of the role of two antilibidinal drugs in the treatment of sex offenders with mental retardation. Ment Retard 1995;33:42–8.
[18] Kaplan MS, Morales M, Becker JV. The impact of verbal satiation of adolescent sex offenders: a preliminary report. J Child Abuse 1993;2:81–8.
[19] Richer M, Crismon ML. Pharmacotherapy of sexual offenders. Ann Pharmacother 1993;27:316–9.
[20] Borduin CM, Henggeler SW, Blaske DM, Stein RJ. Multisystemic treatment of adolescent sexual offenders. Int J Offender Ther Comp Criminol 1990;34:105–13.
[21] Sue R, Carlann W. Juveniles who have sexually offended: a review of the professional literature report. Washington, DC: US Department of Justice, Office of Justice Programs, Office of Juvenile Justice and Delinquency Prevention; 2001 NCJ 184739.
[22] McGuire RJ, Carlise JM, Young BG. Sexual deviation as conditioned behavior: a hypothesis. Behav Res Ther 1965;2:185–90.
[23] Matthews R, Hunter JA, Vuz J. Juvenile female sexual offenders: clinical characteristics and treatment issues. Sex Abuse: J Res Treat 1997;9:187–99.
[24] Widom CS. Victims of childhood sexual abuse—later criminal consequences National Institute of Justice Research in Brief. March 1995. Washington DC: US Department of Justice Office of Justice Programs National Institute of Justice; 1995.
[25] Becker JV, Stein RM. Is sexual erotica associated with sexual deviance in adolescent males? Int J Law Psychiatry 1991;14:85–95.
[26] National Council of Juvenile and Family Court Judges. The revised report from the National Task Force on juvenile sexual offending, The National Adolescent Perpetrator Network. Juv Fam Court J 1993;44(4):5–100.
[27] Snyder HN. Juvenile arrests 2004. Washington, DC: U.S. Department of Justice, Office of Justice Programs, Office of Juvenile Justice and Delinquency Prevention; 2006. NCJ 214562. Available at: www.ojp.usdoj.gov/ojjdp. Accessed May 11, 2007.
[28] Troup-Leasure K, Snyder HN. Statutory Rape Known to Law Enforcement OJJDP: Juvenile Justice Bulletin. Washington, DC: U.S. Department of Justice, Office of Justice Programs, Office of Juvenile Justice and Delinquency Prevention; 2005. Available at: www.ojp.usdoj.gov/ojjdp. Accessed May 11, 2007.
[29] Snyder HN, Sickmund M. National Center for Juvenile Justice Office of Justice Programs 2006. Juvenile justice and delinquency prevention, 2006. Available at: www.ojp.usdoj.gov; www.ojp. Accessed May 11, 2007.

[30] Kole SM. Statute protecting minors in a specified age range from rape o other sexual activity as applicable to defendant minor within protected age groups. American Law Reports (ALR5th) Annotations and Cases 18 ALR 5th: 856–90; 1994.
[31] Office of Juvenile Justice amd Delinquency Prevention: Juvenile transfer to criminal court. Juvenile justice reform initiatives in the States 1994–1996. Washington, DC: U.S. Department of Justice. 1997 NCJ165697. Available at: http://www.ncjrs.gov/pdfiles/reform.pdf. Accessed May 11, 2007.
[32] Myers WC, Burgess AW, Nelson JA. Criminal and behavioral aspects of juvenile sexual homicide. J Forensic Sci 1998;43:340–7.
[33] Berlin FS, Meinecke CF. Treatment of sex offenders with antiandrogenic medication: conceptualization, review of treatment modalities, and preliminary findings. Am J Psychiatry 1981;138:601–7.
[34] Berlin FS. "Chemical castration" for sex offenders. N Engl J Med 1997;336(14):1030–5.
[35] Ryan G, Miyoshi T, Metzner J, Krugman R, et al. Trends in a national sample of sexually abusive youths. J Am Acad Child Adolesc Psychiatry 1996;35:17–25.
[36] Awad G, Saunders E, Levere J. A clinical study of male adolescent sexual offenders. Int J Offender Ther Comp Criminol 1984;28:105–16.
[37] De Jong AR. Sexual interactions among siblings and cousins: experimentation or exploitation? Child Abuse Negl 1989;13:271–9.
[38] Elliott M, editor. Female sexual abuse of children. New York: Guilford Press; 1993.
[39] Saunders EB, Awad GA. Male adolescent sexual offenders: exhibitionism and obscene phone calls. Child Psychiatry Hum Dev 1991;21:169–78.
[40] Bandura A. Social foundations of thought and action: a social cognitive theory. Englewood Cliffs (NJ): Prentice Hall; 1996.
[41] Snyder HN. Juvenile arrests 1996. The Juv Just Bull NCJ 167578, Nov. 1997.
[42] Greenfeld LA. Child victimizers: violent offenders and their victims. Bureau of Justice Statistics U.S. Department of Justice Office of Justice programs and Office of Juvenile Justice and Delinquency Prevention. Washington, DC. 1996 NCJ-153258.
[43] Ryan G, Lane S. Theories on etiology. In: Ryan G, Lane S, editors. Juvenile sexual offending: causes, consequences, and correction. San Francisco: Jossey-Bass Publishers; 1997. p. 267–321.
[44] Blaske DM, Bourduin CM, Henggeler SW, Mann BJ. Individual, family, and peer characteristics of adolescent sex offenders and assaultive offenders. Dev Psychol 1989;25: 846–55.
[45] Bischof GP, Stith SM, Whitley ML. Family environments of adolescent sex offenders and other juvenile offenders. Adolescence 1995;30:157–70.
[46] Kaufman KL, Hilliker DR, Daleiden EL. Subgroup differences in the modus operandi of adolescent sexual offenders. Child Management 1996;1:17–24.
[47] Haapasalo J, Kankkonen M. Self-reported childhood abuse among sex and violent offenders. Arch Sex Behav 1997;26:421–31.
[48] Oliver LL, Hall G, Neuhas SM. A comparison of the personality and background characteristics of adolescent sex offenders and other adolescent offenders. Crim Justice Behav 1993;20: 359–70.
[49] Valliant PM, Bergeron T. Personality and criminal profile of adolescent sexual offenders, general offenders in comparison to nonoffenders. Psychol Rep 1997;81(2):483–9.
[50] Truscott D. Adolescent offenders: comparison for sexual violent, and property offenses. Psychol Rep 1993;73:657–8.
[51] Myers WC, Blashfield R. Psychopathology and personality in juvenile sexual homicide offenders. J Am Acad Psychiatry Law 1997;25:497–508.
[52] American Psychiatric Association. Diagnostic and statistical manual of mental disorders. Fourth edition [DSM-IV-TR]. Washington, DC: American Psychiatric Association; 2000.
[53] Barbaree H, Marshall WL, Hudson SM, editors. The juvenile sex offender. New York: Guilford Press; 1993.

[54] Sexuality Information and Education Council of the United States (SIECUS) Public Policy Department. SIECUS looks at states' sexuality laws and the sexual rights of their citizens. SIECUS Rep 1998;26(6):4–15.
[55] The American Civil Liberties Union. Status of US Sodomy laws. New York: American Civil Liberties Union; 1998.
[56] Erwin CP. Judicial notebook: Tarasoff reconsidered. APA Monitor 2005;36(7):112. Available at: http://www.apa.org/monitor/julaug05/jn.html. Accessed May 11, 2007.

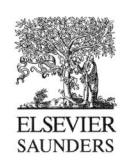

ADHD in Children, Adolescents, and Adults

Sreenivas Katragadda, MD[a],
Howard Schubiner, MD[b,c,d,e,*]

[a]*Department of Psychiatry, Dartmouth Hitchcock Medical Center,
1 Medical Center Drive, Lebanon, NH 03766, USA*
[b]*Department of Internal Medicine, Wayne State University
School of Medicine, Detroit, MI, USA*
[c]*Department of Pediatrics, Wayne State University
School of Medicine, Detroit, MI, USA*
[d]*Department of Psychiatry and Behavioral Neurosciences,
Wayne State University School of Medicine, Detroit, MI, USA*
[e]*Department of Internal Medicine, Providence Hospital, 16001 West Nine
Mile Road, Southfield, MI 48075, USA*

Attention-deficit–hyperactivity disorder (ADHD) and its subtypes are a group of neurobehavioral disorders, characterized by inattention, increased motor activity, and impulsiveness [1]. These disorders are commonly referred to as a single entity, ADHD. ADHD is relatively common in children and adolescents and recent data suggest that it is also fairly common in adults. The prevalence of ADHD is similar in and outside of the United States. Studies using *Diagnostic and Statistical Manual IV* (DSM-IV) criteria have shown prevalence rates of ADHD in preschoolers, school-age children, and adolescents to be as high as 9.5%, 11.4%, and 9.5%, respectively [2–4]. The National Co-morbidity Survey estimated the prevalence of ADHD in adults to be approximately 4.4%, demonstrating that the prevalence is comparable with many common mental health and physical health problems [5]. Recent prevalence data from diverse regions of the world, such as the Ukraine, Australia, India, and Nigeria, using the DSM-IV criteria are broadly comparable with data from the United States [6–9]. These data support the explanation that diagnostic and surveillance inconsistencies rather than the classical behaviors of children account for the differences in prevalence rates

---

* Corresponding author.
E-mail address: howard.schubiner@stjohn.org (H. Schubiner).

of ADHD in different countries [10]. Unlike earlier notions, most children do not out grow ADHD but continue to have symptoms of ADHD as adolescents and adults, especially if they had severe symptoms or were treated with medications [11,12]. A male preponderance has been a typical and consistent finding in many of these United States and international studies across all age groups. If these prevalence rates are applied to United States census data, more than 2 million children and adolescents and more than 7 million adults are expected to meet the diagnostic criteria for ADHD, making it one of the most common clinical entities [13]. Because most of these recent prevalence estimates were based on the DSM-IV criteria, these estimates reflect individuals with significant functional impairments and not just symptom clusters alone. The cost of impairments related to ADHD is only beginning to be appreciated. A recent study by Birnbaum and colleagues [14] estimated the total financial burden of ADHD to patients and families in United States at a staggering $31.6 billion for the year 2000.

Etiology and risk factors

Genetic and developmental factors have been strongly implicated in the etiology of ADHD, and although environmental and social factors are known to contribute, they explain a much smaller proportion of the variance. Some authors have argued, however, that this lack of evidence for social and environmental contribution to ADHD may be secondary to lack of support and enthusiasm for research in this direction [15].

ADHD has been shown to be a highly heritable disorder. The rates of inheritance between 0.85 and 0.90 make ADHD the most heritable disorder among mental health disorders [16]. Family and adoption studies have shown that first-degree relatives of ADHD probands face a 3- to 10-fold increased relative risk of developing ADHD or another comorbid condition [17]. Several twin studies have demonstrated concordance rates of approximately 80% in identical twins versus 40% in fraternal twins [18,19]. Several prenatal and developmental risk factors including maternal smoking during pregnancy, parental alcoholism, and low birth weight have been shown to be independent risk factors for the development of ADHD [20–22]. When prenatal factors and genetic transmission were studied simultaneously, however, genetic factors clearly outweighed prenatal factors [19,23].

Several social and environmental factors have been found to precipitate and worsen ADHD symptoms. Family environments with psychosocial adversities (eg, poverty, high crime, and single parent families), higher levels of conflict, and psychiatric morbidity are significantly associated with levels of impairment in ADHD children [24,25]. Children's perception of marital conflicts has also been shown to be an independent risk factor for inattention and hyperactivity [26]. Divorce and unemployment have been shown to be overrepresented in adults with ADHD in the national comorbidity survey, although these are likely to be consequences of ADHD rather than causal associations [5].

Pathophysiology

There is no single universally accepted explanation for the pathophysiology of ADHD. Several lines of research based on structural imaging, functional imaging, mechanism of action of stimulant medications, genetic studies, psychologic testing, or a combination of these have identified alterations, such as regional cerebral volume differences, reduced functional capacities of certain central nervous system loci, and abnormalities in the catecholamine neurotransmitters, dopamine (DA) and norepinephrine (NE), as being associated with ADHD.

A recent meta-analysis of ADHD structural imaging studies by Valera and colleagues [27] confirmed significant volumetric reductions in total and right cerebral volumes, the right caudate, the cerebellar regions, and the corpus callosum in groups of individuals with ADHD compared with control populations. An important study by Castellanos and colleagues [28] found that the differences in size of brain structures in ADHD were unrelated to stimulant medication treatment. Reduced metabolism in the prefrontal cortex and striatal regions has also been a consistent finding in a number of functional imaging studies [29–32]. The prefrontal cortex may be responsible for suppressing responses to irrelevant stimuli and the basal ganglia may be involved in executing motor responses to these stimuli [29]. Reduced inhibitory activity of the prefrontal cortex may explain the distractibility and motor hyperactivity found in ADHD. Another interesting functional imaging finding has been that when performing the Stroop test, a neurocognitive frontal lobe conflict task, adults with ADHD tended to activate insular cortical pathways as opposed to the anterior cingulate pathways used by controls [33]. Adults with ADHD were also less efficient at cognitive tasks and had longer latencies in processing information.

The neurotransmitter systems thought to be involved in the pathophysiology of ADHD are the catecholamines DA and NE. Most of the evidence to support this comes from mechanisms of action of stimulant medications on releasing catecholamines and their success at reducing symptoms of ADHD. Stimulants, such as methylphenidate (MPH) and amphetamine, block the reuptake of both DA and NE and inhibit monoamine oxidase, an enzyme that plays a role in metabolizing catecholamines. The amphetamines also facilitate the release of DA and NE into the synaptic cleft. The modes of action of nonstimulant medications that treat ADHD (atomoxetine, guanfacine, bupropion) are also ultimately based on their effects on the catecholamines. Evidence from genes involved in ADHD inheritance patterns also points toward involvement of the catecholamine neurotransmitter system. The genetic variations of genes involved in the regulation of catecholamines, including DRD4, DRD5, DAT, DBH, 5-HTT, HTR1B, and SNAP-25, are associated with increased rates of ADHD [34–36].

Diagnosis across the age groups

The diagnosis of ADHD is a clinical process and neither biologic tests nor psychometric instruments are currently available definitively to diagnose ADHD in individual cases. Clinicians to definitively diagnose ADHD based on the results of a comprehensive examination assessing the history and course of ADHD symptoms, functional impairments, pervasiveness of symptoms in different settings, and any associated psychopathology. In the United States, the diagnostic basis of ADHD is the DSM-IV-TR criteria set (Box 1).

The DSM IV-TR criteria for ADHD are a set of 18 criteria, consisting of nine inattention symptoms and nine hyperactivity-impulsivity symptoms. Individuals must display, in two distinct settings, six of nine inattention symptoms or six of nine hyperactivity-impulsivity features for at least 6 months to qualify for a diagnosis. Some of the features must be present before the age of 7 and should interfere with developmentally appropriate social, academic, or occupational functioning. The symptoms may not be better accounted for by another psychiatric or physical disorder. The frequency and severity of these features must be more than what is typically seen in developmentally comparable individuals. DSM-IV-TR characterizes three subtypes of ADHD: (1) predominantly hyperactive, (2) predominantly inattentive, and (3) a combined type based on the predominance of the core symptoms. Although not strictly a subtype, another diagnostic category in the DSM-IV is "ADHD not other wise specified." This category may be useful in diagnosing individuals (especially adults) who have symptoms and impairments of ADHD but do not meet the full criteria for the diagnosis.

The diagnostic process in children should be an integration of a clinical assessment of the child by the clinician and the observations by significant others who interact with the child in two different settings. Careful assessment should be done to rule out hyperactivity that is normally expected in toddlers and preschoolers. Sometimes this may be difficult and some clinicians may choose to wait until school age or there is clear evidence of functional impairment before making a treatment decision. There are several well-validated instruments to assess psychopathology in children (eg, the Child Behavior Check List, and the Conners parent and teacher rating scales) that can be used to obtain detailed ratings by parents, teachers, and other caregivers in various settings [37–40]. The Child Behavior Check List also includes data on other behavioral areas and can help clinicians not only in the diagnosis of ADHD, but also to discern the presence of any

> **Box 1. DSM-IV criteria for diagnosing ADHD in children**
>
> *Inattention features*
> Fails to give close attention
> Difficulty sustaining attention
> Does not listen when spoken to directly
> Difficulty organizing tasks
> Avoids tasks requiring mental effort
> Unable to follow through tasks
> Often loses things
> Easily distracted
> Forgetful
>
> *Hyperactivity and impulsivity features*
> Hyperactivity
>   Fidgeting or squirming
>   Cannot remain seated when required
>   Cannot play quietly
>   Talks excessively
>   Always on the go as if driven by a motor
>   Runs about and climbs excessively
> Impulsivity
>   Blurts out answers
>   Difficulty waiting for turn
>   Often interrupts or intrudes
>
> ---
> *Modified from* American Psychiatric Association. Diagnostic and statistical manual of mental disorders. 4th edition (DSM-IV). Washington: American Psychiatric Association; 2004; with permission.

comorbid conditions and impairments in functioning. An ADHD Rating Scale-IV [41] or SNAP-IV [42] should also be part of the initial diagnostic evaluation. These are DSM-IV–based ADHD scales that can be easily administered to aid in diagnosis and in monitoring symptoms during treatment.

Diagnosing adolescents and adults may be more difficult for several reasons. The ADHD diagnostic criteria are part of the "Disorders usually first diagnosed in infancy, childhood, and adolescence" section of the DSM, and as such reflect the clinical features of ADHD in children. It can be difficult to apply these criteria to adults and older adolescents in their current form. The current DSM criteria are a set of objective observations made by teachers, parents, and clinicians (eg, "makes careless mistakes," "acts as if driven by a motor," and so forth). These are appropriate for children, whereas in diagnosing adolescents and adults one expects to rely on more subjective experiences and subjective difficulties, as in many other adult diagnoses like depression or anxiety [1]. Another issue is that some of the criteria (eg, "climbing excessively," or "difficulty playing quietly") are clearly not appropriate for adults or even adolescents. The DSM-IV age of onset criteria seem to be too restrictive and are not evidence based, as demonstrated in a recent study that found that adults who had onset of ADHD after the age of 7 did not differ from those who had symptom onset before the age of 7 in terms of impairment, comorbidity, or inheritance pattern [43]. Lastly, many adults with ADHD symptoms have functional impairment requiring treatment, yet they may not have the full six out of nine symptoms as required under the DSM-IV criteria [44,45]. To overcome these difficulties, recommendations for a separate set of standardized criteria tailored to adolescents and adults have been made [43,46]. The Utah criteria for ADHD developed by researchers at the University of Utah School of Medicine is one such effort in that direction; however, even these criteria may not be able to identify all the adults with ADHD who are likely to benefit from pharmacotherapy [47].

Nevertheless, clinicians can diagnose adults and older adolescents with ADHD by doing a thorough retrospective assessment of the presence of ADHD symptoms during childhood and then comparing those with current self-reported symptoms, and objective reports from past and present (eg, report cards, school assessments, and parent or spousal reports). The clinical assessment should also determine the level of functional impairment in social or occupational spheres and not just symptom presence, because often this may be the most important consideration in diagnosing and treating adults with ADHD. To do a retrospective assessment of presence of symptoms of ADHD during childhood using patients' own recall, the Wender-Utah Rating Scale-WURS [48] can be used, which has been shown to correlate well with observations made by parents. Once childhood symptoms and impairment is established, the clinician should look for age-appropriate clinical features and impairments of ADHD. The evolution of core symptoms and impairment patterns from childhood through adulthood is described next. An efficient way of assessment of current symptoms is to use a diagnostic scale that assesses developmentally appropriate adult correlates of DSM ADHD symptoms. Examples of such scales include the Conners Adult ADHD rating scales [49], the Brown Attention Deficit Disorder scale [50], and the Conners/Wells Adolescent Self-Report of Symptoms [51].

Evolution of clinical features across the life span

Because ADHD is typically a lifelong affliction, it is important to understand the pattern of symptoms and impairments in all age groups. Inattention is commonly manifested in children as forgetfulness, not paying attention in class, not responding to one's name being called out, inability to organize, inability to focus on tasks at hand, and losing important items. In adults, inattention might manifest differently, as procrastination, poor time management, difficulty in initiating and completing tasks, difficulty shifting attention when needed, and difficulty with multitasking (Box 2).

Hyperactivity in childhood is manifest as excessive fidgeting or squirming, excessive running, excessive climbing, excessive talking, and inability to sit still or play quietly that is inappropriate to the child's developmental background. The purposeless hyperactivity in children often transforms into a pattern of apparently purposeful constant activity in adulthood. In adults, hyperactivity is frequently manifest as adaptive behaviors rather than observed behaviors. For example, adults with hyperactivity may choose a job that requires high levels of activity, may work longer hours, or work two jobs. They may be easily bored and may avoid situations where they are required to be physically inactive and quiet for long periods of time, such as attending plays and meetings. This quest for constant activity and subjective restlessness frequently leads to family tensions and difficulties in relationships. Children with impulsivity often blurt out answers before they completely hear a question, they cannot wait their turn, and they can be very intrusive. Adults with impulsivity may exhibit low frustration tolerance, lose their temper easily, and make snap and irresponsible choices. Impulsivity in adults differs from that in children by the severity of the

---

Box 2. Evolution of inattention

Children
Forgetfulness
Loosing important items
Not responding to name being called out
Not being able to focus on tasks at hand
Avoids tasks requiring mental effort
Easily distracted
Poor organization
Inability to follow through complex acts

Adults
Procrastination
Indecision
Poor time management
Avoiding tasks or jobs that require sustained attention
Difficulty initiating tasks
Difficulty completing tasks
Difficulty multitasking
Difficulty shifting attention from one task to another

consequences. Adults may lose jobs, cause motor vehicle accidents, or break up relationships because of their impulsive actions (Box 3).

Impact of attention-deficit–hyperactivity disorder across the life span

ADHD is associated with significant impairments across the life cycle. Screening, recognition, and treatment are important at all levels of development, not just in childhood. Children with ADHD typically underachieve academically, repeat grades, drop out of school, have difficulties with peer relationships, disrupt family functioning, and are more likely than their peers without ADHD to be delinquent [52]. ADHD in children has also been shown to have a significant impact on family members. Parents of ADHD children are more likely to be depressed, have poor interpersonal relations, and have parenting difficulties [53]. In adolescents, higher rates of school suspensions and dropouts, conduct disorder and oppositional defiant disorder, teenage pregnancy, sexually transmitted diseases, and increased rates of substance use were found by Barkley and colleagues [54] in a recently published study. Compared with adults without ADHD, significantly more adults with ADHD are likely to have a history of

---

Box 3. Evolution of hyperactivity and impulsivity

Children
Squirms and fidgets
Cannot sit still
Cannot play quietly
Talks excessively
Runs and climbs excessively
Always on the go
Cannot wait for their turn
Blurts answers
Intrudes and interrupts

Adults
Chooses highly active job
Avoids situations with low physical activity
May choose to work long hours or two jobs
Seeks constant activity
Easily bored
Impatient
Low frustration tolerance levels
Snap decisions and irresponsible behaviors
Loses temper easily

suspended drivers license, accidents, being arrested, and quitting or being fired from their job. They are also more likely to have a history of multiple marriages and a pattern of poor relationships. They have a greater chance of being substance users and are at higher risk for a diagnosis of antisocial personality disorder (Box 4) [44,55,56].

Comorbidity in attention-deficit–hyperactivity disorder

Psychiatric comorbidity is very common in ADHD, regardless of the age of the individual. In children with ADHD, more than two thirds have a comorbid condition. In the multimodal treatment of ADHD study, the largest, federally funded, multicenter treatment trial ever conducted in the United States, only 31% of ADHD children did not have a comorbid condition. The comorbid conditions that were seen in children included oppositional defiant disorder (40%); conduct disorder (14%); anxiety disorder (31%); and mood disorders (4%). In many children there may be more than one comorbid condition requiring clinical attention [57]. The multimodal treatment of ADHD study also showed that children with comorbid disruptive behaviors responded best to pharmacotherapy alone, whereas children

---

Box 4. Impact of ADHD across the life span

Children
Academic underperformance, poor grades
History of repeating grades
Fewer friends
Disruptive at school
School suspensions
Increased school drop out rates
Delinquency and conduct problems
Disruption of family functioning

Adolescents and adults
Poor employment history
Poor driving record
Academic underachievement
Multiple marriages
Legal problems
Accidents and injuries
Teenage pregnancy
Sexually transmitted diseases
Smoking
Substance use

with ADHD and comorbid anxiety responded better to a combined treatment approach with medication and behavioral therapy [58]. It is imperative for clinicians to cast a wide net in their differential diagnoses to identify comorbidities in children presenting with ADHD symptoms to offer the most effective treatment approach.

Few studies have looked at psychiatric comorbidity in adults, and there seems to be wide variation in the reported comorbidity rates, especially regarding mood disorders. Adult studies do demonstrate, however, that comorbidity is extremely common among adults with ADHD and it may be even rare to find ADHD with no comorbid conditions in an adult. Murphy and Barkley [44] in a study involving 172 ADHD adults found high rates of alcohol abuse or dependence (35%); oppositional defiant disorder (30%); conduct disorder (17%); major depressive disorder (18%); anxiety disorders (32%); drug abuse or dependence (14%); and dysthymia (32%). In a more recent study of ADHD families, McGough and coworkers [59] reported even higher rates of major depression (59%); substance use (47%); and conduct disorder (20%). In this study, 87% adults with ADHD had at least one comorbid condition and 56% had at least two other comorbid conditions.

Substance use disorders (SUD) as comorbid conditions deserve a separate discussion, because the frequency of substance use among adults with ADHD can be as high as 47% [59]. Addressing the issue of comorbidity from the opposite direction, Schubiner and colleagues [60] found the prevalence of ADHD in SUD population to be 24%, and other studies also report a consistently high rate [61]. Considering the frequency with which these conditions co-occur clinicians should consider the possibility of ADHD in all patients with SUD and vice versa. This is also important because it has been found that patients with active ADHD symptoms tend to have higher rates of SUD [62]. Wilens and colleagues [63] have shown that adults with ADHD had a history of substance use starting at an earlier age than controls without ADHD. Indeed, the importance of identifying and treating ADHD at an early age is strengthened by a recent meta-analysis by Wilens and coworkers [64], which showed a 1.9-fold reduction in SUD when ADHD symptoms were pharmacologically treated compared with controls with untreated ADHD symptoms. Identifying comorbidities is important because failing to do so may limit treatment effectiveness for ADHD and contribute to greater overall impairment. In addition, some comorbid conditions are not amenable to ADHD treatments, requiring either other medications or other types of interventions (eg, cognitive behavior therapy for anxiety disorders).

Management of attention-deficit–hyperactivity disorder

Once a diagnosis is made, the management of ADHD should involve patient education, psychosocial interventions, and medication management.

All patients diagnosed with ADHD should be educated about the disorder. Clinicians should share a brief synopsis of the current literature about the epidemiology, etiology, and pathogenesis of ADHD with the patients and their families. A clear understanding that ADHD is a medical problem with a biologic basis may help destigmatize the diagnosis. Family members feel more comfortable accepting the diagnosis and treatment after realizing that ADHD is a heritable disorder and that their family situation or parenting practices did not cause it. ADHD can be explained to patients as a mild disability analogous to having poor eyesight, a mild congenital disability. Patients can readily see that, as in the case of poor eyesight, if ADHD is not appreciated and corrected with the help of aids, it can have a negative impact on social, academic, and occupational functioning. Unfortunately, there exists a lot of misinformation about ADHD and its treatment both in print and on the Internet, which increases the importance of providing patients with a basic understanding of the disorder and with reliable evidence-based print and World Wide Web resources. The information about ADHD in the "parents" section of American Academy of Pediatrics and "facts for families" section of American Academy of Child and Adolescent Psychiatry are World Wide Web–based educational material about ADHD that parents may trust. Web sites of Children and Adults with ADHD (www.chadd.org, www.help4adhd.org) and the Attention Deficit Disorder Association (www.add.org), national support organizations for patients and families with ADHD, are also excellent resources.

In children, psychosocial interventions may include parent training and school-based interventions. Parent training is a cognitive-behavioral approach to help parents manage behavioral issues at home. This can be done on an individual basis or as part of parent training programs. Parent training frequently includes ADHD education, understanding of parent-child relationships, teaching effective communication skills, encouraging positive behaviors, improving motivation of children by using reward systems like tokens, and introducing response costs and time outs for misbehaviors. Parent training may also provide parents with practical management strategies for behavioral issues that can occur in various circumstances, such as in public places. School-based interventions may include teacher education, functional assessment of behaviors, manipulating the antecedents and consequences to achieve behavioral changes, using tokens and rewards programs, preferential seating, teachers providing an overview and summary of the learning exercise, dividing the academic work into smaller chunks, scheduling most academic school work before lunch time, extra planned breaks, computer-aided instruction, and so forth. There should also be collaboration between school and home because consistency in the behavioral approaches is essential for optimal outcomes.

In adolescents who may be more likely to present with behavioral problems and conflicts at home, behavioral family therapy can be helpful. This therapy consists of training parents in behavior management, and training parents and adolescents in effective problem solving, communication, and cognitive restructuring techniques. Here, the adolescent is involved in making decisions regarding house rules, rewards, and consequences. In adults, counseling and practical guidance regarding the management of ADHD-related functional impairments are most helpful for a successful outcome. Counseling should focus on management of the impact of ADHD on the patient, relationships in the family, use of alcohol or other drugs, education, and employment. Many patients also benefit from formal training in organizational skills to improve their academic and employment-related performance. Adults should also be educated about the accommodations that they can receive at their places of employment or education under the Americans with Disabilities Act. Recently, many adults with ADHD have benefited from coaching as a way to help them maintain focus on daily activities and to set priorities. Finally, a variety of Internet-based resources are available including on-line support (http://health.groups.yahoo.com/group/ADD_Advice/).

Pharmacologic treatments

Medications used in the treatment of ADHD can be broadly divided into stimulants and nonstimulants. The stimulants include MPH isomers and amphetamines. The nonstimulants consist of several classes of medications and include atomoxetine, bupropion, modafinil, venlafaxine, clonidine, guanfacine, tricyclic antidepressants, and monoamine oxidase inhibitors. Atomoxetine, however, is the only Food and Drug Administration (FDA)–licensed nonstimulant for use in ADHD in children over the age of 6 years, adolescents, and adults.

Attention-deficit–hyperactivity disorder treatment with stimulants

The first documented use of stimulants in the treatment of behavioral disorders in children was in 1937 by Bradley [65]. He described an immediate improvement in disruptive behaviors of children administered benzedrine, an amphetamine. These children also showed an improvement in attention to task and academic performance. Since then there have been over 200 clinical trials using stimulants in ADHD [66]. Most of these trials were done in school-aged children, but recently there have been several successful trials involving preschoolers, adolescents, and adults using both immediate-release and sustained-release formulations [67–71].

Stimulants have been used with great caution for ADHD symptoms in preschoolers because of difficulties in identification of ADHD in this group and absence of clear evidence supporting their efficacy and safety. In recent years, however, several studies have shown stimulants to be safe and effective in preschool ADHD symptoms. A placebo-controlled study by Short and colleagues [67] using both mixed amphetamine salts (MAS) and MPH in preschoolers showed excellent response to both the stimulants. The Preschool ADHD Treatment Study is the largest multicenter, randomized, controlled trial to date involving preschoolers with ADHD (N = 303). In this study, the researchers used MPH administered as 1.25-, 2.5-, 5-, and 7.5-mg doses three times a day. Compared with placebo, significant decreases in ADHD symptoms were found with MPH at 2.5-mg, 5-mg, and 7.5-mg doses, but not for 1.25-mg dose. The effect sizes of 0.4 to 0.8 were more modest, however, compared with the effect sizes in studies with older children [68]. In addition, side effects were somewhat more common in comparison with older children.

Most of the clinical trials in ADHD performed over the last five decades were short-term trials (usually less than 3 months in duration) in children aged 6 to 12 years using MPH. These studies have shown that between 73% and 77% of children with ADHD respond to stimulant medications. Whereas 25% to 30% of children do not respond to or cannot tolerate an initial stimulant challenge, if a second stimulant medication is tried many of these children do have a clinical response. Studies in this age group using stimulants have not only demonstrated symptom relief but also benefits in terms of overall behavior, academic performance, improved social functioning, and improved interpersonal relationships [66]. The average effect size of stimulants in ADHD in this age group is very strong, varying between 0.91 and 0.95 [72]. The multimodal treatment study of ADHD was a large, federally funded, multicenter, randomized, controlled trial involving 579 children aged 7 to 9.9 years with a DSM-IV ADHD diagnosis. In this study children with ADHD were randomized to one of the four groups and followed for 14 months: (1) medication management alone, (2) behavioral treatments alone, (3) combined medication and behavioral treatments, or (4) standard community care. The study concluded that for core ADHD symptoms, medication management alone was most effective, whereas combined medication and behavioral treatment was more suitable for certain specific groups of children, such as children with comorbid diagnoses (eg, depression or anxiety) [58].

In adolescents and adults, there are far fewer studies compared with children, but these small numbers of studies do provide strong evidence supporting the use of stimulants. Although the response rates and effect sizes in adults are typically lower than those seen in children, there are also some studies where robust responses were seen. Spencer and colleagues [70] conducted a randomized, 6-week, placebo-controlled study of immediate-release MPH in 146 adult patients with DSM-IV ADHD using standardized instruments and an average oral daily dose of 1.1 mg/kg/d and found a therapeutic response in 76% of the subjects receiving MPH, whereas only 19% of the subjects receiving placebo responded. Studies of OROS-MPH (Concerta) and MAS (Adderall XR) in adolescents and adults have been published recently and indicate equivalent response to that of multidosing regimens of immediate-release stimulants [69,71,73]. This is especially significant for this age group, because adults often need coverage for a longer period of time than children, who may only need stimulant action during school hours. Once-a-day regimens are likely to improve adherence because of the simplicity of the regimen and by avoiding the embarrassment of using medications at school or work.

Stimulant formulations and titration

Orally administered MPH, amphetamines, and MAS are licensed by the FDA for ADHD in children over the age of 6 years, adolescents, and in some cases adults. MPH is also available in a transdermal patch form (Daytrana) and is licensed for use only in children over the age of 6 years. Oral formulations of MPH, amphetamines, and MAS are available in immediate-release, intermediate-release, and long-acting preparations. The immediate-release preparations are usually effective for 3 to 4 hours, requiring multiple doses throughout the day. The multiple doses of immediate-release formulations are useful in initial dose titrations and also in situations where long-acting preparations cause insomnia or other undesirable effects late in the evening. The disadvantages of using immediate-release formulations are the need for multiple administrations, decreased adherence, and increased rates of rebound phenomenon when the medication effects wear off. The intermediate-acting formulations are effective for 6 to 8 hours and may be suitable as a once-daily administration for those children where the target duration of action is limited to school hours. The long-acting formulations, such as Concerta, Focalin XR, Metadate CD, and Adderall XR, have durations of action of over 10 hours and are suitable to be administered once a day in the morning even when medication effects are needed well into the evening. Even with these longer-acting medications, however, some patients require two doses per day. Daytrana is a transdermal MPH patch that has been shown to be equipotent to long-acting oral formulations, and when used according to the manufacturer's recommendation is effective for 12 hours a day [74,75]. Clinicians should be aware of the patterns of duration of behavioral action of individual formulations to titrate a medication regimen accurately on an individual basis. Table 1 provides an overview of stimulant formulations and the length of their action.

The titration process is essentially determining the optimal dose for each individual, which is the dose at which they achieve maximum therapeutic benefit with a minimum of side effects. A simple approach to the titration of stimulants is to start with small doses of stimulants, which are increased in dose every 3 to 5 days until a desirable effect occurs or side effects preclude using higher doses. Dosing limits noted in many publications may be lower than necessary for a good clinical response in some adolescents and adults. Common side effects from stimulant use include insomnia, feeling anxious, anorexia, dry mouth, headaches, abdominal pain, and mild

Table 1
Durations of action of stimulant formulations

Medications generic descriptions	Examples of commercial formulations	Approximate duration of action in hours
Methylphenidate	Ritalin, Methylin, Metadate	3–4
Methylphenidate	Ritalin SR, Methylin ER, Metadate ER	6–8
Methylphenidate	Ritalin LA, Metadate CD	8–9
Methylphenidate	Concerta	12
Methylphenidate patch	Daytrana	12
Dextromethylphenidate	Focalin	4
Dextromethylphenidate	Focalin XR	12
Dextroamphetamine	Dexedrine, Dextrostat	4–6
Mixed amphetamine salts	Adderall	4–6
Mixed amphetamine salts	Adderall XR	12

increases in heart rate and blood pressure. Contraindications to stimulants include coronary artery disease, structural heart disease, cardiomyopathy, history of arrhythmias, glaucoma, untreated hypertension, severe tic disorders, Tourette's syndrome, active SUD, and a concurrent prescription with monoamine oxidase inhibitors. Stimulants can exacerbate psychosis and hence should not be prescribed in patients with psychotic conditions or known vulnerability to develop psychosis. Patients with bipolar disorder should only be treated with stimulants once the bipolar disorder is well controlled. Seizure disorders when co-occurring in children with ADHD should not preclude clinicians from using MPH if the seizure disorder is under control. A growing number of studies attest to the safety of MPH in children with electroencephalogram abnormalities and seizure disorders [76–78].

Common concerns with stimulant use

Some clinicians are reluctant to use stimulant medications because of specific concerns of growth retardation, tics, addictive potential, and sudden cardiac death that have been raised as potential consequences of stimulant use. These concerns are discussed next. Growth retardation or failure to achieve ultimate potential height are two of the commonest concerns with stimulant use. Anorexia and weight loss are common side effects of stimulant use; hence, weight and eating patterns of children on stimulants should be closely monitored. If a child starts to lose significant amounts of weight, alteration of regimen to allow some drug holidays to allow the child to catch up with the weight loss may be helpful. Another strategy is to feed the child late in the evening, taking advantage of the rebound from the anorectic effects of the stimulants. In many short-term studies some decreased growth rate is noticed during the stimulant phases of the trials. For example, in the

Preschool ADHD Treatment Study in preschoolers taking MPH, annual growth rates were 20.3% less than expected for height [79]. Most long-term follow-up studies seem to show a temporary reduction in growth rate during childhood and early adolescent periods in active stimulant treatment followed by a growth pattern ultimately leading to the full expected adult height [80,81]. Some studies found the growth reduction to be inherent to ADHD and not caused by psychotropic medication use [81]. A study by Kramer and colleagues [82] reported some small ultimate growth decrements (approximately 0.25 in) in a minority of cases and these individuals were predicted on the basis of anorectic symptoms during treatment phase. Further evidence may be needed to quantify the risks of growth reduction from using stimulants continuously from preschool years through adulthood, because studies of this nature and such lengths are not yet available. Considering the available evidence, however, it is reasonable to assume a very small risk to potential adult height or weight from stimulant use during childhood or adolescence.

Sudden cardiac death is another concern that has been raised after Health Canada, the Canadian regulatory authority equivalent to the US FDA, suspended the sale of Adderall XR between February and August, 2005. This was after a total of 12 cases of sudden cardiac death in children were reported to the FDA between 1999 and 2003. Most of these cases occurred in children with structural and congenital heart defects, with a family history of cardiac arrhythmias, and other situations where the risk of sudden cardiac death was elevated independent of the use of Adderall. Further investigation by the FDA led to this statement: "it does not appear that the number of deaths reported is greater than the number of sudden deaths that would be expected to occur in this population without treatment" [83]. The sudden cardiac death rate in those taking MPH or amphetamines is approximately 0.2 to 0.4 per 100,000 patient-years and is between 1.5 and 8.3 per 100,000 patient-years in children not taking any medications [84]. The FDA has issued a "black box" warning for the use of Adderall in patients with known cardiac problems. Clinicians should be aware that some individuals may have silent cardiac abnormalities predisposing them to sudden cardiac death. Thorough screening for family histories of early myocardial infarctions, serious arrhythmias, congenital cardiac defects, and sudden cardiac death should be a part of the evaluation of ADHD. The clinician should also ask about a personal history of heart disease, hypertension, heart murmur, palpitations and arrhythmias, syncope, dizziness with exertion, chest discomfort, and shortness of breath. An ECG and cardiac work-up is not routinely indicated but should be done in children or adults suspected of cardiac abnormalities.

Development of new-onset tics or exacerbation of pre-existing tics has been of particular concern to some clinicians. There is a paucity of evidence, however, implicating stimulant use with these risks. In a recent study by Lipkin and colleagues [85], the risk of developing chronic tics after stimulant use was estimated at approximately 1%. Interestingly, in this study personal or family tic history, medication selection, or dosage was not related to onset of tics or dyskinesias. In a longitudinal study comparing children treated with stimulants with children treated with placebo over 1 year, Law and Schachar [86] did not find significant differences between the groups in terms of development of new-onset tics even though the rates of development of tics were relatively high (19.6% versus 16.7%). In a multicenter, randomized, controlled trial by the Tourette's Syndrome Study Group involving 136 children with chronic tics and ADHD, the proportion of individual subjects reporting a worsening of tics as an adverse effect was no higher in those treated with MPH (20%) than those being administered clonidine (26%) or placebo (22%) [87]. It seems that children with ADHD have a high risk of developing tics with or without stimulant treatment. The attributable risk of developing new-onset tics caused by stimulant use is very small and the risk of developing intractable tics despite withdrawing stimulant treatment is negligible. In children presenting with a mild tic disorder, stimulants with close monitoring can be considered as a first-line treatment option after a careful risk-benefit discussion with the family. For those children with problematic tics, the combination of clonidine or guanfacine with stimulants may also be considered [88].

Some clinicians are deterred from using stimulants because of the perceived risk of developing SUD as an adolescent. There is little evidence, however, to support that concern. In 14 studies addressing this issue to date, only one study reported an increased future risk of SUD in children treated with stimulants, and that study did not control for conduct disorder, which is a known predictor of SUD [66]. The best evidence available on this issue is from the meta-analysis performed by Wilens and colleagues [64] showing a twofold decrease in SUD when ADHD symptoms were pharmacologically treated in comparison with a control group that did not receive stimulant medications. Most clinicians believe that early treatment of ADHD is likely to prevent, rather than promote, SUD in the future. There has been concern about recent increases in the abuse and diversion of stimulant medications among adolescents and young adults. Most patients prescribed stimulants for ADHD do not abuse them. McCabe and colleagues [89–91] in their recently published large college surveys found that two thirds of college students prescribed stimulants used stimulants as medically prescribed. Approximately 6% of college students have been reported to use stimulants without a prescription. Of this group, about two thirds state that they used stimulants to study and concentrate, whereas one third used stimulants to "get high." They also reported that students abusing prescribed stimulants were likely also to be abusing other illicit drugs. If abuse or diversion is a concern, using long-acting formulations, such as Concerta, may be helpful in reducing the risk of abuse as shown in a recent study by Spencer and colleagues [92]. Newer agents, such as the MPH patch (Daytrana), and a soon to be approved product, lis-dexamphetamine (a prodrug that is converted to amphetamine in the intestinal tract) seem to have lower risk for abuse potential. In patients with active SUD or a high risk for diversion, treatment with alternative medications, such as atomoxetine or bupropion, should also be considered. Despite the potential complications of stimulant use, they remain the choice of most clinicians for ADHD therapy because of the magnitude of the effects, the fact that they are so well tolerated, and the paucity of serious side effects over time. A recent review of the treatment of adolescents and adults with ADHD and comorbid SUD provides a model for treatment for these individuals [93].

Nonstimulant medications

Atomoxetine, a potent inhibitor of the NE transporter system, is the only nonstimulant medication that is approved by the FDA for ADHD in patients over the age of 6 years. Atomoxetine is especially useful for ADHD patients who do not respond or develop unacceptable side effects to stimulant use. It is also helpful in ADHD patients with comorbid tics, anxiety, and SUD. Atomoxetine has been shown to be effective in treating the core ADHD symptoms in children, adolescents, and adults [94–96]. Several recently reported long-term studies have shown improved functioning, better quality of life measures, and good long-term safety after 2 years of continuous atomoxetine use [97–100]. Atomoxetine has also been shown to be an effective treatment for ADHD patients with comorbid anxiety and depression and it may be a good initial choice for these patients [101].

Atomoxetine is typically administered once daily, although twice daily dosing can also be used. Atomoxetine should be initiated at doses of about 0.5 mg/kg body weight for about 2 weeks and then titrated upward based on clinical response to 1.2 to 1.4 mg/kg or a maximum total dose of approximately 100 mg/day. Although doses above this are not approved by the FDA, clinical trials have established safety with the use of doses up to 1.8 mg/kg [94]. It may take several weeks before the benefits from atomoxetine become apparent; therefore, it is important to inform patients about this to ensure continued compliance despite apparently little impact on symptoms during the initial stages of treatment. Common adverse effects with atomoxetine use include gastrointestinal upset, headaches, fatigue, and mild increases in heart rate and blood pressure. Rare but important adverse effects that should be discussed with patients include liver toxicity and increased suicidal thoughts. Two cases of liver toxicity out of an estimated 2 million prescriptions were reported by the manufacturer, and in both these patients the liver damage was completely reversible after stopping the atomoxetine [102]. An analysis of clinical trials by the manufacturer showed increased suicidal thoughts in 4 (0.4%) out of 1000 patients, but there were no attempted or completed suicides [102]. Nevertheless, the FDA warns clinicians to counsel patients about this potential risk.

Bupropion is an antidepressant that has agonist effects on noradrenergic and dopaminergic systems [103]. Although it has been shown to be efficacious in the treatment of ADHD symptoms in children and adults, it is not currently approved by FDA for use in ADHD [104,105]. Bupropion may be particularly useful in ADHD patients with comorbid SUD and depression [106,107]. Several other antidepressants have been shown to be efficacious in the treatment of ADHD symptoms. Tricyclic antidepressants inhibit reuptake of NE and have a large body of evidence supporting their use in ADHD in both children and adults [108,109]. Because of their effect on cardiac conduction and the reported excessive sudden deaths, however, they should not be routinely used in children with ADHD [110]. Monoamine oxidase inhibitors and venlafaxine are other antidepressants that have been reported to be effective in ADHD in some open trials and case reports.

Clonidine and guanfacine are α_2-adrenergic receptor agonists, which have been shown modestly to be effective in the treatment of core ADHD symptoms, when used as monotherapy [111–114]. Traditionally these agents have been used as adjuvant to stimulants in treating aggression or tics that are sometimes comorbid with ADHD, or as an aid to sleep [88]. Modafinil is a new wakefulness-promoting agent that is licensed for use in cases of daytime sleepiness associated with sleep apnea and narcolepsy. Its mechanism of action is not well understood. Modafinil at doses of 300 to 400 mg per day in divided doses has been shown to have efficacy in the treatment of core ADHD symptoms in children [115,116]. In clinical trials of modafinil involving children, the most common side effects included insomnia, abdominal pain, and headaches. A case of Stevens-Johnson syndrome was reported by a clinical trial, prompting the FDA to issue a nonapprovable letter for its use in children with ADHD in June 2006.

Summary

ADHD is a commonly occurring, heritable neurobehavioral disorder. It is now clear that it is distributed worldwide and does not typically resolve after childhood. The significant impact of ADHD on an individual's family, relationships, educational performance, and performance at work is now well established. Potentially dangerous outcomes of untreated ADHD, such as accidents (motor vehicle and others), SUD, and legal problems, are also now known. It is also becoming clear, however, that medical treatment of ADHD is effective not only in alleviating symptoms but also in improving overall functioning. It is imperative that primary care physicians be well versed in this disorder and its clinical features across the age groups. The primary care physician should be able to screen, diagnose, educate, and initiate medication management in patients with uncomplicated ADHD. Because many patients with ADHD have comorbid psychiatric disorders, such as depression and anxiety, adjunctive treatments or referrals are often necessary. The clinician should also be aware of local referral mechanisms for psychosocial interventions, such as parent training, individual and family therapy, coaching, and educational support. Finally, reasonable accommodations are allowable by law for students and employees, and physicians can help their ADHD patients by documenting the disorder and writing letters on their behalf.

References

[1] American Psychiatric Association. Diagnostic and statistical manual of mental disorders. 4th edition (DSM-IV). Washington, DC: American Psychiatric Association; 2004.
[2] Gimpel GA, Kuhn BR. Maternal report of attention deficit hyperactivity disorder symptoms in preschool children. Child Care Health Dev 2000;26:163–76.
[3] Wolraich ML, Hannah JN, Pinnock TY, et al. Comparison of criteria for attention deficit hyperactive disorder in a country wide sample. J Am Acad Child Adolesc psychiatry 1996; 35:319–24.
[4] Barbaresi WJ, Katusic SK, Colligan RC, et al. How common is attention-deficit/hyperactivity disorder? Incidence in a population-based birth cohort in Rochester, Minn. Arch Pediatr Adolesc Med 2002;156:217–24.
[5] Kessler RC, Adler L, Barkley R, et al. The prevalence and correlates of adult ADHD in the United States: results from the national co morbidity survey replication. Am J Psychiatry 2006;163:716–23.
[6] Gadow KD, Nolan EE, Litcher L, et al. Comparison of attention-deficit/hyperactivity disorder symptom subtypes in Ukrainian school children. J Am Acad Child Adolesc Psychiatry 2000;39(12):1520–7.
[7] Graetz BW, Sawyer MG, Hazell PL, et al. Validity of DSM–IV ADHD subtypes in a nationally representative sample of Australian children and adolescents. J Am Acad Child Adolesc psychiatry 2001;40:1410–7.
[8] Adewuya AO, Famuyiwa OO. Attention deficit hyperactivity disorder among Nigerian primary school children: prevalence and co-morbid conditions. Eur Child Adolesc Psychiatry 2006 [Published online 28 November 2006].
[9] Mukhopadhyay M, Misra S, Mitra T, et al. Attention deficit hyperactivity disorder. Indian J Pediatr 2003;70(10):789–92.
[10] Taylor E, Sandberg S. Hyperactive behavior in English schoolchildren: a questionnaire survey. J Abnorm Child Psychol 1984;12(1):143–55.
[11] Kessler RC, Adler L, Barkley R, et al. Patterns and predictors of attention-deficit/hyperactivity disorder persistence into adulthood: results from the national comorbidity survey replication. Biol Psychiatry 2005;57(11):1442–51.
[12] Biederman J, Faraone S, Milberger S, et al. Predictors of persistence and remission of ADHD into adolescence: results from a four-year prospective follow-up study. J Am Acad Child Adolesc Psychiatry 1996;35:343–51.
[13] US Census 2005. Available at: http://www.census.gov/popest/national/asrh/NC-EST2006/NC-EST2006-01.xls. Accessed November 19, 2006.
[14] Birnbaum HG, Kessler RC, Lowe SW, et al. Costs of attention deficit hyperactivity disorder in the United States: excess costs of persons with ADHD and their family members in 2000. Curr Med Res Opin 2005;47(6):565–72.
[15] Ruff ME. Attention deficit disorder and stimulant use: an epidemic of modernity. Clin Pediatr (Phila) 2005;44(7):557–63.
[16] Rhee SH, Waldman ID, Hay DA, et al. Sex differences in genetic and environmental influences on DSM-III-R attention-deficit/hyperactivity disorder. J Abnorm Psychol 1999;108:24–41.

[17] Biederman J, Faraone SV, Keenan K, et al. Further evidence for family-genetic risk factors in attention deficit hyperactivity disorder: patterns of comorbidity in probands and relatives psychiatrically and pediatrically referred samples. Arch Gen Psychiatry 1992;49(9): 728–38.
[18] Gilger JW, Pennington BF, DeFries JC. A twin study of the etiology of co morbidity: attention deficit hyperactivity disorder and dyslexia. J Am Acad Child Adolesc Psychiatry 1992;31:343–8.
[19] Goodman R, Stevenson J. A twin study of hyperactivity. II: The aetiological role of genes, family relationships and perinatal adversity. J Child Psychol Psychiatry 1989;30:691–709.
[20] Linnet KM, Wisborg K, Obel C, et al. Smoking during pregnancy and the risk for hyperkinetic disorder in offspring. Pediatrics 2005;116(2):462–7.
[21] Knopik VS, Sparrow EP, Madden P, et al. Contributions of parental alcoholism, prenatal substance exposure, and genetic transmission to child ADHD risk: a female twin study. Psychol Med 2005;35(5):625–35.
[22] Linnet KM, Wisborg K, Agerbo E. Gestational age, birth weight, and the risk of hyperkinetic disorder. Arch Dis Child 2006;91(8):655–60 [Epub 2006].
[23] Knopik VS, Heath AC, Jacob T. Maternal alcohol use disorder and offspring ADHD: disentangling genetic and environmental effects using a children-of-twins design. Psychol Med 2006;36(10):1461–71.
[24] Biederman J, Faraone SV, Monuteaux MC. Differential effect of environmental adversity by gender: Rutter's index of adversity in a group of boys and girls with and without ADHD. Am J Psychiatry 2002;159(9):1556–62.
[25] Pressman LJ, Loo SK, Carpenter EM. Relationship of family environment and parental psychiatric diagnosis to impairment in ADHD. J Am Acad Child Adolesc Psychiatry 2006;45(3):346–54.
[26] Counts CA, Nigg GT, Stawicki JA, et al. Family adversity in DSM-IV ADHD combined and inattentive subtypes and associated disruptive behavior problems. J Am Acad Child Adolesc Psychiatry 2005;44:690–8.
[27] Valera EM, Faraone SV, Murray KE, et al. Meta-analysis of structural imaging findings in attention-deficit/hyperactivity disorder. Biol Psychiatry 2006 [epublication ahead of print accessed on 25th November 2006].
[28] Castellanos FX, Lee PP, Sharp W, et al. Developmental trajectories of brain volume abnormalities in children and adolescents with attention-deficit/hyperactivity disorder. JAMA 2002;288(14):1740–8.
[29] Casey BJ, Castellanos FX, Giedd JN, et al. Implication of right frontostriatal circuitry in response inhibition and attention-deficit/hyperactivity disorder. J Am Acad Child Adolesc Psychiatry 1997;36(3):374–83.
[30] Zametkin AJ, Nordahl TE, Gross M, et al. Cerebral glucose metabolism in adults with hyperactivity of childhood onset. N Engl J Med 1990;323:1361–6.
[31] Rubia K, Overmeyer S, Taylor E, et al. Hypofrontality in attention deficit hyperactivity disorder during higher-order motor control: a study with functional MRI. Am J Psychiatry 1999;156:891–6.
[32] Zang YF, Jin Z, Weng XC, et al. Functional MRI in attention deficit hyperactivity disorder: evidence for hypofrontality. Brain Dev 2005;27(8):544–50.
[33] Bush G, Frazier JA, Rauch SL, et al. Anterior cingulate cortex dysfunction in attention deficit/hyperactivity disorder revealed by f MRI and the Counting Stroop. Biol Psychiatry 1999;45(12):1542–52.
[34] Kent L, Doerry U, Hardy E, et al. Evidence that variation at the serotonin transporter gene influences susceptibility to attention deficit hyperactivity disorder (ADHD): analysis and pooled analysis. Mol Psychiatry 2002;7:908–12.
[35] Hawi Z, Lowe N, Kirley A, et al. Linkage disequilibrium mapping at DAT1, DRD5 and DBH narrows the search for ADHD susceptibility alleles at these loci. Mol Psychiatry 2003;8(3):299–308.

[36] Li D, Sham PC, Owen MJ, et al. Metaanalysis shows significant association between dopamine system genes and attention deficit hyperactivity disorder (ADHD). Hum Mol Genet 2006;15(14):2276–84 E pub 2006 Jun.
[37] Achenbach TM. Manual for the Child Behavior Checklist/4-18 and 1991 Profile. Burlington (VT): University of Vermont, Department of Psychiatry; 1991.
[38] Achenbach TM. Manual for the Teacher's Report Form and 1991 profile. Burlington (VT): University of Vermont, Department of Psychiatry; 1991.
[39] Conners CK, Sitarenios G, Parker JD, et al. Revision and restandardization of the Conners Teacher Rating Scale (CTRS-R): factor structure, reliability, and criterion validity. J Abnorm Child Psychol 1998;26(4):279–91.
[40] Conners CK, Sitarenios G, Parker JD, et al. The revised Conners' Parent Rating Scale (CPRS-R): factor structure, reliability, and criterion validity. J Abnorm Child Psychol 1998;26(4):257–68.
[41] DuPaul GJ, Power TJ, Anastopoulos AD, et al. ADHD rating scale-IV. New York: Guilford Press; 1998.
[42] Swanson JM. School based assessments and interventions for ADD students. Irvine (CA): KC publishing; 1992.
[43] Faraone SV, Biederman J, Spencer T, et al. Diagnosing adult attention deficit hyperactivity disorder: are late onset and subthreshold diagnoses valid? Am J Psychiatry 2006;163(10): 1720–9.
[44] Murphy K, Barkley RA. Attention deficit hyperactivity disorder adults: comorbidities and adaptive impairments. Compr Psychiatry 1996;37:393–401.
[45] Barkley RA, Fischer M, Smallish L, et al. The persistence of attention-deficit/hyperactivity disorder into young adulthood as a function of reporting source and definition of disorder. J Abnorm Psychol 2002;111:279–89.
[46] McGough JJ, Barkley RA. Diagnostic controversies in adult attention deficit hyperactivity disorder. Am J Psychiatry 2004;161(11):1948–56.
[47] Wender PH. Attention deficit hyperactivity disorder in adults. New York: Oxford University Press; 1995.
[48] Wender PH, Ward MF, Reimherr FW. The Wender Utah Rating Scale: an aid in the retrospective diagnosis of childhood attention deficit hyperactivity disorder. Am J Psychiatry 1993;150:1280.
[49] Conners C, Erhardt D, Sparrow E. The Conners Adult ADHD Rating Scale (CAARS). Toronto (Canada): Multi-Health Systems Inc; 1998.
[50] Brown TE. Brown attention-deficit disorders scales: manual. San Antonio (TX): Psychological Corp; 1996.
[51] Conners CK, Wells KC, Parker JD, et al. A new self-report scale for assessment of adolescent psychopathology: factor structure, reliability, validity, and diagnostic sensitivity. J Abnorm Child Psychol 1997;25(6):487–97.
[52] Barkley RA. Attention deficit hyperactivity disorder: handbook for diagnosis and treatment. 3rd edition. New York: The Guildford Press; 2006.
[53] Brown RT, Pacini JN. Perceived family functioning, marital status, and depression in parents of boys with attention deficit disorder. J Learn Disabil 1989;22(9):581–7.
[54] Barkley RA, Fischer M, Smallish L, et al. Young adult outcome of hyperactive children: adaptive functioning in major life activities. J Am Acad Child Adolesc Psychiatry 2006; 45(2):192–202.
[55] Biederman J, Faraone SV, Spencer TJ, et al. Functional impairments in adults with self-reports of diagnosed ADHD: a controlled study of 1001 adults in the community. J Clin Psychiatry 2006;67(4):524–40.
[56] Mannuzza S, Klein RG, Bessler A, et al. Adult outcome of hyperactive boys: educational achievement, occupational rank, and psychiatric status. Arch Gen Psychiatry 1993;50(7): 565–76.

[57] Jensen PS, Hinshaw SP, Kraemer HC, et al. ADHD comorbidity findings from the MTA study: comparing comorbid subgroups. J Am Acad Child Adolesc Psychiatry 2001;40(2): 147–58.
[58] The MTA cooperative group. Multimodal treatment study of children with ADHD: a 14-month randomized clinical trial of treatment strategies for attention-deficit/hyperactivity disorder. Arch Gen Psychiatry 1999;56(12):1073–86.
[59] McGough JJ, Smalley SL, McCracken JT, et al. Psychiatric comorbidity in adult attention deficit hyperactivity disorder: findings from multiplex families. Am J Psychiatry 2005;162: 1621–7.
[60] Schubiner H, Tzelepis A, Milberger S, et al. Prevalence of attention-deficit/hyperactivity disorder and conduct disorder among substance abusers. J Clin Psychiatry 2000;61(4):244–51.
[61] Levin FR, Evans SM, Keleber HD, et al. Prevalence of adult attention-deficit hyperactivity disorder among cocaine abusers seeking treatment. Drug Alcohol Depend 1998;52(1):15–25.
[62] Upadhyaya HP, Rose K, Wang W, et al. Attention deficit/hyperactivity disorder, medication treatment, and substance use patterns among adolescents and young adults. J Child Adolesc Psychopharmacol 2005;15:799–809.
[63] Wilens TE, Biederman J, Mick E, et al. Attention deficit hyperactivity disorder (ADHD) is associated with early onset substance use disorders. J Nerv Ment Dis 1997;185(8):475–82.
[64] Wilens TE, Faraone SV, Biederman J, et al. Does stimulant therapy of attention-deficit/ hyperactivity disorder beget later substance abuse? A meta-analytic review of the literature. Pediatrics 2003;111(1):179–85.
[65] Bradley C. The behavior of children receiving benzedrine. Am J Psychiatry 1937;94:577–85.
[66] Connor DF. Stimulants. In: Barkley RA, editor. Attention-deficit hyperactivity disorder: a handbook for diagnosis and treatment. New York: Guilford Press; 2006. p. 608–37.
[67] Short EJ, Manos MJ, Findling RL. A prospective study of stimulant response in preschool children: insights from ROC analyses. J Am Acad Child Adolesc Psychiatry 2004;43(3): 251–9.
[68] Greenhill L, Kollins S, Abikoff H, et al. Efficacy and safety of immediate-release methylphenidate treatment for preschoolers with ADHD. J Am Acad Child Adolesc Psychiatry 2006;45(11):1284–93.
[69] Wilens TE, McBurnett K, Bukstein O, et al. Multisite controlled study of OROS methylphenidate in the treatment of adolescents with attention deficit/hyperactivity disorder. Arch Pediatr Adolesc Med 2006;160:82–90.
[70] Spencer T, Biederman J, Wilens T, et al. A large, double blind, randomized clinical trial of methylphenidate in the treatment of adults with attention deficit/hyperactive disorder. Biol Psychiatry 2005;57:456–63.
[71] Biederman J, Mick E, Surman C, et al. A randomized, placebo-controlled trial of OROS methylphenidate in adults with attention-deficit/hyperactivity disorder. Biol Psychiatry 2006;59:829–35.
[72] Faraone SV. Understanding the effect size of ADHD medications: implications for clinical care. Medscape Psychiatry Mental Health 2003;8(2).
[73] Spencer T, Biederman J, Wilens T, et al. Efficacy and safety of mixed amphetamine salts extended release (Adderall XR) in the management of attention-deficit/hyperactivity disorder in adolescent patients: a 4-week, randomized, double-blind, placebo-controlled, parallel-group study. Clin Ther 2006;28(2):266–79.
[74] Pelham WE, Manos MJ, Ezzell CE, et al. A dose-ranging study of a methylphenidate transdermal system in children with ADHD. J Am Acad Child Adolesc Psychiatry 2005; 44(6):522–9.
[75] Shire Pharma. Daytrana product information from Shire pharmaceuticals Wayne, PA 19087-5367. Available at: www.Daytrana.com. Accessed on September 12, 2006.
[76] Gucuyener K, Kemal Erdemogu A, Senol S, et al. Use of methylphenidate for attention-deficit hyperactivity disorder in patients with epilepsy or electroencephalographic abnormalities. J Child Neurol 2003;18:109–12.

[77] Feldman H, Crumrine P, Handen BL, et al. Methylphenidate in children with seizures and attention deficit disorder. Am J Dis Child 1989;143:1081–6.
[78] Van der Feltz-Cornelis CM, Aldenkamp AP. Effectiveness and safety of methylphenidate in adult attention deficit hyperactivity disorder in patients with epilepsy: an open treatment trial. Epilepsy Behav 2006;8(3):659–62.
[79] Swanson J, Greenhill T, Wigal J, et al. Stimulant-related reductions of growth rates in the PATS. J Am Child Adolesc Psychiatry 2006;45(11):1304–13.
[80] Klein RG, Mannuzza S. Hyperactive boys almost grown up. III. Methylphenidate effects on ultimate height. Arch Gen Psychiatry 1988;45:1131–4.
[81] Spencer TJ, Biederman J, Harding M, et al. Growth deficits in ADHD children revisited: evidence for disorder-associated growth delays? J Am Child Adolesc Psychiatry 1996; 35(11):1460–9.
[82] Kramer JR, Loney J, Ponto LB, et al. Predictors of adult height and weight in boys treated with methylphenidate for childhood behavior problems. J Am Child Adolesc Psychiatry 2000;39(4):517–24.
[83] Public Health Advisory for Adderall and Adderall XR, US Food and Drug Administration, Center for Drug Evaluation and Research, Feb. 9, 2005. Available at: http://www.fda.gov/cder/drug/advisory/adderall.htm. FDA website Accessed on November 19, 2006.
[84] Wilens TE, Prince JB, Spencer TJ, et al. Stimulants and sudden death: what is a physician to do? Pediatrics 2006;118(3):1215–9.
[85] Lipkin PH, Goldstein IJ, Adesman AR. Tics and dyskinesias associated with stimulant treatment in attention-deficit hyperactivity disorder. Arch Pediatr Adolesc Med 1994; 148(8):859–61.
[86] Law SF, Schachar R. Do typical clinical doses of methylphenidate cause tics in children treated for attention-deficit hyperactivity disorder? J Am Child Adolesc Psychiatry 1999; 38(8):944–51.
[87] Tourette syndrome study group. Treatment of ADHD in children with tics: a randomized controlled trial. Neurology 2002;58(4):527–36.
88] Scahill L, Chappelll PB, Kim YS, et al. A placebo controlled study of Guanfacine in the treatment of children with tic disorders and attention deficit hyperactivity disorder. American Journal of Psychiatry 2001;158(7):1067–74.
[89] McCabe SE, Teter CJ, Boyd CJ. Medical use, illicit use, and diversion of abusable prescription drugs. J Am Coll Health 2006;54(5):269–78.
[90] Teter CJ, McCabe SE, LaGrange K, et al. Illicit use of specific prescription stimulants among college students: prevalence, motives, and routes of administration. Pharmacotherapy 2006;26(10):1501–10.
[91] Teter CJ, McCabe SE, LaGrange K, et al. Prevalence and motives for illicit use of prescription stimulants in an undergraduate student sample. J Am Coll Health 2005; 53(6):253–62.
[92] Spencer TJ, Biederman J, Ciccone PE, et al. PET study examining pharmacokinetics, detection and likeability, and dopamine transporter receptor occupancy of short- and long-acting oral methylphenidate. Am J Psychiatry 2006;163:387–95.
[93] Schubiner H. Treatment of individuals with ADHD and substance use disorders. CNS Drugs 2005;19(8):643–55.
[94] Michelson D, Faries DE, Wernicke J, et al. Atomoxetine in the treatment of children and adolescents with attention-deficit/hyperactivity disorder: a randomized, placebo controlled, dose-response study. Pediatrics 2001;108(5):E83.
[95] Michelson D, Allen AJ, Busner J, et al. Once-daily atomoxetine treatment for children and adolescents with attention deficit hyperactivity disorder: a randomized, placebo-controlled study. Am J Psychiatry 2002;159:1896–901.
[96] Michelson D, Adler L, Spencer T, et al. Atomoxetine in adults with ADHD: two randomized, placebo-controlled studies. Biol Psychiatry 2003;53:112–20.

[97] Adler LA, Spencer TJ, Milton DR, et al. Long-term, open-label study of the safety and efficacy of atomoxetine in adults with attention-deficit/hyperactivity disorder: an interim analysis. J Clin Psychiatry 2005;66(3):294–9.
[98] Adler LA, Sutton VK, Moore RJ, et al. Quality of life assessment in adult patients with attention-deficit/hyperactivity disorder treated with atomoxetine. J Clin Psychopharmacol 2006;26(6):648–52.
[99] Wilens TE, Newcorn JH, Kratochvil CJ, et al. Long-term atomoxetine treatment in adolescents with attention-deficit/hyperactivity disorder. J Pediatr 2006;149(1):112–9.
[100] Kratochvil CJ, Wilens TE, Greenhill LL, et al. Effects of long-term atomoxetine treatment for young children with attention-deficit/hyperactivity disorder. J Am Acad Child Adolesc Psychiatry 2006;45(8):919–27.
[101] Kratochvil CJ, Newcorn JH, Arnold LE. Atomoxetine alone or combined with fluoxetine for treating ADHD with comorbid depressive or anxiety symptoms. J Am Acad Child Adolesc Psychiatry 2005;44(9):915–24.
[102] Safety and side effect information in children, teens and adults. Available at: http://www.strattera.com/ Accessed on January 9, 2006.
[103] Horst WD, Preskorn SH. Mechanisms of action and clinical characteristics of three atypical antidepressants: venlafaxine, nefazodone, bupropion. J Affect Disord 1998;51:237–54.
[104] Conners CK, Casat CD, Gualtieri CT, et al. Bupropion hydrochloride in attention deficit disorder with hyperactivity. J Am Acad Child Adolesc Psychiatry 1996;35:1314–21.
[105] Wilens TE, Spencer TJ, Biederman J, et al. A controlled clinical trial of bupropion for attention deficit hyperactivity disorder in adults. Am J Psychiatry 2001;158(2):282–8.
[106] Solhkhah R, Wilens TE, Daly J, et al. Bupropion SR for the treatment of substance-abusing outpatient adolescents with attention-deficit/hyperactivity disorder and mood disorders. J Child Adolesc Psychopharmacol 2005;15(5):777–86.
[107] Levin FR, Evans SM, Mc Dowell DM, et al. Bupropion treatment for cocaine abuse and adult attention-deficit/hyperactivity disorder. J Addict Dis 2002;21(2):1–16.
[108] Biederman J, Baldessarini RJ, Wright V, et al. A double-blind placebo controlled study of desipramine in the treatment of attention deficit disorder: I. Efficacy. J Am Acad Child Adolesc Psychiatry 1989;28:777–84.
[109] Wilens TE, Biederman J, Prince J, et al. Six week double-blind, placebo-controlled study of desipramine for adult attention deficit hyperactivity disorder. Am J Psychiatry 1996;153:1147–53.
[110] Amitai Y, Frischer H. Excess fatality from desipramine in children and adolescents. J Am Acad Child Adolesc Psychiatry 2006;45(1):54–60.
[111] Connor DF, Barkley RA, Davis HT. A pilot study of methylphenidate, clonidine, or the combination in ADHD comorbid with aggressive oppositional defiant or conduct disorder. Clin Pediatr (Phila) 2000;39(1):15–25.
[112] Hunt RD, Minderaa RB, Cohen DJ. Clonidine benefits children with attention deficit disorder and hyperactivity: report of a double-blind placebo-crossover therapeutic trial. J Am Acad Child Adolesc Psychiatry 1985;24:617–29.
[113] Hunt RD, Arnsten AFT, Asbell MD. An open trial of guanfacine in the treatment of attention deficit hyperactivity disorder. J Am Acad Child Adolesc Psychiatry 1995;34:50–4.
[114] Horrigan JP, Barnhill LJ. Guanfacine for treatment of attention-deficit hyperactivity disorder in boys. J Child Adolesc Psychopharmacol 1995;5:215–23.
[115] Greenhill LL, Biederman J, Boellner SW. A randomized, double-blind, placebo-controlled study of modafinil film-coated tablets in children and adolescents with attention-deficit/hyperactivity disorder. J Am Acad Child Adolesc Psychiatry 2006;45(5):503–11.
[116] Swanson JM, Greenhill LL, Lopez FA, et al. Modafinil filmcoated tablets in children and adolescents with attention deficit/hyperactivity disorder: results of a randomized, double-blind, placebo-controlled fixed-dose study followed by abrupt discontinuation. J Clin Psychiatry 2006;67(1):137–47.

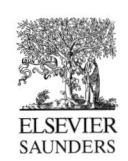

Autism Spectrum Disorders in Early Childhood: An Overview for Practicing Physicians

James E. Carr, PhD*, Linda A. LeBlanc, PhD

Department of Psychology, Western Michigan University, 1903 West Michigan Avenue, Kalamazoo, MI 49008-5439, USA

The term *autism spectrum disorder* (ASD) (termed *pervasive developmental disorders* [PDDs] in the *Diagnostic and Statistical Manual of Mental Disorders*, 4th edition [text revision] (DSM-IV-TR) [1]) refers to developmental disorders of varying clinical presentation that share a core feature of pervasive and qualitative impairments in reciprocal social interaction [1–3]. In the past decade, researchers and clinicians have broadened the diagnostic concept to include milder and atypical forms of autism and autism-related disorders that are represented as a spectrum [4]. These disorders are estimated to occur at a much higher rate than previously thought, making it likely for the average physician to encounter patients with ASDs in his or her practice. Thus, the purpose of this article is to review the recent literature on ASDs in early childhood to prepare physicians for the critical role they can take in identification, referral, and intervention for children with ASDs.

Current diagnostic criteria and course

Three PDDs are typically considered ASDs: autism, Asperger's disorder, and PDD not otherwise specified (NOS) [5]. Although all ASDs involve impairments in reciprocal social interaction skills, the degree of impairment in communication skills and cognitive abilities and the form and degree of stereotyped behavior, interests, and activities vary. Each

---

* Corresponding author.
  E-mail address: jim.carr@wmich.edu (J.E. Carr)

disorder is associated with a slightly different set of diagnostic criteria as described in this article.

Autism

Current diagnostic criteria for autism specify multiple impairments in social functioning and communication as well as restricted and repetitive behavior present before the age of 3 years [1,2]. To qualify for a diagnosis, individuals must meet six criteria, including at least two criteria in the realm of impaired social interaction and one criterion each in the areas of communication impairment and restricted, repetitive, or stereotyped patterns of behavior. The manifestations of this disorder vary greatly in terms of the degree of impairment, ranging from early estimates of 75% of individuals having comorbid mental retardation [6,7] to recent reviews suggesting as few as 30% to 60% of individuals with this specific comorbidity [8,9].

People with autism experience substantial social impairments that have an impact on almost every aspect of their interactions with others. Peer interactions are often avoided, and play behaviors often remain stereotypic and lacking in pretense [10,11]. Even within the first 12 to 18 months of life, parents often note difficulties in joint attention, social responsiveness, and eye contact; these have been confirmed by retrospective videotaped studies [12]. These social impairments contribute greatly to subsequent language delays by dramatically limiting the number of meaningful learning opportunities during a critical developmental period.

Communication is another core deficit of autism. Moderate to profound language impairments typically are the first symptoms to draw the pediatrician's notice. Many children with autism fail to develop language at all unless dramatic intervention procedures are pursued [13,14]. Those who do develop speech often engage in echolalia (ie, repeating words or phrases heard previously) or fail to speak for social purposes, such as engaging in conversation [15]. Effective language intervention is a critical component of effective intervention, because one of the best predictors of outcome for children with autism is the development of spontaneous language before 6 years of age [16].

Restricted and repetitive behavior is the third domain affected in children with autism, occurring more commonly in older preschool- and school-aged children than in young children or adolescents and adults [17–19]. Common repetitive motor behaviors observed in children with autism include hand flapping, toe walking, and rocking [18]. Restricted interests are often evident, with strong preferences for only a few or unusual items and distress and problem behavior when those items are not readily available. Insistence on sameness in routines and rituals or compulsions can be observed in most aspects of daily activities, taking the form of rigid sequences of actions or extreme distress in the face of relatively minor changes in the environment or scheduled events [4].

Asperger's disorder

Although first described in 1944 by Asperger [20], the disorder drew virtually no attention from the scientific and clinical communities until Lorna Wing [21] translated Asperger's work and began a line of research on the disorder. The disorder was not classified as a PDD along with autism until the *DSM-IV* was published in 1994 [22,23]. The criteria for Asperger's disorder share some similarities with autism. To qualify for a diagnosis of Asperger's disorder, an individual must demonstrate at least two characteristic criteria in the area of impaired social interaction and one characteristic criterion in the area of restricted, repetitive, and stereotyped patterns [1]. Individuals with Asperger's disorder do not have clinically significant delays in language skills, cognitive development, or age-appropriate self-help skills or adaptive behavior [1]. In fact, individuals with Asperger's disorder are often verbally fluent and have above-average intelligence in many areas, whereas clear deficits and learning disabilities may be evident in other areas [23,24]. The restricted and repetitive patterns are often manifested as abnormally intense interest and factual knowledge about unusual and age-inappropriate topics and strong emotional responses to change in routine or environment [23]. Finally, developmental milestones are often within normal to advanced limits; thus, identification of these children typically occurs at a later age as difficulties develop on entry into preschool or daycare or into general education environments [24].

Pervasive developmental disorder not otherwise specified

A diagnosis of PDD-NOS is used for milder problems on the spectrum when an individual displays a severe impairment in the development of reciprocal social interaction associated with verbal or nonverbal communication skills or with the presence of stereotyped behavior, interests, and activities but without meeting criteria for another PDD [1]. Thus, an individual diagnosed with PDD-NOS may exhibit behavior similar to individuals diagnosed with autism or Asperger's disorder but not to the extent that he or she meets the criteria for one of those disorders.

Prevalence

The most recent evaluation of the prevalence of ASDs conducted by the US Centers for Disease Control and Prevention (CDC) estimates that among children aged 4 to 17 years, 5 to 6 of 1000 are affected [25]. Previous estimates were much lower, at approximately four to five cases per 10,000 individuals [26]. The CDC estimates are based on parental report of a child having received a diagnosis, however. Other recent articles using different methodologies have produced estimates in the range of 1 in 1000 children for autism and 1.6 in 1000 children for all other ASDs [9,27,28].

Approximately 20% of children with autism experience a skill regression around the age of 18 months after relatively typical development, including acquisition of language and play skills [29,30]. This regressive subtype has been validated using home videotapes in which children who had regressed were no different than typically developing children in joint attention and communicative behaviors at 1 year of age but were indistinguishable from children with autism in these deficit areas by 24 months of age [31]. The unfortunate timing of most regressions (around 18 months of age) was the basis for two controversial publications that sparked relatively widespread concern among laypersons about the possibility of vaccinations [32] or mercury-based preservatives [33] as a cause of autism. Consequently, the rate of measles vaccinations has decreased, and infections have increased [34], in spite of the subsequent publication of multiple well-controlled studies that have found no differences in rates of autism among children who are vaccinated and those who are not [35–42]. Currently, there is no scientific evidence to support a link between vaccination and autism [43].

Screening and referral

It is generally believed that early identification and early intervention are associated with the best outcomes for children with ASDs [44]. In the United States, however, the average age of identification is still older than 4 years of age [27,45], despite the ability to identify ASDs as early as 2 years of age. In a recent survey of licensed pediatricians in Maryland and Delaware, 82% screened for general delays but only 8% screened for ASDs [46]. Thus, researchers and clinicians in recent years have endeavored to develop screening procedures and screening tools that pediatricians can use as part of typical "well child" visits at 18 to 24 months to identify children who may be at risk of developing ASDs. Researchers can now reliably identify children as early as 24 months of age [5,47]; however, ASD symptoms can appear much earlier. Although these early symptoms are often insufficient for reliable diagnosis, they highlight the importance of early screening and comprehensive follow-up. Pediatricians should screen all children for ASDs at least once at well-child visits, with follow-up interview for those children scoring higher than the cutoff. At-risk children should be screened at every visit between the ages of 18 and 36 months, and if scores are greater than the cutoff, children should be referred for a comprehensive diagnostic evaluation, including such tools as the Autism Diagnostic Interview-Revised [48], Autism Diagnostic Observation Schedule [49], and measures of developmental and adaptive functioning.

One of the most common screening tools is the Checklist for Autism in Toddlers (CHAT) [50]. This tool uses parent report for 9 items plus medical staff administration of 5 direct-observation test items to identify at-risk children. The sensitivity is 38% when children at medium and high risk are included, with milder cases of autism generally missed. A recent 2-year follow-up study from a different sample indicates that the CHAT criteria for medium to high risk for autism predicted classification with autism 2 years later 83% of the time [51]. Researchers in the United States have modified the tool and tested it in pediatric practice with children 18 months and older under the name of Modified CHAT (M-CHAT) [52]. This 23-item tool is based entirely on parent report and has resulted in a sensitivity of 0.87 and specificity of 0.99, suggesting that the M-CHAT identified most children who subsequently developed ASDs and did not falsely identify children. A follow-up interview has since been developed that further reduces the false-positive rate of the checklist [53]. The CHAT and M-CHAT are freely available on the First Signs Web site [54].

There are also several commercially available alternatives to the CHAT and M-CHAT. The Social Communication Questionnaire was developed primarily for research purposes and is most appropriate for children older than the age of 48 months [55]. This 40-item scale is available from Western Psychological Services. The Pervasive Developmental Disorders Screening Test-II (PDDST-II) [56] is a 23-item parent report screening measure useful with children older than 18 months of age. The PDDST-II is available from Harcourt Assessment. Children with Asperger's disorder may not show substantial difficulties until later (ie, 4 years of age and older), but cases in which parents report problems similar to those described previously should be screened using a checklist, such as the Gilliam Asperger's Disorder Scale [57], which is appropriate for those aged 3 to 22 years.

Treatment of early childhood autism

There currently exists an abundance of treatment options for early childhood autism. These treatments vary in their modality (eg, psychoeducational, biomedical), in how thoroughly they have been disseminated, and in the degree to which they are supported by well-controlled research. Physicians should be aware that professional workshops and the Internet have resulted in widespread dissemination of treatments for ASDs. This proliferation of information, combined with the perseverance with which a parent is likely to pursue treatment options, sometimes leads to ineffective or iatrogenic treatment.

Ten treatments for early childhood autism are presented here [58].[1] These specific treatments were selected because they have been demonstrated to be effective, are relatively common, or are likely to be presented to a physician for opinion. Each treatment is described, and a summary of its supporting empiric evidence is presented. When counseling parents, the authors recommend, at the least, that they are made aware of the National Research

---

[1] See also the web site of the Association for Science in Autism Treatment in which dozens of treatments for ASD are critically analyzed with respect to their supporting evidence [58].

Council's recommendations for early intervention. The National Research Council recommends the following, regardless of the specific treatment approach: (1) entry into a treatment program as soon as the diagnosis is seriously considered, (2) intensive treatment delivery (at least 25 hours per week), (3) treatment that comprehensively addresses the disorder's key deficit areas, (4) formal parent involvement in treatment delivery, (5) low student/teacher ratios, and (6) ongoing evaluation of the program's effectiveness [44].

Psychoeducational treatment

Early and intensive behavioral intervention

Early and intensive behavioral intervention (EIBI) is a skills-based treatment approach based on the science of applied behavior analysis. Although various EIBI models exist, they all share the same three primary characteristics: (1) intensive treatment delivery (eg, 30–40 hours per week for 2 years); (2) a hierarchically organized curriculum that focuses on learning readiness, communication, social, and preacademic repertoires [59,60]; and (3) the use of teaching methods based on the principles of operant conditioning [61]. Although multiple well-controlled investigations have been conducted on EIBI, the most well known is the investigation of the University of California at Los Angeles (UCLA) Young Autism Project, in which nearly half of experimental group participants with ASDs achieved normal intellectual functioning after 2 to 3 years of one-to-one treatment delivered for 40 hours per week [14,62]. This outcome has since been replicated several times by independent investigators [63–65]. To date, no other treatment approach has been able to produce this magnitude of effect for children with ASDs [15]. In addition, the US Surgeon General has recommended EIBI as an effective treatment [66]. Parents who are interested in pursuing this treatment approach should be referred to the Behavior Analyst Certification Board [67] to locate a professional qualified to oversee such a program.

Treatment and education of autistic and related communication-handicapped children

Project TEACCH (Treatment and Education of Autistic and Related Communication-Handicapped Children) is a classroom model for the instruction of children with ASDs. Rather than attempting to intensively remediate the core deficits of autism, the goal of Project TEACCH is to accommodate the learning styles of children with autism by using a variety of strategies, such as visual stimuli to prompt skills, individual workstations to minimize distraction, and picture activity schedules to assist with transition, among others [68]. The TEACCH model has been widely disseminated in classrooms across the United States. Although the National Research Council considers Project TEACCH a plausible intervention with positive program evaluation data [44], there are currently no well-controlled studies of its effects.

Developmental and relationship approaches

The relationship development intervention (RDI) and developmental, individual-difference, relationship-based model (DIR) are treatment packages that are based on developmental theory. In RDI, which is based on a relatively new theory of "dynamic intelligence," children are taught to make "authentic social connections" through numerous parent-led treatment sessions [69]. The social deficits of autism seem to be RDI's primary targets for change. DIR is based on a stage-based developmental theory of child development [70]. During DIR, a caregiver participates in interactive "floor time" sessions with the child, in which he or she follows the child's lead. Over time, the caregiver attempts to influence the child to participate in more sophisticated interactions. Like RDI, social deficits seem to be the primary focus of DIR treatment. Despite the popularity of these two approaches and their relatively widespread dissemination, no well-controlled studies have been published to document their effects. Furthermore, the developmental theories on which RDI and DIR are based are untested. Thus, the authors recommend that these factors be included in any deliberation regarding the use of these approaches.

Sensory integrative therapy

Sensory integrative therapy (SIT) is a common treatment for ASDs that is often administered by occupational therapists in school settings. SIT is based on the theory that many problems associated with developmental disability are a result of improper neurologic processing because of dysfunction of the sensory systems (eg, vestibular, proprioceptive, tactile). Treatment comprises a series of exercises and activities (eg, joint compression, body brushing, spinning) designed to stimulate and help reorganize the sensory systems. To date, there have been relatively few studies published on SIT, and they have generally used poor experimental controls. The findings of this small body of literature are equivocal in support of SIT [71]. In addition, the theory on which SIT is based is not supported by the literature [72]. Nevertheless, SIT is ubiquitous in the school system as a treatment for ASDs. Therefore, the authors' recommendation is for the effects of SIT to be carefully and objectively assessed to determine its benefit at the individual level when it is implemented.

Biomedical treatment

Gluten-free/casein-free diet

Gluten and casein are groups of proteins that are found in cereals (eg, wheat, rye) and dairy products (eg, milk, cheese), respectively. A gluten-free/casein-free (GFCF) diet is a popular form of treatment of childhood autism. One of the rationales for this treatment involves abnormal gastrointestinal (GI) functioning in individuals with autism. Gluten and casein are broken down into metabolites that act as opiate agonists. It is hypothesized that children with autism have "leaky guts," such that the compounds seep out of the stomach and enter the central nervous system, where they facilitate opioid activity in the brain [73]. To date, the evidence for the use of the GFCF diet in children with autism is equivocal. The results of a randomized single-blind experiment in 20 children with autism showed statistically significant differences between experimental and control group participants on measures of autistic behavior [74]. The results of a subsequent double-blind experiment showed no differences between experimental and control group participants, however [75]. Despite the absence of convincing evidence of the effectiveness of the GFCF diet, the treatment has been heavily disseminated, most likely because it is viewed as nutritional and noninvasive. Children with autism often have food selectivity, however, which can be exacerbated with overly restrictive diets [76,77]. Thus, the authors do not recommend the use of the GFCF diet, especially for children who already have demonstrated food selectivity.

Vitamin therapy

Vitamin supplements, such as vitamin C, vitamin B_6, and vitamin B_{12}, represent a relatively common form of treatment for ASDs [78]. These supplements are generally used because it is thought that they enhance neurotransmitter function in ways beneficial to individuals with ASDs. The most prevalent vitamin supplement for ASDs is a combination of vitamin B_6 and magnesium (Mg). This combination has also received the most research attention of all the vitamin supplements for ASDs. Although numerous early reports indicated a positive effect of vitamin B_6 and Mg on ASD symptoms, these investigations were generally methodologically flawed [79]. Several more recent and better controlled investigations have produced equivocal findings [80]. Given the lack of convincing evidence for the effects of vitamin B_6 and Mg and the dearth of research on other vitamin supplements, the authors recommend that physicians help parents who choose this treatment approach to monitor dosage and adverse effects [77].

Risperidone

Risperidone (Risperdal) is an atypical antipsychotic medication used to treat symptoms of schizophrenia, bipolar disorder, and Tourette's syndrome. In 2006, the US Food and Drug Administration (FDA) approved risperidone for the treatment of problem behavior (eg, aggression, self-injury, tantrums) associated with autism. The basis for this approval was a series of recent investigations, most of which were methodologically sound. In one randomized clinical trial, it was shown that 69.4% of 48 children with ASDs who received risperidone had a mean reduction in reported irritability scores of 56.9%. At 6 months, most participants demonstrated sustained benefits [81] and minor improvements in adaptive behavior [82], although the core features of autism remained unchanged [83]. The most common adverse effects of risperidone are weight gain and sleepiness [84,85]. It has already been well established in the literature that the problem behavior of individuals with developmental disabilities (including autism) serves as a way to communicate for attention, escape from unpleasant situations, and gain access to preferred toys and activities [86,87]. Functional assessment, the process by which these communicative intentions are identified, has been shown to be effective in selecting psychoeducational interventions (eg, functional communication training, noncontingent reinforcement) that result in substantial reductions in problem behavior without medication [88]. Thus, the authors recommend the use of risperidone as a treatment for problem behavior associated with autism only after a function-based approach has been shown ineffective.

Chelation therapy

Chelation therapy is the removal of toxic metals, such as lead, from soft tissues in the body through the use of substances (chelators) that bind with the metals. Common methods of chelation include the oral or intravenous administration of dimercaptosuccinic or lipoic acids. Although the FDA has not approved chelation therapy for autism, its use and dissemination have been facilitated by the unsupported notion that vaccines containing thimerosal (mercury) are causally related to the onset of autism [43]. Based on the invasiveness of the chelation procedure, the lack of any published empiric support, and the fact that at least one child with autism has died during the procedure [89], the authors advise against recommending chelation therapy as a treatment for autism.

Secretin

Secretin, a hormone secreted by the duodenum in response to increased acidity in the stomach, was approved by the FDA in 1981 for use in the diagnosis of GI disorders. Secretin was used as a treatment for autism after a case series was published in which three children with ASDs received a single infusion of intravenous porcine secretin during diagnostic GI endoscopy for chronic diarrhea [90]. Within 5 weeks, all children evidenced amelioration of their GI symptoms and their parents reported dramatic improvement in their children's communication and social behavior. A recent literature review found that 12 of 13 placebo-controlled experiments found no reliable symptomatic relief of autism from the hormone secretin beyond that which could be expected from a placebo, however [91]. Given the overwhelming evidence against the effectiveness of secretin and the invasiveness of the procedure, the authors advise against using intravenous secretin as a treatment for autism.

Hyperbaric oxygen therapy

Hyperbaric oxygen therapy (HBOT) involves the inhalation of pure oxygen inside a pressurized chamber. Although originally developed to treat diving disorders, such as decompression sickness, HBOT has since been successfully used to treat a wide range of medical problems, such as malignant tumors [92] and chronic diabetic wounds [93]. HBOT is now available for home treatment as a result of the advent of portable pressurized chambers. HBOT has not yet been experimentally evaluated for the treatment of autism. The only evidence for the use of HBOT in autism treatment is a preliminary case series that suggests positive outcomes [94]. The Internet includes numerous anecdotal reports and commercial applications. Given the lack of well-controlled experimentation on HBOT, however, the authors advise against pursuing this form of therapy until more convincing data emerge.

Common medical problems associated with autism spectrum disorders

Several commonly observed medical problems in children with ASDs are worthy of discussion, although they are not formally considered as part of the autism spectrum, per se. These problems occur so frequently in children with ASDs and can produce such substantial negative effects on quality of life that all practitioners should screen for them when serving this population.

Sleep problems

Studies have reported sleep disturbances in 44% to 83% of children with autism, with the highest rates of sleep disturbances among preschool-aged children [95,96]. Most children with sleep problems begin having problems in infancy, with the most common problems being difficulty in falling asleep and night and early morning awakenings [97,98]. It is less clear to what degree total hours of sleep per night is lower for children with autism than for typically developing children because of the equivocal findings reported in the literature [95,96,99]. A recent study investigated sleep problems in adolescents and young adults and found evidence of substantial sleep disturbances in the form of low sleep efficiency and long latencies to sleep onset for 80% of the participants, even when self-report and parent report suggested only moderate impairments [100]. Thus, sleep problems seem to persist into adulthood and to have an impact on the daily functioning of individuals with ASDs [101].

It is critically important for the primary care physician to screen for sleep disturbances because of the everyday ramifications of fatigue for children with autism. Several studies suggest that fatigue can worsen such problem behaviors as aggression, self-injurious behavior, and even food refusal [102–104]. In addition, safety issues may arise when children with ASDs are awake but unsupervised. Parents often resort to such strategies as cosleeping or light sleeping, increasing their own fatigue, which may result in less consistency in parenting and problem solving. Parents also use locks to ensure that the child cannot exit his or her room, which presents fire safety concerns.

Physicians are encouraged to inquire about sleep issues and ill-advised strategies that the parents may be using to cope with them. Intervention resources should be recommended if families are struggling with sleep problems. Electronic alerting systems (eg, WanderGuard, WanderGuard UK, London, England) provide a safe alternative to locks in the short term. Secretin has proven ineffective in reducing sleep problems [105], but an open-label study has shown positive effects of controlled-release melatonin in children with autism [106]. The evidence base for melatonin is limited, however, and caution is advised. Durand's parent-friendly guide to long-term treatment of sleep problems in children with disabilities [107] and Schreck's review of empirically supported behavioral treatment strategies for sleep disturbances in children with autism [108] are excellent resources for environmental and behavioral strategies.

Feeding disorders

Feeding disorders are common among children with ASDs and often take the form of food or texture selectivity, refusal of liquids, and problem behaviors associated with mealtimes [109]. A survey of parents with typically developing children and parents of children with autism found that feeding problems are relatively common for all children (50% had a problem at some time) but are nearly ubiquitous for children with ASDs (90% had a problem at some time) [110]. This discrepancy has since been confirmed in an empiric study that revealed significantly more feeding problems for children with autism than for typically developing children [111]. A recent investigation found that only 4 of 30 students with autism willingly accepted most foods [109]. The others exhibited a wide range of patterns of food selectivity, including selectivity by type (eg, starch, protein) and by texture. Thus, the typical child with an ASD experiences food refusal and selectivity concerns at some point, making it critical that physicians counsel parents about the importance of establishing an effective mealtime routine, consistently presenting new foods, and addressing food refusal at its earliest presentation.

Kedesdy and Budd's overview of assessment and treatment of feeding problems from a biobehavioral perspective [112] and Kerwin's review of empirically supported treatments for pediatric feeding disorders [113] are excellent resources. In addition to selectivity attributable to strong preferences, physiologic problems, such as esophageal reflux and nausea, are sometimes responsible for initial food refusal and should be evaluated before attempting other interventions. Refusal problems may persist even when these problems have been resolved, however, because of behavioral factors. Assessment typically involves the use of functional assessment and preference assessments to investigate the variables associated with food refusal [114,115]. Subsequent treatment by a pediatric psychologist with behavioral training and experience in feeding disorders typically involves a combination of several behavioral interventions designed to increase the child's motivation to consume novel foods and to minimize the aversiveness of the feeding experience [113,116].

Gastrointestinal problems

Chronic GI problems are common for children with ASDs and result in such symptoms as abdominal pain, chronic diarrhea, bloating, and irritability. Two studies have found that approximately 70% of their participants with autism had inflammation of the GI tract and evident symptoms [117,118]. Two other studies found only 23% [119] and 17% [42] of children with autism exhibiting GI symptoms, however. Another investigation found no difference in the history of GI problems of children with autism and matched controls before the date of diagnosis, suggesting that the GI problems are neither causally related to autism nor particularly associated with regression [120]. Severe food selectivity may account for many of the GI problems that these children develop throughout their lifetimes. For the children who do experience substantial GI problems, their discomfort and diarrhea may have a great impact on their adaptive and social functioning and may contribute to overall behavior problems. Thus, children with ASDs should be screened for GI problems and treated accordingly.

Summary

The authors hope that the summary and recommendations provided here are helpful in designing more sensitive and effective medical services for individuals with ASDs and their families. Given the importance of treating ASDs as early as possible, the authors recommend that primary care physicians adopt universal screening practices and evaluate parental reports regarding possible ASD-related deficits rather liberally. Furthermore, establishing a relationship with local diagnosticians before they are needed can help to expedite the diagnostic process for families. Even without universal screening, recent estimates of the prevalence of ASDs suggest that it is likely for primary care physicians, pediatricians, and pediatric neurologists to come into contact with individuals with ASDs in their practice. To maintain consistency with trends in evidence-based medicine, the authors encourage physicians to make recommendations and referrals for treatment that are informed by the available empiric support. Finally, the authors recommend that physicians who have individuals with ASDs in their practice educate patients and their families about comorbid medical conditions (eg, sleep, feeding, GI problems) and assess whether they are present in their patients.

References

[1] American Psychiatric Association. Diagnostic and statistical manual of mental disorders, 4th edition [text revision]. Washington, DC: American Psychiatric Association; 2000.
[2] Tidmarsh L, Volkmar FR. Diagnosis and epidemiology of autism spectrum disorders. Can J Psychiatry 2003;48:517–25.

[3] Zager D, editor. Autism spectrum disorders: identification, education, and treatment. 3rd edition. Mahwah (NJ): Lawrence Erlbaum Associates; 2005. p. 3–46.
[4] Bregman J. Definitions and characteristics of the spectrum. In: Zager D, editor. Autism spectrum disorders: identification, education, and treatment. Mahwah (NJ): Lawrene Erlbaum Associates; 2005. p. 3–46.
[5] Volkmar FR, Lord C, Bailey A, et al. Autism and pervasive developmental disorders. J Child Psychol Psychiatry 2004;45:135–70.
[6] Fombonne E. The epidemiology of autism: a review. Psychol Med 1999;29:769–86.
[7] Rutter M. Autistic children: infancy to adulthood. Semin Psychiatry 1970;2:2–22.
[8] Chakrabarti S, Fombonne E. Pervasive developmental disorder in preschool children: confirmation of high prevalence. Am J Psychiatry 2005;162:1133–41.
[9] Fombonne E. Epidemiological surveys of autism and other pervasive developmental disorders: an update. J Autism Dev Disord 2003;33:365–82.
[10] Carter AS, Davis NO, Klin A, et al. Social development in autism. In: Volkmar FR, Paul R, Klin A, et al, editors. Handbook of autism and pervasive developmental disorders, vol. 1. 3rd edition. Hoboken (NJ): Wiley; 2005. p. 312–34.
[11] Rogers SJ, Cook I, Meryl A, et al. Imitation and play in autism. In: Volkmar FR, Paul R, Klin A, editors. Handbook of autism and pervasive developmental disorders, vol. 1. 3rd edition. Hoboken (NJ): Wiley; 2005. p. 382–405.
[12] Osterling JA, Dawson G, Munson JA. Early recognition of 1-year-old infants with autism spectrum disorder versus mental retardation. Dev Psychopathol 2002;12:239–51.
[13] Eikeseth S, Smith T, Jahr E, et al. Intensive behavioral treatment at school for 4-7 year old children with autism: a 1-year comparison controlled study. Behav Modif 2002;26:49–68.
[14] Lovaas OI. Behavioral treatment and normal educational and intellectual functioning in young autistic children. J Consult Clin Psychol 1987;55:3–9.
[15] Smith T. Outcome of early intervention for children with autism. Clinical Psychology: Science and Practice 1999;6:33–49.
[16] Satzmari P, Bryson SE, Boyle MH, et al. Predictors of outcome among high-functioning children with autism and Asperger syndrome. J Child Psychol Psychiatry 2003;44:520–8.
[17] Charman T, Baird G. Practitioner review: diagnosis of autism spectrum disorders in 2- and 3-year-old children. J Child Psychol Psychiatry 2002;43:289–305.
[18] Lord C, Pickles A, McLennan J, et al. Diagnosing autism: analyses of data from the autism diagnostic interview. J Autism Dev Disord 1997;30:205–23.
[19] Moore V, Goodson S. How well does early diagnosis of autism stand the test of time? Follow-up study of children assessed for autism at age 2 and development of an early diagnostic service. Autism 2003;7:47–63.
[20] Asperger H. Die 'Autistichen Psychopathen' im Kindesalter. Arch Psychiatr Nervenkr 1944;117:76–136.
[21] Wing L. Asperger's syndrome: a clinical account. Psychol Med 1981;11:115–29.
[22] American Psychiatric Association. Diagnostic and statistical manual of mental disorders. 4th edition. Washington, DC: American Psychiatric Association; 1994.
[23] Myles BS, Simpson RL. Asperger syndrome: an overview of characteristics. Focus Autism Other Dev Disabl 2002;17:132–7.
[24] Klin A, McPartland J, Volkmar FR, et al. Asperger syndrome. In: Volkmar FR, Paul R, Klin A, editors. Handbook of autism and pervasive developmental disorders, vol. 1. 3rd edition. Hoboken (NJ): Wiley; 2005. p. 88–125.
[25] Centers for Disease Control. Parental report of diagnosed autism in children aged 4–17 years, United States, 2003-2004. MMWR Morb Mortal Wkly Rep 2006;55:481–6.
[26] Fombonne E. The prevalence of autism. JAMA 2003;289:87–9.
[27] Croen LA, Grether JK, Hoogstrate J, et al. The changing prevalence of autism in California. J Autism Dev Disord 2002;32:207–15.
[28] Fombonne E, Du Mazaubrun C, Cans C, et al. Autism and associated medical disorders in a French epidemiological survey. J Am Acad Child Adolesc Psychiatry 1997;36:1561–9.

[29] Luyster R, Richler J, Risi S, et al. Early regression in social communication in autism spectrum disorders: a CPEA study. Dev Neuropsychol 2005;27:311–36.
[30] Volkmar FR, Steir DM, Cohen DJ. Age of recognition of pervasive developmental disorder. Am J Psychiatry 1985;142:1450–2.
[31] Werner E, Dawson G. Validation of the phenomenon of autistic regression using home videotapes. Arch Gen Psychiatry 2005;62:889–95.
[32] Wakefield AJ. MMR vaccination and autism. Lancet 1999;354:949–50.
[33] Bernard S, Enayati A, Redwood L, et al. Autism: a novel form of mercury poisoning. Med Hypotheses 2001;56:462–71.
[34] Ramsay M. Time to review policy on contraindications to vaccination. Lancet 2000;356:1459–60.
[35] Dales L, Hammer SJ, Smith NJ. Time trends in autism and in MMR immunization coverage in California. JAMA 2001;285:1183–5.
[36] Fombonne E, Chakrabarti S. No evidence for a new variant of measles-mumps-rubella induced autism. Pediatrics 2001;108:e58.
[37] Honda H, Shmizu Y, Rutter M. No effect of MMR withdrawal on the incidence of autism: a total population study. J Child Psychol Psychiatry 2005;46:572–9.
[38] Kaye JA, der Mar Meler-Montes M, Jick H. Mumps, measles, and rubella vaccine and the incidence of autism recorded by general practitioners: a time trend analysis. BMJ 2001;322:460–3.
[39] Madsen KM, Hviid A, Vestergaard M, et al. A population-based study of measles, mumps, and rubella vaccination and autism. N Engl J Med 2002;347:1477–82.
[40] Smeeth L, Cook C, Fombonne E, et al. MMR vaccination and pervasive developmental disorders: a case-control study. Lancet 2004;364:963–9.
[41] Taylor B, Miller E, Farrington CP, et al. Autism and measles, mumps, and rubella vaccine: no epidemiological evidence for a causal association. Lancet 1999;353:2026–9.
[42] Taylor B, Miller E, Lingam R, et al. Measles, mumps, and rubella vaccination and bowel problems or developmental regression in children with autism: population study. BMJ 2002;324:393–6.
[43] Parker SK, Schwartz B, Todd J, et al. Thimerosal-containing vaccines and autistic spectrum disorder: a critical review of published original data. Pediatrics 2004;114:793–804.
[44] National Research Council. Educating children with autism. Washington, DC: National Academy Press; 2001.
[45] Wiggins LD, Baio J, Rice C. Examination of the time between first evaluation and first autism spectrum diagnosis in a population-based sample. J Dev Behav Pediatr 2006;27:S79–89.
[46] Dosreis S, Weiner CL, Johnson L, et al. Autism spectrum disorder screening and management practices among general pediatric providers. J Dev Behav Pediatr 2006;27:S88–97.
[47] Lord C. Follow-up of two-year olds referred for possible autism. J Child Psychol Psychiatry 1995;36:1365–82.
[48] Lord C, Rutter M, Le Couteur A. Autism Diagnostic Interview-Revised: a revised version of a diagnostic interview for caregivers of individuals with possible pervasive developmental disorders. J Autism Dev Disord 1994;24:659–85.
[49] Lord C, Rutter M, DiLavore P, et al. Autism Diagnostic Observation Schedule (ADOS). Los Angeles (CA): Western Psychological Services; 1999.
[50] Baird G, Charman T, Baron-Cohen S, et al. A screening instrument for autism at 18 months of age: a 6-year follow-up study. J Am Acad Child Adolesc Psychiatry 2000;39:694–702.
[51] Scambler DJ, Hepburn SL, Rogers SJ. A two-year follow-up on risk status identified by the checklist for autism in toddlers. J Dev Behav Pediatr 2006;27:S104–7.
[52] Robins DL, Fein D, Barton ML, et al. The Modified Checklist for Autism in Toddlers: an initial study investigating the early detection of autism and pervasive developmental disorders. J Autism Dev Disord 2001;31:131–44.

[53] Robins DL, Dumont-Mathieu TM. Early screening for autism spectrum disorders: update on the Modified Checklist for Autism in Toddlers and other measures. J Dev Behav Pediatr 2006;27:S111–9.
[54] Available at: www.firstsigns.org. Accessed May 15, 2007.
[55] Rutter M, Bailey A, Lord C. Social communication questionnaire. Los Angeles (CA): Western Psychological Services; 2003.
[56] Siegal B. Pervasive developmental disorders screening test II. San Antonio (TX): Harcourt Publishers; 2004.
[57] Gilliam J. Gilliam Asperger disorder scale. Austin (TX): Pro Ed; 2001.
[58] Available at: www.asatonline.org. Accessed May 15, 2007.
[59] Lovaas OI. Teaching individuals with developmental delays: basic intervention techniques. Austin (TX): PRO-ED; 2003.
[60] Sundberg ML, Partington JW. Teaching language to children with autism or other developmental disabilities. Pleasant Hill (CA): Behavior Analysts, Inc.; 1998.
[61] Smith T. Discrete trial training in the treatment of autism. Focus Autism Other Dev Disabl 2001;16:86–92.
[62] McEachin JJ, Smith T, Lovaas OI. Long-term outcome for children with autism who received early intensive behavioral treatment. Am J Ment Retard 1993;97:359–72.
[63] Cohen H, Amerine-Dickens M, Smith T. Early intensive behavioral treatment: replication of the UCLA model in a community setting. J Dev Behav Pediatr 2006;27:S145–55.
[64] Howard JS, Sparkman CR, Cohen HG, et al. A comparison of intensive behavior analytic and eclectic treatments for young children with autism. Res Dev Disabil 2005; 26:359–83.
[65] Sallows GO, Graupner TD. Intensive behavioral treatment for children with autism: four-year outcome and predictors. Am J Ment Retard 2005;110:417–38.
[66] Department of Health and Human Services. Mental health: a report of the surgeon general. Rockville (MD): Department of Health and Human Services; 1999.
[67] Available at: www.bacb.com. Accessed May 15, 2007.
[68] Mesibov GB, Shea V, Schopler E. The TEACCH approach to autism spectrum disorders. New York: Springer; 2005.
[69] Gutstein SE, Sheely RK. Relationship development intervention with young children: social and emotional development activities for Asperger syndrome, autism, PPD and NLD. London: Jessica Kingsley Publishers; 2002.
[70] Wieder S, Greenspan SL. The DIR (developmental, individual-difference, relationship-based) approach to assessment and intervention planning. Zero to Three 2001;21:11–9.
[71] Smith T, Mruzek DW, Mozingo D. Sensory integrative therapy. In: Jacobson JW, Foxx RM, Mulick JA, editors. Controversial therapies for developmental disabilities: fad, fashion and science in professional practice. Mahwah (NJ): Laurence Erlbaum Associates; 2005. p. 331–50.
[72] Arendt RE, MacLean WE, Baumeister AA. Critique of sensory integration therapy and its application in mental retardation. Am J Ment Retard 1988;92:401–11.
[73] Christison GW, Ivany K. Elimination diets in autism spectrum disorders: any wheat amidst the chaff? J Dev Behav Pediatr 2006;27:S162–71.
[74] Knivsberg A, Reichelt KL, Hoien T, et al. A randomized, controlled study of dietary intervention in autistic syndromes. Nutr Neurosci 2002;5:251–61.
[75] Harrison Elder J, Shankar M, Shuster J, et al. The gluten-free, casein-free diet in autism: results of a preliminary double blind clinical trial. J Autism Dev Disord 2006;36:413–20.
[76] Ahearn WH. Is eliminating casein and gluten from a child's diet a viable treatment for autism? Available at: http://www.behavior.org/autism/ahearn.cfm. Accessed January 13, 2007.
[77] Levy SE, Hyman SL. Novel treatments for autistic spectrum disorders. Ment Retard Dev Disabil Res Rev 2005;11:131–42.
[78] Green VA, Pituch KA, Itchon J, et al. Internet survey of treatments used by parents of children with autism. Res Dev Disabil 2006;27:70–84.

[79] Pfeiffer SI, Norton J, Nelson L, et al. Efficacy of vitamin B6 and magnesium in the treatment of autism: a methodology review and summary of outcomes. J Autism Dev Disord 1995;25:481–93.
[80] Nye C, Brice A. Combined vitamin B6-magnesium treatment in autism spectrum disorder. Cochrane Database Syst Rev 2005;4:CD003497.
[81] McCracken JT, McGough J, Shah B, et al. Risperidone in children with autism and serious behavioral problems. N Engl J Med 2002;347:314–21.
[82] Williams SK, Scahill L, Vitiello B, et al. Risperidone and adaptive behavior in children with autism. J Am Acad Child Adolesc Psychiatry 2006;45:431–9.
[83] McDougle CJ, Scahill L, Aman MG, et al. Risperidone for the core symptom domains of autism: results from the study by the Autism Network of the Research Units on Pediatric Psychopharmacology. Am J Psychiatry 2005;1(62):1142–8.
[84] Aman MG, Arnold LE, McDougle CJ, et al. Acute and long-term safety and tolerability of risperidone in children with autism. J Child Adolesc Psychopharmacol 2005;15:869–84.
[85] Hellings JA, Zarcone JR, Reese RM, et al. A crossover study of risperidone in children, adolescents and adults with mental retardation. J Autism Dev Disord 2006;36:401–11.
[86] Iwata BA, Pace GM, Dorsey MF, et al. The functions of self-injurious behavior: an experimental-epidemiological analysis. J Appl Behav Anal 1994;27:215–40.
[87] Reese RM, Richman DM, Belmont JM, et al. Functional characteristics of disruptive behavior in developmentally disabled children with and without autism. J Autism Dev Disord 2005;35:419–28.
[88] Kahng S, Iwata BA, Lewin AB. The impact of functional assessment on the treatment of self-injurious behavior. In: Schroeder SR, Oster-Granite ML, Thompson T, editors. Self-injurious behavior: gene-brain-behavior relationships. Washington, DC: American Psychological Association; 2002. p. 119–31.
[89] Centers for Disease Control. Deaths associated with hypocalcemia from chelation therapy Texas, Pennsylvania, and Oregon, 2003-2005. MMWR Morb Mortal Wkly Rep 2006;55:204–7.
[90] Horvath K, Stefanatos G, Sokolski KN, et al. Improved social and language skills after secretin administration in patients with autistic spectrum disorders. J Assoc Acad Minor Phys 1998;9:9–15.
[91] Esch BE, Carr JE. Secretin as a treatment for autism: a review of the evidence. J Autism Dev Disord 2004;34:543–56.
[92] Daruwalla J, Christophi C. Hyperbaric oxygen therapy for malignancy: a review. World J Surg 2006;30:2112–31.
[93] Roeckl-Wiedmann I, Bennett M, Kranke P. Systematic review of hyperbaric oxygen in the management of chronic wounds. Br J Surg 2005;92:24–32.
[94] Rossignol DA, Rossignol LW. Hyperbaric oxygen therapy may improve symptoms in autistic children. Med Hypotheses 2006;67:216–28.
[95] Hering E, Epstein R, Elroy S, et al. Sleep patterns in autistic children. J Autism Dev Disord 1999;29:143–7.
[96] Richdale AL, Prior MR. The sleep/wake rhythm in children with autism. Eur Child Adolesc Psychiatry 1995;4:175–86.
[97] Richdale AL. Sleep problems in autism: prevalence, cause and intervention. Dev Med Child Neurol 1999;41:60–6.
[98] Taira M, Takase M, Sasaki H. Development and sleep: sleep disorder in children with autism. Psychiatry Clin Neurosci 1998;52:182–3.
[99] Clements J, Wing L, Dunn G. Sleep problems in handicapped children: a preliminary study. J Child Psychol Psychiatry 1986;27:399–407.
[100] Oyane NMF, Bjorvatn B. Sleep disturbances in adolescents and young adults with autism and Asperger syndrome. Autism 2005;9:83–94.

[101] Malow BA, McGrew SG. Sleep and autism spectrum disorders. In: Tuchman R, Rapin I, editors. Autism: a neurological disorder of early brain development. London: Mac Keith Press; 2006. p. 189–201.
[102] Fisher WW, Piazza CC, Roane HS. Sleep and cyclical variables related to self-injurious and other destructive behaviors. In: Schroeder SR, Oster-Granite ML, Thompson T, editors. Self-injurious behavior: gene-brain-behavior relationships. Washington, DC: American Psychological Association; 2002. p. 205–21.
[103] Kennedy CH, Meyer KA. Sleep deprivation, allergy symptoms, and negatively reinforced problem behavior. J Appl Behav Anal 1996;29:133–5.
[104] Reed GK, Dolezal DN, Cooper-Brown LJ, et al. The effects of sleep disruption on the treatment of a feeding disorder. J Appl Behav Anal 2005;38:243–5.
[105] Honomichl RD, Goodlin-Jones BL, Burnham MM, et al. Secretin and sleep in children with autism. Child Psychiatry Hum Dev 2002;33:107–23.
[106] Giannotti F, Cortesi F, Cerquiglini A, et al. An open-label study of controlled-release melatonin in treatment of sleep disorders in children with autism. J Autism Dev Disord 2006; 36:741–52.
[107] Durand VM. Sleep better!: a guide to improving sleep for children with special needs. Baltimore (MD): Paul H Brookes; 1999.
[108] Schreck KA. Behavioral treatments for sleep problems in autism: empirically supported or just universally accepted? Behavioral Interventions 2001;16:265–78.
[109] Ahearn WH, Castine T, Nault K, et al. An assessment of food acceptance in children with autism or pervasive developmental disorder-not otherwise specified. J Autism Dev Disord 2001;31:505–11.
[110] DeMeyer MK. Parents and children in autism. New York: Wiley; 1979.
[111] Schreck K, Williams K, Smith AF. A comparison of eating behaviors between children with and without autism. J Autism Dev Disord 2004;34:433–8.
[112] Kedesdy JH, Budd KS. Childhood feeding disorders: biobehavioral assessment and intervention. Baltimore (MD): Paul H Brookes; 1998.
[113] Kerwin ME. Empirically supported treatments in pediatric psychology: severe feeding problems. J Pediatr Psychol 1999;24:193–214.
[114] Patel MR, Piazza CC, Layer SA, et al. A systematic evaluation of food textures to decrease packing and increase oral intake in children with pediatric feeding disorders. J Appl Behav Anal 2005;38:89–100.
[115] Piazza CC, Fisher WW, Brown KA, et al. Functional analysis of inappropriate mealtime behaviors. J Appl Behav Anal 2003;36:187–204.
[116] Ledford JR, Gast DL. Feeding problems in children with autism spectrum disorders: a review. Focus Autism Other Dev Disabl 2006;21:153–66.
[117] Horvath K, Papadimitriou JC, Rabsztyn A, et al. Gastrointestinal abnormalities in children with autistic disorder. J Pediatr 1999;135:559–63.
[118] Valicenti-McDermott M, McVicar K, Rapin I, et al. Frequency of gastrointestinal symptoms in children with autistic spectrum disorders and association with family history of autoimmune disease. J Dev Behav Pediatr 2006;27:S128–36.
[119] Molloy CA, Manning-Courtney P. Prevalence of chronic gastrointestinal symptoms in children with autism and autism spectrum disorders. Autism 2003;7:165–71.
[120] Black C, Kaye JA, Jick H. Relation of childhood gastrointestinal disorder to autism: nested case-control study using data from the UK General Practice Research Database. Prim Care 2002;325:419–21.

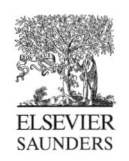

Learning Disorders in Children and Adolescents

Helen D. Pratt, PhD*, Dilip R. Patel, MD

Division of Behavioral-Developmental Pediatrics, Michigan State University, Kalamazoo Center for Medical Studies, 1000 Oakland Drive, Kalamazoo, MI 49008, USA

In many societies, the ability successfully to navigate the educational system means access to success, wealth, and power. In every educational system there is a subset of learners who are unable to engage in academic exercises because of deficits in sustaining attention, recalling and manipulating information, mastering specific cognitive processes, or demonstrating conceptual learning. These deficits may be the result of some type of intellectual, emotional, behavioral, physical, or environmental factor. Any combination of these factors can result in school failure [1]. Nearly 4 million school-age children have learning disabilities (LD). Of these, at least 20% have a type of disorder that leaves them unable to focus their attention [2].

Presentation

Parents most often ask for help with learning problems when they have been confronted by a family member or teacher about their child's difficulties. By this time in the process, the parents and teachers are often frustrated and may not be receptive to suggestions for rehabilitation. Parents who present with a child who has mild symptoms may be less able to articulate their concerns. They may describe their child as messy, unfocused, disorganized, unmotivated, clumsy, or odd. As their child grows up and the disability impacts the child's life in a more significant manner, teachers may describe him or her as a daydreamer, being zoned out, intentionally ignoring the teacher, or maybe even as being disturbed [3–5]. A well-behaved,

---

This article is adapted with permission from: Pratt HD, Patel DR, Greydanus DE. Learning disorders. In: Greydanus DE, Patel DR, Pratt HD, editors. Behavioral pediatrics, vols. 1 and 2. 2nd edition. New York: iUniverse; 2006. p. 143–160.

* Corresponding author.

E-mail address: pratt@kcms.msu.edu (H.D. Pratt).

nondisruptive, polite child with an attention or language disorder may not come to the attention of the physician until a critical threshold of academic demand is reached. Parents of a child who has more serious deficits in functioning (eg, cognitive, communication, hearing, attention, motor skills) often bring their child into the physician's office with concerns about their child's development, instruction following, and academic skills [3,4].

Normal learning abilities: a developmental perspective

Cognitive development

A child's or adolescent's ability to perform simple to complex mental tasks, including sustaining attention, mental processing (speed or alertness), thinking skills, problem solving skills, and judgment all combine to define the cognitive domain [5–15]. Learning begins in utero and progresses in a fairly predictable fashion throughout life. Very young children (ages 3–5 years) learn through repetition and trial and error [6,7,13]. By the age of 6 to 10 years, children are considered as "concrete thinkers," wherein they usually see things as "here and now," "right or wrong," and "black or white" [7,13,14]. They generally cannot predict the outcomes of their behaviors and may not understand the consequences of their behavior or actions.

Young adolescents (ages 11–13 years) have developed a more refined cognitive ability that includes critical thinking, problem solving, and rapid decision making. They can understand the intent of and can follow oral and written directions, and can adopt another person's perspective [8,9,11,13,14]. They may have difficulty generalizing or extrapolating rules and concepts from familiar to unique or novel situations [8,9]. Inductive and deductive reasoning abilities, prepositional logic, a sense of morality and altruism, abstract thinking, analytical abilities, and transitional skills are all in the early stages of development [6,11,14–17].

Language development

Preschool children (ages 3–5 years) typically use speech that is 100% intelligible to strangers [7,11]. Telegraphic speech and three-word sentences are a part of a normal child's speech learning behaviors. By the age of 5 years they have a vocabulary of about 2500 words, can speak sentences of up to five words, can use future tense, can name four colors, and can count 10 or more objects. By age 6 their vocabulary increases to about 5000 words [7,11]. They have some difficulty understanding homonyms and their ability to comprehend complex or compound sentences is limited. Some children may misuse sounds, words, or not always use correct grammar, which may also be within the norm, but if it persists after consistent correction, then a speech evaluation may be warranted.

By middle adolescence (ages 13–15 years) youth can understand and give complex directions; they have the cognitive ability to understand a broader range of words and their symbolic use [7–11]. They understand homonyms and synonyms. Cognitively, youth move away from acquisition to the cognitive aspects of language development; they understand the semantics of language and have the ability to use language to convey different types of information of varying levels of quality. They can use symbols, signs, and coded words to understand games and directions [10,14–16].

Sensory-perceptual development

Attention

The ability to pay attention and to discriminate between relevant and irrelevant stimuli increases with normal growth and maturation of the child's physical, neurologic, cognitive, and emotional systems. Infants learn to attend by gazing into their mother's eyes while feeding, watching objects placed in front of them, and listening to familiar sounds in their environments. This process requires a sophisticated interaction between the following domains: visual, auditory, kinesthetic, and cognitive processing. During early adolescence selective attention and memory are more soundly established [6,10]. For youth to learn to speak, read, and write, they must be able to detect relevant stimuli and sustain that attention long enough to recognize essential aspects of the stimulus.

Visual-motor

Visual motor ability refers to the normal development of visual acuity, color vision, visual discriminatory ability, and tracking ability. Children younger than 6 or 7 are farsighted. Their limited ability to track objects and judge the speed of moving objects is caused by their limited vision, and not by a lack of coordination [13]. By age 10 children have improved visual acuity, tracking ability, and have a more mature level of visual-perceptual motor integration; however, their sense of directionality may not yet be fully developed [7,13,18]. Prepubescent youth may have problems with eye-hand coordination. By late adolescence visual-motor abilities are well developed and highly sophisticated [18].

Auditory

Normal hearing helps children locate the source and direction of the auditory stimuli; follow essential instructions or advice (from teachers, parents, or other adults); and communicate with friends. All academic activities require a sophisticated level of auditory listening skills. The ability to listen selectively matures as the child grows [6,7,13,19]. By middle adolescence children have acquired well-developed listening skills.

Perceptual motor

The child's auditory, cognitive, kinesthetic, language, physical, and visual domains, and the ability to plan complex motor functions, are influenced by his or her level of perceptual motor development [7,10,13,18,20–22]. This domain involves fine motor responses, gross motor responses (including co-ordination, balance, and agility), reaction time, and visual-motor responses and involves the ability to perceive, interpret, and execute an appropriate neuromotor response to a stimulus [7,13,21–23].

Psychosocial-emotional development

Developmental deficits in relationship building and maintenance skills can impact youth once they are required to interact with siblings or peers. Children who do not learn how to engage in healthy reciprocal play activities do not develop the necessary friendships that help them develop the ability to initiate healthy intimate peer relationships. The convergence of body image and motor skills occurs during early adolescence and youth begin to worry over perceived physical differences, and sexual relationships may occupy much of their time [8,9,11,13,15,17,24]. During middle adolescence (ages 13–15 years) youth actively seek to develop increased levels of independence from parents and authority figures [14,15].

Role of deficits in domains of function

The impact of abnormal development in the previously mentioned domains can be severe enough to impede a child or adolescent's ability to learn. It is important for clinicians to understand what role each domain plays in a child or adolescent's ability to learn to communicate expressively and understand language, read, write, and calculate mathematical problems. Clinicians who know what an individual should be able to do (with allowance for variation) at a specific developmental level are better prepared to detect problem learners. Not all learning problems are necessarily LD. Many children are simply slower in developing certain skills. Because children show natural differences in their rate of development, sometimes what seems to be a LD may simply be a delay in maturation. To be diagnosed as a LD, specific criteria must be met.

Defining learning disorders

The term "learning disability" only describes a constellation of symptoms and does not represent a group of independent symptoms, nor does it represent a single entity; the term should be thought of as a label. LD is defined as a discrepancy between the actual academic achievement of a student and that student's intellectual potential. Individuals who have LD experience seriously impaired functioning in one or more of the following areas: (1) reading (comprehension); (2) language (expression, comprehension); (3) written expression; (4) mathematics (calculation, reasoning); (5) sustained attention; and (6) goal-directed behavior [25–28]. The LD must be the primary cause of problems in functioning even in the presence of other disabilities (physical, mental, behavioral) [25–28].

Many aspects of speaking, listening, reading, writing, and arithmetic overlap and build on the same brain capabilities. Individuals can be diagnosed as having more than one area of LD. For example, the ability to understand language underlies learning to speak. Any disorder that hinders the ability to understand language also interferes with the development of speech, which in turn hinders learning to read and write. A single gap in the brain's operation can disrupt many types of activity [2].

Diagnosis

Students who perform substantially below grade level and obtain lower scores on standardized achievement tests (eg, reading, mathematics, or written expression) may meet criteria for a LD. This disability must significantly interfere with the student's ability to function in these subjects. "Significant" is defined as having standard scores on achievement tests that are more than 2 standard deviations below scores obtained in intelligence tests. Youth who have multiple impairments that produce the same outcome may also be diagnosed with a LD. Some associated problems include cognitive processing deficits, comorbid mental disorders, general medical conditions, or the individual's ethnic or cultural background. The presence of a sensory deficit does not preclude diagnosis if the learning problems are in excess of those usually associated with the deficit [2,25].

Reading disorder (dyslexia)

Impaired ability to read accurately or fully comprehend written words and text is called reading disability or dyslexia. The impairment must substantially interfere with academic achievement and result in performance that is substantially below that expected from the individual's age, intelligence, and educational level. Its prevalence is estimated to be 2% to 8% of school-age children and is more common in boys [2,25]. Children who are poor readers or have associated attention-deficit–hyperactivity disorder (ADHD) symptoms share a common generalized deficit in phonologic processing and word recognition [2,25,27,28].

Developmental speech and language disorders

Speech and language problems are often the earliest indicators of a LD. Children with developmental speech and language disorders have difficulty producing speech sounds, using spoken language to communicate, or understanding what other people say. Depending on the problem, the specific diagnosis may be one of the following. (1) Developmental articulation disorder: youth with this disorder may have trouble controlling their rate of speech and have problems with production ("wabbit" instead of "rabbit" and "thwim" for "swim."). Most youth out grow this disorder by age 8 if they receive speech therapy. (2) Developmental expressive language disorder: these youth have problems with expressing themselves in speech. (3) Developmental receptive language disorder: these youth have difficulty in comprehending [2,25].

Developmental receptive language disorders

Some people have trouble understanding certain aspects of speech. It is as if their brains are set to a different frequency and the reception is poor. There's the toddler who does not respond to his name, a preschooler who hands you a bell when you asked for a ball, or consistently cannot follow simple directions. Their hearing is fine, but they cannot make sense of certain sounds, words, or sentences they hear. They may even seem inattentive. Using and understanding speech are strongly related; many people with receptive language disorders also have an expressive language disability [2,25].

During attempts to read, these youth often focus undue emphasis on the critical process of attempting to decode the phonetic sounds of individual words. In doing so, however, they lose actual comprehension of the concepts that the words and groups of words convey, which is the very purpose of the decoding. Organizational skills, sequential memory, and planning abilities are badly disrupted. This disruption in turn seriously affects both spoken and written receptive and expressive functioning [25]. Girls are somewhat less frequently identified with this group of disorders than are boys [2].

Developmental writing disorder

Writing, too, involves several brain areas and functions. The brain networks for vocabulary, grammar, hand movement, and memory must all be in good working order. A developmental writing disorder may result from problems in any of these areas. For example, a child who is unable to distinguish the sequence of sounds in a word has problems with spelling. A child with a writing disability, particularly an expressive language disorder, might be unable to compose complete, grammatically correct sentences [2].

Disorders of written expression

Disorder of written expression refers to an impaired ability to use written language skills. The deficits cause the child to perform at a level that is substantially lower than those skills expected of that child based on age, intelligence, and education [2,5,25].

Developmental arithmetic disorder (dyscalculia)

Developmental arithmetic disorder refers to an impaired ability to perform mathematical functions, specifically in the critical arenas of calculation, and of handling the stepwise logic of word—based problems [2,5,25]. Arithmetic is a complex mental process that requires the student to recognize numbers and symbols; memorize facts, such as the multiplication table; align numbers; understand abstract concepts, such as place value and fractions; and recall that information. Any of these may be difficult for children with developmental arithmetic disorders. Most students are also required to use fine and visual motor skills when performing academic work in mathematics. This means that problems in visual tracking and fine motor control, and executive functions of planning and execution, are also involved. Problems with numbers or basic concepts are likely to show up early. Disabilities that appear in the later grades are more often tied to problems in reasoning [1,2,25].

Motor skills disorder (dysgraphia)

Motor skills disorders refer to coordination disorders that can lead to poor penmanship, and certain spelling and memory disorders. Problems with pinscher grasp, fine motor control, and visual motor coordination can add to the student's inability to learn. Additionally, delays in acquiring motor skills that can affect the ability to learn, but do not meet the criteria for a specific LD, are included in this category [2,25].

Specific learning disorder not otherwise specified

Specific learning disorders not otherwise specified refers to delays in acquiring language, academic, and motor skills that can affect the ability to learn, but do not meet the criteria for a specific LD (eg, difficulties telling time and poor sequencing abilities, visual perceptual reversals) [2,25].

Etiology

Learning disorders are caused by a variety of neurocortical deficits and areas of neurologic dysfunction; however, exact etiologies have not been completely elucidated. Normal brain functioning is characterized by consistent brain—side dominance of one side over the other [1]. One theory postulates that such lateralization may be replaced by discoordinate or competitive dominance shared by both sides of the brain, resulting in learning difficulties [1].

Current research indicates that a neural quadrant picture involving the two prefrontal cortical regions and the two temporo—parieto—occipital cortical regions may be more accurate theater for such deficits [5,29]. This model supports the more specifically observed deficits and helps one begin to understand the basis of such problems whose origins seem to be located primarily in the prefrontal and frontal areas of either side of the brain rather than in a small area of the right hemisphere, such as attention deficit disorder and certain types of mathematical difficulties [2]. Cognitive disorders are caused by a number of factors that can include unexplained trauma; infections (congenital and postnatal); chromosomal abnormalities; genetic abnormalities and inherited metabolic disorders; exposures to toxins; malnutrition; and environmental causes (poverty, low socioeconomic status). Evidence shows that most LD do not stem from a single, specific area of the brain, but from difficulties in bringing together information from various brain regions [2].

A current leading theory is that LD stems from subtle disturbances in brain structures and functions. Some scientists believe that, in many cases, the disturbance begins before birth and includes errors in fetal brain development; genetic factors; tobacco, alcohol, and other drug use (eg, cocaine); complications during pregnancy or delivery; toxins in the child's environment (eg, cadmium); chemotherapy; and radiation.

Comorbidity

Although children with LD can manifest problems in attention and communication, those impairments may not be the primary result of a learning disorder. Problems in communication, language, behavior, or emotions can also be significant enough to be diagnosed independently.

Distinction between LD and ADHD is often difficult because of overlapping features and because ADHD often coexists with LD [26]. The shared symptoms include distractibility, disorganization, impulsivity, poor social skills, poor frustration tolerance, impulsiveness, poor self-control, poor self—concept, and lack of self—esteem [30]. Children diagnosed with LD show higher rates of anxiety. Youth with LD, by contrast, characteristically demonstrate phonologic, logic, and language problems not seen in children with anxiety disorders [1].

Although the underlying basis of learning disorders and attention deficits may be a neurophysiologic defect in cognitive processing, the overall effect is a cascade that seriously affects many other critical areas of function [3,31]. Research indicates youth rarely experience single or isolated disability. More than one of these disabilities, each with its retinue of secondary problems, may occur in a given child, and is the presentation most frequently seen [5,26].

Youth with learning disorders may drop out of school (nearly 40%); be demoralized; have low self esteem; and suffer from social skills deficits [25]. The high drop out rates (roughly 1.5 times higher than for the general population) and learning deficits also limit later employment [25]. Conduct, oppositional defiant disorders, ADHD, dysthymic disorders, major depressive disorders, and developmental language delays are each associated disorders (10%–25%) with LD. Evidence suggests that developmental delays in language may occur in association with LD, especially reading disorder [2,25]. LD may also be associated with a higher rate of developmental coordination disorder. Individuals with LD may have underlying abnormalities in cognitive processes (visual-perceptual, linguist processes, attention, memory, or a combination of these); however, measure of these processes is generally less reliable and valid than other psychoeducational tests [25]. LD is frequently found in association with a variety of general medical conditions, including lead poisoning, fetal alcohol syndrome, and fragile X syndrome [25]. Although genetic predisposition and perinatal injury and various neurologic or general medical conditions may be associated with the development of LD, the presence of such conditions does not invariably predict an LD.

Differential diagnosis

Differential diagnoses of LD include normal academic variation in attainment, impairment in vision and hearing, mental retardation, and pervasive developmental disorders; chromosomal anomalies and genetic disorders; neurologic disorders; congenital malformations; inborn errors in metabolism; developmental disorders; severe toxic exposure; chronic mental illness; severe infectious; chronic disease; side effects of medication used to treat other conditions; and psychoemotional trauma and psychologic trauma [2,25].

Assessment

Assessment should always begin with (1) a comprehensive general physical that includes a neurologic screening examination, (2) a comprehensive medical history, (3) a mental status examination, and (4) a psychosocial history. A good psychosocial history includes (1) developmental history (including prenatal and birth data); (2) history of unusual behaviors or habits; (3) family history (including screening for history of mental illness, alcoholism, child abuse or spousal abuse, neglect, incarceration, learning disorders, communications disorders, and attention disorders); and a thorough behavioral observation (minimum includes at school in several different activities or classes and in the physician's or psychologist's office; optimal includes home setting). This data gathering should include three additional types of information on problem behaviors or issues: (1) the onset, frequency, duration, and intensity of problem issues or behaviors; (2) anecdotal information (parental and teacher observations); and (3) school records and teacher observations.

Psychologic evaluation

A qualified psychologist administers several basic tests to determine if a child has a problem in a specific area that is significant enough to warrant a mental health diagnosis. Those tests can range from screening sessions to comprehensive examinations and include an assessment of intellectual ability (intelligence quotient) and function; behavioral; academic (math, reading, spelling, classroom behavior); language (expressive and receptive); neuropsychologic (gross and fine motor, sequencing, visual motor, coordination and balance, hearing, and visual spacial); emotional (affective disorders); adaptive (social, emotional, independence, maturity); and personality (psychopathology) functioning. The decision to use a screening test versus a comprehensive test battery is governed by the type of question asked at the time of referral and the severity of the child's problems. Only a few of these tests provide appropriate norms for individuals with different sociocultural backgrounds.

Consultation for language, motor, vision, and auditory deficits

Youth who evidence problems with vision should be referred to an ophthalmologist. Those with language or hearing delays should be referred to a speech pathologist and audiologist. Those with gross or fine motor, coordination, balance, or visual motor problems should be referred to an occupational therapist. Each of these individuals conducts more comprehensive evaluations to identify specific deficits and provide treatment recommendations. Results from such evaluations require the physician to organize clinical findings in a manner that facilitates patient management and allows the physician to advocate on behalf of the child.

Treatment principles

The primary care clinician should identify and appropriately treat any underlying neurologic or medical disorder, and assist in the medical management of any comorbid disorders, such as **ADHD**, anxiety disorder, and so forth. Physicians who expect to manage children with learning disorders effectively must collect relevant information that allows them to arrive at an accurate diagnosis. This is a complex and time-consuming venture that requires the input of multiple professionals; he or she must work at developing a network of health care professionals and educators in the community who can provide specific diagnostic evaluations, treatment recommendations, and implement treatment interventions. Early diagnosis is very important for effective intervention and academic success of the child. It is important to note that the underlying deficits of specific learning disorders persist for life and any management plan must take a life span perspective starting from early childhood to workplace. The clinician should familiarize himself or herself with the specific laws pertaining to education of children with LD.

Specific LDs require specific individualized intervention strategies and in broad terms encompass some form of remedial and accommodative interventions. During elementary and early school years remedial instructions play a key role in the management (eg, in children with reading disability specific instructions in phonemic awareness, vocabulary, comprehension, and so forth are integrated in the plan). During later years (secondary school and college years) the strategy shifts from remediation to accommodations, such as allowing more reading time and allowing use of hand-held computer devices or laptops, tape recorders, and recorded books. In children with specific problems with writing methods can be used that bypass writing, such as recorded books, prewritten assignments where the students has only to enter answers, and occupational therapy for young children [32]. Special education in each local school district is protected and regulated by strong legislative and judicial safeguards created by the federal Education for All Handicapped Children Act (PL 94-142) [33,34].

The law provides for youth with disabilities severe enough to impair their ability to learn and function at age, grade, and developmentally appropriate levels. Educational systems must provide those youth diagnosed with LD special accommodation. The special accommodations are generally managed by multidisciplinary teams (comprised of educators, school psychologists and social workers, the involved parents, speech therapist, occupational therapists, and other specialists as necessary). School systems are usually very interested in having the youth's physician involved in the planning. Such planning activities are referred to as an "Individual Education Plan" and the committee is referred to as the "Individual Education Planning Committee." Youth who are suspected of having a LD are referred to the committee by their teachers or other school personnel. The youth is then evaluated in the classroom and a decision is made as to whether testing (psychologic, speech, occupational) should occur. Once the testing is completed, the results are evaluated to determine if the youth meets criteria for receiving special accommodation or if special education services are required. If the youth does not meet criteria to receive services from the school, parents can appeal and can seek services and supports through the local or state protection and advocacy group. The clinician can also refer the child for independent evaluation to determine if the youth does indeed have multiple disabilities or problems more severe than the school determined. All clinicians should refer to their professional organization's policy statements dealing with children with LD.

Prognosis

Even though a LD does not disappear, given the right types of educational experiences, people have a remarkable ability to learn. The brain's flexibility to learn new skills is probably greatest in young children and may diminish somewhat after puberty. This is why early intervention is so important. Nevertheless, the ability to learn is retained throughout one's life. Because certain learning problems reflect delayed development, many children do eventually catch up. Of the speech and language disorders, children who have an articulation or an expressive language disorder are the least likely to have long-term problems. For people with dyslexia, the outlook is mixed, but an appropriate remedial reading program can help learners make great strides.

Summary

Findings indicate that students with severe LD can profit from instruction geared toward abstract higher-order comprehension when it is designed according to their particular instructional requirements [35]. Early intervention improves outcomes for most children with disorders of learning, attention, and cognition [26,36,37]. Impairment in the physical, language, sensory, or mental domains is usually harder to diagnose before a child's entry into the school system, but they are easier to treat if caught early. Children with more severe disorders are easier to detect, but children with milder disorders may not be easy to recognize [29]. Delayed detection often results in greater problems in academic, social, emotional, and psychologic functioning and even can result in a child dropping out of school. Most authors agree that although individuals may never outgrow their disabilities, children with above-average intellectual abilities often have the ability to compensate or master appropriate coping mechanisms to minimize greatly their overall negative outcomes [36]. Parental attitudes and commitment, availability of resources, and the presence of associated neurologic deficit or medical disorder can also significantly impact outcomes [38,39].

References

[1] Pratt HD. Neurodevelopmental issues in the assessment and treatment of deficits in attention, cognition, and learning during adolescence. Adolesc Med 2002;13(3):579–98.
[2] Neuwirth S. Learning disorders. U.S. Department of Health and Human Services, Public Health Service, National Institutes of Health, National Institute of Mental Health; 1993. NIH Publication No. 93-3611. Bethesda (MD).
[3] Schachter DC, Pless IB, Burk M. The prevalence and correlates of behavioral problems in disabled children. Can J Psychiatry 1991;36(6):323–31.
[4] Stanley PD, Dai Y, Nolan RF. Differences in depression and self esteem reported by learning disabled and behavior disordered middle school students. J Adolesc 1997;20(2):219–22.
[5] Blumsack J, Lewandowski L, Waterman B. Neurodevelopmental precursors to learning disabilities: a preliminary report from a parent survey. J Learn Disabil 1997;30(2):228–37.
[6] Capute AJ, Accardo PJ. A neurodevelopmental perspective on the continuum of developmental disabilities. In: Capute AJ, Accardo PJ, editors. Developmental disabilities in infancy and childhood. 2nd edition. Baltimore (MD): Paul H. Brooks Publishing; 1996. p. 1–24.
[7] Dixon SD, Stein MT, editors. Encounters with children: pediatric behavior and development. 3rd edition. Philadelphia: Mosby; 2000.
[8] Erickson E. Childhood and society. New York: W.W. Norton and Co.; 1963.

[9] Erickson E. Identity, youth and crisis. New York: W.W. Norton and Co.; 1968.
[10] Gemelli R. Normal child and adolescent development. Washington, DC: American Psychiatric Press; 1996.
[11] Gesell A, Ilg FL, Ames LB. The child from five to ten. New York: Harper and Row Publishers; 1946.
[12] Illingworth R. The development of the infant and young child. 7th edition. London: Churchill Livingstone; 1980.
[13] Levine MD. Neurodevelopmental dysfunction in the school age child. In: Behrman RE, Kliegman RM, Jenson HB, editors. Nelson textbook of pediatrics 16th edition. Philadelphia: WB Saunders Company; 2000. p. 94–100.
[14] Piaget J. Intellectual evaluation from adolescence to adulthood. Hum Dev 1969;1–12.
[15] Piaget J, Inhelder B. The psychology of the child. New York: Basic Books; 1969.
[16] Abe JA, Izard CE. A longitudinal study of emotion, expression and personality relations in early development. J Pers Soc Psychol 1999;77(3):566–77.
[17] Hofmann AD. Adolescent growth and development. In: Hofmann AS, Greydanus DE, editors. Adolescent medicine. 3rd edition. Stamford (CT): Appleton and Lange; 1997. p. 11–22.
[18] Gomez JE. Growth and maturation. In: Sullivan AJ, Anderson SJ, editors. Care of the young athlete. Park Ridge (IL): American Academy of Orthopaedic Surgeons; 2000. p. 25–33.
[19] Needleman RD. Growth and development. In: Behrman RE, Kliegman RM, Jenson HB, editors. Nelson textbook of pediatrics. 16th edition. Philadelphia: W.B. Saunders; 2000. p. 23–65.
[20] Feldman H, Bauer RE. Developmental-behavioral pediatrics. In: Zitelli BJ, Davis HW, editors. Atlas of pediatric physical diagnosis. 3rd edition. ST. Louis (MO): Mosby-Wolfe; 1997. p. 47–74.
[21] Fagard J. Skill acquisition in children: a historical perspective. In: Bar Or O, editor. The child and adolescent athlete. Oxford (England): Blackwell Science; 1996. p. 74–91.
[22] Rieser JJ, Pick HL, Ashmead DH, et al. Calibration of human locomotion and models of perceptual-motor organization. J Exp Psychol Hum Percept Perform 1995;21(3):480–97.
[23] Branta C, Haubensticker J, Seefeldt V. Age changes in motor skills during childhood and adolescence. Exerc Sport Sci Rev 1984;12:467–520.
[24] Kreipe RE. Normal somatic adolescent growth and development. In: McAnarney ER, Kreipe RE, Orr DP, editors. Textbook of adolescent medicine. Philadelphia: W.B.Saunders; 1994. p. 44–67.
[25] American Psychiatric Association. Disorders first diagnosed in infancy, childhood and adolescence. Diagnostic and statistical manual of mental disorders fourth edition. Washington, DC: American Psychological Association; 1994. p 46–52.
[26] Lyon GR. Learning disabilities. The future of children–special education for students with disabilities. The Future of Children—Special Education for Students with Disabilities 1996;(1):54–76.
[27] Swanson HL, Mink J, Bocian KM. Cognitive processing deficits in poor readers with symptoms of reading disabilities and ADHD. More alike than different? J Educ Psychol 1999;91(2):321–33.
[28] World Health Organization. International statistical classification of diseases and related health disorders ICD-10. Geneva (Switzerland): World Health Publications; 1997.
[29] Branch WB, Cohen MJ, Hynd GW. Academic achievement and attention—deficit/hyperactivity disorder in children with left or right—hemisphere dysfunction. J Learn Disabil 1995;28(1):35–43.
[30] Tsatsani KD, Fuerst DR, Rourke BP. Psychosocial dimensions of learning disabilities: external validation and relationship with age and academic functioning. J Learn Disabil 1997;30(5):490–502.
[31] Rock EE, Fessler MAS, Church RP. The concomitance of learning disabilities and emotional/behavioral disorders: a conceptual model. J Lear Disabil 1997;30(3):245–63.

[32] Mason A, Pratt HD, Patel DR, et al. Psychology of prejudice and discrimination towards persons with disabilities. In: Chin JL, editor. The psychology of prejudice and discrimination. Praeger Press; 2004. p. 51–93.
[33] American Academy of Pediatrics. Committee on children with disabilities: provision of educationally-related services for children and adolescents with chronic diseases and disabling conditions policy statement. Pediatrics 2000;105(2):448–51.
[34] American Academy of Pediatrics. Committee on children with disabilities: the pediatrician's role in development and implementation of an individual education plan (IEP) and/or an Individual Family Service Plan (IFSP) policy statement. Pediatrics 1999;104(1):124–7.
[35] Wilder AA, Williams JP. Students with severe learning disabilities can learn higher order comprehension skills. J Educ Psychol 2001;93(2):268–79.
[36] Denckla MB. The child with developmental disabilities grown up: adult residua of childhood disorders. Neurol Clin 1993;11(1):105–25.
[37] Spreen O. Prognosis of learning disability. J Consult Clin Psychol 1988;56(6):836–42.
[38] Barga N. Students with learning disabilities in education: managing a disability. J Learn Disabil 1996;29(4):413–21.
[39] Greydanus DE, Pratt HD, Patel DR. Attention deficit hyperactivity disorder across the lifespan. Dis Mon 2007;53(2):65–132.

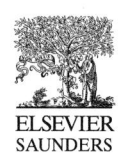

Intellectual Disability (Mental Retardation) in Children and Adolescents

Helen D. Pratt, PhD*, Donald E. Greydanus, MD

Michigan State University College of Human Medicine, Pediatrics Program, MSU/Kalamazoo Center for Medical Studies, 1000 Oakland Drive, Kalamazoo, MI 49008-1284, USA

Mental retardation (MR) (current term, *intellectual disability* [ID]) is a label used to describe a constellation of symptoms that includes severe deficits or limitations in an individual's developmental skills in several areas or domains of function: *cognitive, language, motor, auditory, language, psychosocial, moral judgment, and specific integrative adaptive* (*activities of daily living*) (Appendix 1) [1–14]. Individuals diagnosed with MR/ID will require various levels of support to learn how to engage in self-care activities, develop healthy reciprocal intimate relationships, obtain appropriate employment, and acquire other important activities of daily living. Basic skill attainment may take longer to learn (ie, speaking, walking, and taking care of personal needs such as dressing or eating). Academic, social, and self-regulatory functioning may be the most significantly affected areas [15,16]. The current label suggested for the term *mental retardation* by The American Association on Intellectual and Development Disabilities (AAIDD formerly AAMR) is *intellectual disability (ID)*.

A general description from multiple sources refers to ID as a developmental, cognitive, or intellectual deficit that: 1) occurs concurrently with deficits (mild to severe) in adaptive behavior, academic performance, adaptive functioning and 2) is manifested during the developmental period (birth to late adolescence or before age 18) [15–22].

---

* Corresponding author.
 E-mail address: pratt@kcms.msu.edu (H.D. Pratt).

Prevalence

ID is the most common developmental disorder. On average, about 1% of children ages 3 to 10 years have ID. ID is more common in older children (ages 6–10 years) than in younger children (ages 3–5 years). ID was also more common in boys than in girls and more common in black children than in white children [16,17]. As many as three of every 100 people in the country have ID [17,19,23]. Nearly 613,000 children ages 6 to 21 have some level of ID and need special education in school [23]. In fact, 1 of every 10 children who need special education has some form of ID [17].

Etiology

Current literature supports that the following represent common causes of ID: (1) genetic conditions (fragile X syndrome, Down syndrome, certain infections [such as congenital cytomegalovirus]); (2) problems during pregnancy or birth (Cri-du-chat syndrome or Prader-Willi syndrome, fetal alcohol syndrome [FAS]); (3) birth defects that affect the brain (such as hydrocephalus or cortical atrophy [such as asphyxia]) that occur while a baby is being born or soon after birth; and (4) problems during infancy, childhood, and adolescence (ie, injury, disease, or a brain abnormality, serious head injury, stroke, or certain infections such as meningitis) [16,22]. These listed causes are not all inclusive.

Certain causes of ID are preventable, such as FAS, which is prevented by having pregnant women refrain from drinking alcohol [22]. Another cause of ID, phenylketonuria (PKU), galactosemia, and congenital hypothyroidism, can be prevented if babies with these conditions begin appropriate treatment soon after birth [22].

Signs of intellectual disability

Infants and children who have ID diagnosed generally do not reach developmental milestones within the expected age range for other infants and children of their same ages and cultural environments (eg, sitting up, crawling or walking, talking, or using coherent language). Other symptoms may include cognitive delays, such as problems with short-term memory, concept formation, understanding social rules or how to solve problems, using logic, or understanding cause and effect relationships [18].

Diagnosis

The diagnostic criteria for determining the presence of ID requires that an individual must *first*, manifest serious to severe deficits in more than one domain of functioning: (1) cognitive, (2) language, (3) self care, (4) motor, and (5) adaptive–integrative functioning (Appendix 1) [15–23]. *Next*, they must obtain a score that is two or more standard deviations (70 or less) below the mean (100 on most standardized intelligence quotient [IQ] tests) of at least one standardized intellectual assessment (Box 1) [22–33].

Box 1. Examples of standardized intellectual assessments

Infants
Bayley Scales of Infant and Toddler Development–Third Edition
  (Bayley–III™) [25] (ages 1 to 42 months)
- Addresses IDEA 2004 regulations thatrequire infants
  and toddlers to receive developmental services in the areas
  of physical, cognitive, communication, social–emotional,
  and adaptive development.

Toddlers
Wechsler's Pre-school and Primary Scale of Intelligence,
  Forth Edition (WPPSI-IV®) [26] (ages 2 years, 6 months
  to 7 years, 3 months)
- Assesses cognitive abilities (verbal, perceptual, working
  memory, and processing speed).
McCarthy Scales of Children's Abilities [27] (ages 2 years,
  6 months to 8 years, 6 months)
- Provides broad picture of abilities.

Children and Adolescents (Early to Mid)
Wechsler's Intelligence Scale for Children, Forth Edition
  Integrated (WISC-IV®) [28] (ages 6 years to 16 years, 11
  months)
- Assesses cognitive abilities (verbal, perceptual, working
  memory, and processing speed).
Wechsler Intelligence Scale for Children®-Fourth Edition
  Integrated (WISC IV®) [29].
- Assesses cognitive abilities (verbal, perceptual, working
  memory, and processing speed).
- Examiner can determine if underlying processing problems are
  affecting WISC-IV® core test results.

Nonverbal Assessment
Leiter International Performance Scale: Revised [30] (ages 2 years
  to 21 years)
Assesses the cognitive abilities of children with low academic
  performance (visualization, reasoning, attention, and memory).

These standardized tests yield scores that are called Intelligence Quotients (IQs). The mean score for most is 100 with a standard deviation of 15. IQ scores of 70 are two standard deviations below the mean (considering the standard error of measurement for the specific assessment instrument used and the instruments strengths and limitations). The obtained scores on the standardized test must be the result of a valid administration and a true estimate of the person's intellectual abilities; the degrees of ID range from mild to profound [19]. Assessment of intellectual functioning is only one component of an assessment for ID.

Severity levels

Degrees of intellectual deficits are determined by deviations from the mean scores. IQ scores that are two standard deviations from the mean (obtained scores of 50–70) combined with concurrent deficits in adaptive functioning in at least two domains of function and clinical observations and overall assessment that support such deficits may result in an individual being labeled with *mild* mental retardation. Obtained scores of 35 to 55 and the same additional factors listed above may result in a diagnosis of *moderate* mental retardation. Scores between 20 and 40 combined with concurrent deficits in adaptive functioning and factors as listed above may result in a diagnosis of *severe* mental retardation. *Profound* mental retardation is based on those same deficits and scores below 20 to 25. If standardized testing is unable to be conducted with an individual, but all other deficits are present, a diagnosis of mental retardation, *severity unspecified* may be used [19].

ID is an Axis II on the multiaxial coding system used in the American Academy of Psychiatry's Diagnostic and Statistical Manual of Mental Disorders or *DSM-IV-TR* [19]. ID is a pervasive and lifelong condition that is used as part of the DSM classification systems and identifies individuals who will need various degrees of social, academic, and work life supports to carry out tasks of everyday living. The American Association of Mental Retardation states that there essential factors that must be considered when working to develop an accurate diagnosis of ID in an individual child or adolescent; these factors include: (1) cultural issues, (2) environmental conditions (ie, prematurity, neglect, intellectual deprivation), (3) linguistic issues (eg, comprehension and usage or English as a second language), and (4) physical and motor developmental issues, and the individual's personal strengths and weaknesses [17–24].

Differential diagnosis

ID can and often does co-exist with other deficits or disabilities in any domain of function (see Appendix 1); ID can also co-occur with other mental health conditions. The risk of comorbid disabilities is higher for youth with severe mental retardation than for youth with mild mental retardation [17,19,21,31–33]. Appropriate psychological assessments should clearly differentiate between youth who appear to have significant intellectual deficits and those who are manifesting these symptoms because of psychological trauma (cognitive and psychomotor functioning) or conditions that have limited an individual's ability to learn (ie, neglect or onset of major physical illness regardless of etiology).

Prognosis

The clinical impact of having sufficient deficits to receive a diagnosis of ID depends on many factors, including level of severity, access to resources, and environmental conditions.

Mild mental retardation

Individuals with mild ID may have problems reaching developmental milestones and acquiring language. With adequate training, most of these persons will achieve full independence in most domains of function but may have some problems with adaptive integrative domain [31–33]. As with many youth, most problems occur when they are matriculating through the educational system (especially with reading, writing, and timed tests) and interpersonal relationship skills with peers. Job coaches or aides may be necessary to help these youth learn work routines and develop solid employment skills. Most individuals (87%) with ID will exhibit barely noticeable problems of learning; however, as the demands of academic work become more complex, differences will become more pronounced. The more impaired the individual's functioning, the earlier those differences will become problematic for the child or adolescent.

Youth who have mild ID often do not experience major psychosocial problems until they enter the adolescent years, when abstract thinking, problem solving, critical thinking, and developing the ability to engage in sustained employment and mutually healthy intimate relationships become the goals of development. These executive functioning skills become more essential to one's successful navigation through social, academic, and emotional situations. Individuals with mild to moderate ID can successfully live independently as adults and have very normal lives; however, the guidance, training, and support they receive as children and adults will determine the level of success a specific individual achieves [15,17,19,20,24].

Moderate mental retardation

In addition to the deficits and needs of the individuals above, those with moderate mental retardation have more serious deficits in language expression and comprehension. They will need guidance and support throughout their lives. Their academic skills will always be limited and may not develop beyond a basic level. Semi-independent living conditions are usually best and safest. They will need close supervision in employment endeavors but can be very dependable and loyal employees if given the appropriate structured tasks, training, and support. They can develop simple friendships and engage in appropriately supervised and developed physical activities [15,17,20,24].

Severe mental retardation

As the degree of functioning decreases, the degree of needed support and supervision increases. Limitations in expected levels of achievement also increase. Problems with marked degrees of motor impairment or other associated deficits are prevalent. Clinically significant damage to or maldevelopment of the central nervous system is also often a factor [32,33]. These youth will need care and supervision to perform most activities of daily living [15,17,19,20,30–33].

Profound mental retardation

Youth who manifest symptoms or behaviors that meet criteria for profound ID have severe limitations (rudimentary level) in language comprehension, expression, and ability to comply with requests or instructions; they are primarily immobile or severely restricted in mobility, are incontinent, and require constant help and supervision [15,17,19,20,24]. Expectations for attaining developmental milestones and matriculating through infancy, childhood, and adolescence to adulthood are severely limited.

Summary

Intellectual disability is a disorder that first develops during pregnancy, birth, infancy, childhood, or adolescence; diagnosis must occur before age 18. Youth who manifest these symptoms may have significant delays in their domains of function during development (see Appendix 1). Diagnosis must be made based on multiple sources of evidence that include attainment of developmental milestones and cognitive or intellectual disability (two standard deviations below the mean on standardized intellectual assessments [Box 2]) and that concurrently occur with (1) deficits (mild to severe) in adaptive behavior, (2) academic performance, and (3) adaptive functioning. The majority of youth with ID can live independent or semi-independent lives as adults if they have received the appropriate personalized support over a sustained period, especially during the formative years [32,33]. A list of resources is provided in Box 2.

Box 2. Resources

The Arc of the United States
1010 Wayne Avenue, Suite 650
Silver Spring, MD 20,910
301.565.3842
Info@thearc.org (E-mail)
www.thearc.org (Web)
www.TheArcPub.com *Web* (Publications)

American Association on Intellectual and Developmental Disabilities (formerly the American Association on Mental Retardation, AAMR)
444 North Capitol Street NW, Suite 846
Washington, DC 20001-1512
202.387.1968; 800.424.3688 (outside DC)
www.aaidd.org (Web)

Division on Developmental Disabilities
The Council for Exceptional Children
1110 North Glebe Road, Suite 300
Arlington, VA 22,201-5704 888.232.7733; 703.620.3660
866.915.5000 *TTY*
cec@cec.sped.org (E-mail)
www.dddcec.org (Web)

The Genetics Home Reference: Your guide to understanding genetic problems
Genetic Disorders A to Z and related genes and chromosomes
Concepts & Tools for understanding human genetics
http://ghr.nlm.nih.gov/ghr/page/Home

Appendix 1. Domains of function [1–16]

1. Cognitive Domain
   - Attention and responses focus generally and selectively
   - Ability to sustain focus generally and selectively
   - Ability to respond to stimuli
   - Ability to respond effectively to environmental cues and stimuli resulting in appropriate behavioral adaptation to optimize positive outcomes and minimize negative outcomes Ability to acquire, store, retrieve relevant information on demand
   - Conceptual learning
     - Ability to understand concepts based on familiar information or situations

- o Ability to understand concepts based on combination of old and new information
- o Ability to develop concepts based on new information
- Reasoning inductive, deductive
- Reasoning knowledge of specific facts
- Comprehension of information
- Application of knowledge
- Concrete thinking (here and now, black and white)
- Critical thinking skills
  - o Compare facts or information
  - o Contrast facts or information
  - o Analysis of that knowledge
  - o Synthesis of that knowledge
  - o Evaluation of information
  - o Ability to generate creative strategies from that knowledge
  - o Abstract thinking
  - o Insight
  - o Futuristic thinking
- Problem solving
  - o Ability to use basic thinking skills to generate a solution to a problem
  - o Ability to use basic and critical thinking skills to generate solution to a problem and make changes in behavior based on that solution
- Basic decision-making skills
  - ■ Ability to use basic thinking and problem solving skills to make a decision
- Complex decision-making skills
  - ■ Ability to use basic and critical thinking as well as problem solving skills to make an appropriate and effective decision
  - ■ Ability to change decision based on new information mental flexibility ability to adopt another's perspective
- Basic planning skills
  - o Ability to recognize situation in which action is required
  - o Ability to engage in basic thinking skills
  - o Ability to engage in basic decision-making skills
  - o Ability to select a course of action or plan a strategy
- Complex planning skills
  - o Ability to recognize situation in which action is required
  - o Ability to analyze the circumstances
  - o Ability to evaluate a situation
  - o Ability to use rest of critical thinking skills
  - o Ability to engage in complex decision-making skills
  - o Ability to select a course of action
  - o Ability to plan a strategy
- Basic execution skills

- Ability to execute the basic plan
- Complex execution skills
  - Ability to execute the complex plan
  - Ability to engage in multitasking
  - Ability to perform multiple tasks simultaneously
2. Motor domain
   - Fine motor
     - Pinscher grasp precise
     - Specific neuromotor responses
     - coordination of fine motor responses
     - Drawing objects
     - Manipulating object
     - Holding objects
   - Gross motor
     - Head and trunk control
     - Purposeful movement of arms and legs
     - Crawling, walking
     - Running, jumping, skipping, hopping
     - Throwing, catching, ability to hit an object (ball) with a bat or racket
     - Total postural control (coordination of skeletal muscles)
   - Planning ability
     - Ability to balance body during activities
   - Muscular strength
   - Muscular endurance and agility
   - Visual motor tracking
     - Extraocular muscle control
     - Resting balance control of eye movement
     - Visuo-motor coordination
   - Perceptual motor
     - Integrated stimulus-specific fine motor and gross motor responses
     - Visuo-spatial discrimination eye–hand coordination
     - Stereognosis judgment of speed
     - Judgment of direction
     - Judgment of spatial orientation of moving objects
     - Awareness of sequential ordering time and sequence of events
   - Proprioceptive sense
   - Kinesthetic sense time elapsed between stimulus perception and initial neuromotor responses
3. Auditory
   - Hearing acuity
     - Processing selective discrimination of sounds
     - Selective discrimination of written language
4. Language
   - Receptive language: comprehension

- Oral
  - Symbolic
  - Semantic
  - Syntax
- Written
  - Symbolic
  - Semantic
  - Syntax
- Expressive language
  - Oral
  - Symbolic
  - Semantic
  - Syntax
- Written
  - Symbolic
  - Semantic
  - Syntax
- Prepositional logic

5. Psychosocial
  - Emotional ability to exhibit affect that is appropriate to situation or set of circumstances
    - Ability to monitor emotions
    - Ability to regulate emotions
  - Social ability to develop friendships
    - Ability to sustain friendships
    - Ability to develop healthy interpersonal relationships
    - Ability to establish mutually beneficial intimate relationships
    - Ability to maintain mutually intimate relationships
    - Ability to be altruistic

6. Moral judgment
  - Discriminate right from wrong
  - Sense of morality

7. Specific integrative and adaptive skills
  - Ability to coordinate, integrate, and adapt various domains to meet specific demands of a given task.
  - Ability to integrate skills in domains of function to effectively engage in self-care skills
  - Ability to integrate skills in domains and adapt those skills to effectively meet demands of activities of daily living

References

[1] Gesell A, Ilg FL, Ames LB. The child from five to ten. New York: Harper and Row Publishers; 1946.

[2] Gomez JE. Growth and maturation. In: Sullivan AJ, Anderson SJ, editors. Care of the young athlete. Park Ridge (IL): American Academy of Orthopaedic Surgeons; 2000. p. 25–32.
[3] Blumsack J, Lewandowski L, Waterman B. Neurodevelopmental precursors to learning disabilities: a preliminary report from a parent survey. J Learn Disabil 1997;30(2):228–37.
[4] Branta C, Haubensticker J, Seefeldt V. Age changes in motor skills during childhood and adolescence. Exerc Sport Sci Rev 1984;12:467–520.
[5] Capute AJ, Accardo PJ. A neurodevelopmental perspective on the continuum of developmental disabilities. In: Capute AJ, Accardo PJ, editors. Developmental disabilities in infancy and childhood. 2nd edition. Baltimore (MD): Paul H. Brooks Publishing; 1996. p. 1–24.
[6] Erickson E. Childhood and society. New York: W.W. Norton and Co., Inc.; 1963.
[7] Erickson E. Identity, youth and crisis. New York: W.W. Norton and Co., Inc.; 1968.
[8] Fagard J. Skill acquisition in children: a historical perspective. In: Bar-Or O. The child and adolescent athlete. Oxford (UK): Blackwell Science, 1996. p. 74–91.
[9] Gemelli R. Normal child and adolescent development. Washington, DC: American Psychiatric Press, 1996.
[10] Levine MD. Neurodevelopmental dysfunction in the school age child. In: Behrman RE, Kliegman RM, Jenson HB, editors. Nelson textbook of pediatrics. 16th edition. Philadelphia: W.B. Saunders Company; 2000. p. 94–100.
[11] Piaget J. Intellectual evaluation from adolescence to adulthood. Hum Dev 1972;15(1):1–12.
[12] Piaget J, Inhelder B. The psychology of the child. New York: Basic Books; 1969.
[13] Rieser JJ, Pick HL, Ashmead DH, et al. Calibration of human locomotion and models of perceptual-motor organization. J Exp Psychol Hum Percept Perform 1995;21(3):480–97.
[14] Seefeldt V, Haubenstricker J. Patterns, phases, or stages: an analytical model for the study of developmental movement. In: Kelso JAS, Clark JE, editors. The development of movement control and coordination. New York: John Wiley and Sons; 1982. p. 309–18.
[15] National. Dissemination Center for Children with Disabilities (NICHCY). Mental Retardation Fact Sheet 8 (FS8) 2004 Available at: http://www.nichcy.org/pubs/factshe/fs8txt.htm#whatis. Accessed May 21, 2007.
[16] Luckasson R, Schalock RL, Spitalnik DM, et al. Mental retardation: definition, classification, and systems of support. 10th edition. Washington, DC: American Association on Mental Retardation; 2002. p. 250.
[17] American Association on Mental Retardation (AAMR) (2002). Mental retardation: definition, classification, and systems of support. 10th edition. Washington, DC: American Association on Mental Retardation (AAMR) Available at: http://www.aamr.org/. Accessed May 21, 2007.
[18] World Health Organization. Mental retardation division of mental health and prevention of substance abuse world health organization icd-10 guide for mental retardation. Geneva (Switzerland): World Health Organization; 1996. p. 1–74. Available at: http://www.who.int/mental_health/media/en/69.pdf. Accessed May 21, 2007.
[19] American Psychiatric Association: Disorders first diagnosed in infancy, childhood and adolescence. Diagnostic and statistical manual of mental disorders. 4th edition, [text revision] [DSM-IV-TR]. Washington, DC: American Psychiatric Association, 2000. p. 39–134.
[20] World Health Organization: International classification of diseases and related health problems (10th edition) [ICD 10]. Geneva (Switzerland): World Health Organization, 1993.
[21] Wolraich MD, Felice ME, Drotar D. The classification of child and adolescent mental diagnoses in primary care: diagnostic and statistical manual for primary care (DSM-PC) child and adolescent version. Elk Grove Village (IL): American Academy of Pediatrics; 1996. p. 59–110.
[22] Department of Health and Human Services, Centers for Disease Control and Prevention. Developmental disabilities: mental retardation. Atlanta (GA): Department of Health and Human Services, Centers for Disease Control and Prevention, 2005 Available at: http://www.cdc.gov/ncbddd/dd/ddmr.htm. Accessed May 21, 2007.

[23] United States Department of Education. Twenty-fourth Annual Report to Congress, to assure the free appropriate public education of all children with disabilities individuals with disabilities education Act, Section 618. Jessup (MD): United States Department of Education; 2002. Available at: http://www.ed.gov/about/reports/annual/osep/2002/toc-execsum.pdf. Accessed March 7, 2007.

[24] Department of Health and Human Services, Centers for Disease Control and Prevention. Developmental disabilities: fetal alcohol spectrum disorders. Atlanta (GA): Department of Health and Human Services, Centers for Disease Control and Prevention, 2007 Available at: http://www.cdc.gov/ncbddd/fas/default.htm.

[25] Bayley N. Bayley–III™ screening test. San Antonio (TX): Psychological Corp; 2005. Available at: http://harcourtassessment.com/hai/Images/pdf/catalog/2007PsychologicalCatalog.pdf. Accessed May 21, 2007.

[26] Wechsler D. Wechsler's pre-school and primary scale of intelligence. 4th edition. (WPPSI-IV®). San Antonio (TX): Psychological Corp., Harcourt Brace; 1991. Available at: http://harcourtassessment.com/hai/Images/pdf/catalog/2007PsychologicalCatalog.pdf. Accessed May 21, 2007.

[27] McCarthy D: McCarthy scales of children's abilities. Harcourt assessment; 1972, San Antonio (TX): Psychological Corp., Harcourt Brace. Available at: http://harcourtassessment.com/hai/Images/pdf/catalog/2007PsychologicalCatalog.pdf. Accessed May 21, 2007.

[28] Wechsler D. Wechsler intelligence scale for children. 4th edition. San Antonio (TX): Psychological Corp., Harcourt Brace; 1991. Available at: http://harcourtassessment.com/hai/Images/pdf/catalog/2007PsychologicalCatalog.pdf. Accessed May 21, 2007.

[29] Wechsler D, Kaplan K, Delis D, et al. Wechsler intelligence scale for children®. 4th edition. Integrated (WISC — IV®). Antonio (TX): Psychological Corp., Harcourt Brace. Available at: http://harcourtassessment.com/HaiWeb/Cultures/enus/harcourt/Community/Psychology/results.htm?Community=CognitionIntelligence. Accessed May 21, 2007.

[30] Roid G, Miller L. Leiter international performance scale: revised. London: nfer-nelson, Granada Learning Group. Available at: http://shop.nfer-nelson.co.uk/icat/leiterinternationalperfor. Accessed May 21, 2007.

[31] Sulkes SB. "Mental retardation in children and adolescents". In: Greydanus DE, Patel DR, Pratt HD, editors. Behavioral pediatrics. 2nd edition. Lincoln (NE): iUniverse Publishers; 2006. p. 66–82.

[32] Greydanus DE, Bhave S. Adolescents with mental retardation. Recent Advances in Pediatrics 2006;17(14):174–92.

[33] Greydanus DE, Pratt HD. Syndromes and disorders associated with mental retardation: selected comments. Indian J Pediatr 2005;72(10):27–32.

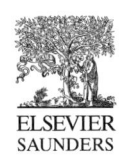

Psychological Impact of Trauma on Developing Children and Youth

C. Richard Spates, PhD[a,*], Nishani Samaraweera, MA[a], Brian Plaisier, MD[b], Theresa Souza, MA[a], Kanako Otsui, PhD[c]

[a]Department of Psychology, Western Michigan University, 3500 Wood Hall, Kalamazoo, MI 49008, USA
[b]Trauma Program, Bronson Healthcare Group, Bronson Methodist Hospital, Mailbox #67, 601 John Street, Kalamazoo, MI 49007, USA
[c]Department of Integrated Psychological Science, Kwansei Gakuin University, 1-1555 Ichibancho, Uegahara, Nishinomya City, 662-8501 Japan

This report introduces the primary care professional to the psychological impact of trauma on the developing child. It identifies common types of trauma likely to be seen in primary care, their potential immediate and long-term effects, practical means of assessing their psychological impact, and evidence-based treatment options. In identifying these treatment options, our intent is to familiarize primary care practitioners (PCPs) with effective professional interventions that may serve as a basis for successful referral and follow-up monitoring. We begin by addressing the nature of trauma and its effects in the immediate and near-term for children and youth.

Overview of children's traumatic experience

Exposure to traumatic events is common, and posttraumatic stress disorder (PTSD) is not rare. In a community sample of adolescents, Giaconia and colleagues [1] found that 43% had experienced "qualifying" traumas, placing subjects at great risk for PTSD. Of those with "qualifying" traumas, 14.5% met PTSD criteria, as did 6.3% of the entire sample. Cuffe and colleagues [2] found the prevalence of PTSD was 1% in boys and 3% in girls in another community sample of adolescents.

---

* Corresponding author.
 E-mail address: rspates@wmich.edu (C.R. Spates).

Common traumas encountered by children and youth include physical abuse, maltreatment, automobile crashes, bullying, sexual abuse, stalking, corporal punishment, life-threatening diagnoses, accidents, terrorism, and displacement caused by political and natural disasters. They also include witnessing life-threatening events that happened to loved ones. Whatever the source, when a trauma occurs in a child's life, it affects a developmental progression that is fully underway. The stage of development has implications for the near-term trauma reaction and how later developmental stages are successfully transitioned. Learning, memory, emotions, and behavior are all potential impact zones, ultimately leading to negative alterations in a developing personality if the psychological reactions go untreated.

Three clusters of symptoms are associated with PTSD: reexperiencing, avoidance, emotional numbing, and hyperarousal. Initial trauma symptoms lasting up to a period of 4 weeks receive a diagnosis of acute stress disorder (ASD). A diagnosis of ASD (which precedes PTSD) requires evidence of dissociation either during or immediately after the traumatic event, and at least one symptom from each of the three symptom clusters. When the number of symptoms of ASD increases and symptoms persist for longer than 4 weeks, the diagnosis is changed to PTSD [3].

Because children often are not likely to have developed a ready repertoire of effective coping skills or in many instances an effective vocabulary with which to describe their own complex reactions, their capabilities for overcoming the effects of traumatic exposure while meeting developmental challenges are limited. Thus, they will require at least support and, for some, serious psychological or medical intervention to ameliorate enduring damaging effects.

Effects on cognitive development

Cognitive and academic impairments among traumatized youth, including language delay [5] and lower IQ scores [6], have been reported consistently in a number of studies [4].

An association between traumatic experiences and the development of aggressive behaviors is well documented [7,8]. This increase in aggressive behavior after exposure to traumatic events appears to be correlated with emotion dysregulation, especially hyperarousal and agitation. Maltreatment too has been shown to result in affect dysregulation and aggressive behavior [9].

Other studies have found that nearly 80% of maltreated children exhibited dysregulated emotion patterns in response to witnessed anger, compared with approximately 36% of nonmaltreated children. The findings suggest that within the context of maltreating environments, dysregulated emotion patterns may serve an adaptive function by helping children maintain a sense of safety while meeting the demands of their unpredictable and frightening home life [10]. Other research has found that maltreated children also have deficits in recognizing facial expressions [11], developing expressive vocabularies [12], and responding appropriately to peers' distress [13]. Smith and Walden [14] also reported these abnormalities, along with deficits in social problem solving strategies, and suggested that these problems may be caused by impairment in cognitive–language development caused by maltreatment.

Trauma's relationship to brain function in children

Previous studies have shown the effect of traumatic experience on children's central nervous system functions. Traumatic stress can precipitate chemical imbalance (and aberrations in functional circuitry) in the central nervous system, such as low serotonin levels and increased testosterone, both of which are linked to impulsive aggression [15,16]. The elevation of amygdala corticotrophin releasing factor (CRF) is also an important stress response [17]. Amygdala CRF is known to be involved in stress-induced anxiety behaviors [18,19].

A very recent study by Richert and colleagues [20] found that children with PTSD symptoms exhibited a significantly larger volume of gray matter in the middle-inferior and ventral regions of the prefrontal cortex (PFC) than did healthy control children. The ventral PFC is involved in social–emotional functioning including emotion regulation [21] and learning of positive and negative reinforcements [22]. The middle-inferior PFC is also implicated in social functioning and fear conditioning [23]. Regions within the inferior PFC are involved in the neural modulation of emotional responses to aversive stimuli, and therefore aberrant morphology of these areas suggests biological mechanism by which emotional inhibition may be impaired in children with PTSD [20]. Although the adult PTSD literature has focused on aberrant hippocampal morphology, these reports of PFC impairment of children with PTSD symptoms are something unique to this early developmental stage.

The clinical encounter with trauma in primary care practice

A lifetime of potentially traumatic exposures and their perceptions must be taken into account when evaluating the child or adolescent who displays symptoms that have resulted in an office visit. The primary care practitioner (PCP) often is the first person sought out to begin a professional assessment. This clinical encounter is a valuable opportunity to raise the suspicion for PTSD and begin a therapeutic endeavor. If unrecognized or untreated, PTSD may lead to potentially lifelong changes in brain development and predispose patients to depression, suicide, substance abuse, and conduct disorders [24,25], and chronic fatigue syndrome in adulthood [26,27].

Recognition that symptoms may be resulting from traumatic events, either acute or chronic, is the most important step. Such symptoms, although readily identifiable by the PCP, may overlap, with other anxiety disorders, mood disorders, or substance abuse [28,29]. Although symptoms may begin soon after the offending incident, onset may not occur for several months and, if untreated, may persist for years or even decades [1,30–32]. Therefore, unexplained symptoms or behavior, such as problems with sleep, somatic complaints, poor perceived health, anxiety, anger, or poor academic performance, should prompt further questioning about traumatic experiences, even those from the distant past [1,29].

Failing to ask specifically about traumatic events, therefore, is a pitfall that must be avoided. Every effort must be made to allow disclosure of these events, because patients may be reluctant to reveal things that involve shame or secrecy. Children and parents should be asked about interpersonal violence, motor vehicle crashes, animal bites, acute illnesses, emergency department evaluations, and hospitalizations. Whether there has been witnessing of violence must be a part of the trauma history because these patients are 85 times more likely to satisfy diagnostic criteria for PTSD than controls [2]. More than 50% of school-age children in certain urban centers of the United States report directly observing violence [33].

The mechanism of injury must be explored carefully because each may have unique effects depending on patient circumstances. The incidence of PTSD in children after motor vehicle crashes is 12% to 35% [34,35]. Predictors of PTSD in these investigations included previous trauma, perceived threat, and female gender [36,37]. Nearly 55% of children have been found to have either full or partial PTSD after dog bites [38]. Sanders and colleagues [39] found that one third of children had PTSD after minor orthopedic injuries, and the risk was increased if hospital admission was required. Long-term PTSD was seen in 27% of children after trauma center admission with risks including perceived threat to life, death of family member at the scene, no control over the event, and violence [40]. PTSD was in turn statistically associated with poor quality of life [40].

The PCP should also seek out events not associated with kinetic energy. In a noninjured cohort of children admitted to the intensive care unit, 21% fulfilled criteria for PTSD compared with 0% of children admitted to the general floor [41]. Risks for PTSD in this sample included perceived illness severity, perceived threat to life, and total length of hospital stay [41]. In a group of adolescent transplant patients, 16.3% displayed full PTSD criteria, and 14.4% had partial PTSD with subjective appraisal of threat having a greater contribution than objective measures of illness severity [42]. It should also be remembered that treatment procedures themselves might be perceived as traumatic [43].

Refugee children displaced as a result of natural disaster or warfare have unique needs and may have never received a formal evaluation. Children displaced after the December 26, 2004 tsunami in Thailand were more likely to have PTSD than those not displaced, and the prevalence of PTSD did not decline between 2 and 9 months [44]. Extreme fear increased the risk for

PTSD nine times, and if family members were in danger the risk increased sixfold [44]. An investigation of youths 10 years after the Rwandan genocide found that more than 40% displayed PTSD, and two thirds had never spoken with anyone about their problems [45]. Independent predictors of PTSD in Sudanese child refugees included ever being injured, foster care with an American family (no Sudanese people), and thoughts of loneliness [30].

When suspicion of trauma arises in the primary care physician

Once suspicion for PTSD has been raised, decisive action should be taken, because early identification and referral will likely improve outcome [24,32]. The PCP should do whatever possible to ensure an environment of safety and support for the child. Both parent(s) and child should be educated concerning normal and abnormal responses after a traumatic event, and care should be taken to guard against excessive trauma-relevant media exposure [46]. Referral should be made to the appropriate mental health specialist even for children with subthreshold criteria as they may exhibit similar impairments as those with all three of the PTSD symptom clusters [47].

The integrity of the family unit itself can also be affected by childhood injury, and assistance should be provided to the entire group [48]. Montgomery and coworkers [49] found that among families of children with severe traumatic brain injury, 40% reported that the injury had a moderate to profound effect on the family as a whole. Almost one third of families had experienced financial deterioration, and 28% reported that an adult was fired or forced to quit a job because of requirements imposed by their injured child's care. Fifty-five percent of families reported behavioral changes in patients' siblings that included increased fear, decreased school performance, and difficulty with peer relationships.

It is within the purview of the PCP to begin pharmacotherapy while arranging a mental health referral [29,50]. Medications may be used to target disabling symptoms so the child may pursue normal growth and development [47]. Pharmaceutical intervention may also provide relief of distressing material encountered within psychotherapy and daily life [51]. Despite the absence of controlled medication trials, many (95%) child psychiatrists use psychotropic medication with selective serotonin reuptake inhibitors being used as first-line agents [47,51,52]. These drugs have broad-spectrum activity in anxiety, mood, and obsessive–compulsive disorders [51]. Adrenergic agents may be used to specifically target re-experiencing and hyperarousal symptoms [47,51]. Dopaminergic compounds should be reserved for cases in which psychotic symptoms, severe aggression, and self-harm are not controlled with first-line agents [51]. It should be emphasized, however, that currently there are no adequate empirical data to conclude that any pharmacologic therapies effectively treat childhood PTSD [24]. And for this reason, the PCP should remain open to consultation from mental health specialists, once psychological therapy has been initiated, concerning the need or utility of continued pharmaceutical intervention.

Although open-label drug trials are guided by respectable professional judgment, there must be a thoughtful, individualized approach because there may be no comparison group (Table 1) [24,25,53–64]. Informed consent should be obtained from parents or legal guardians. Because of the lack of randomized, controlled trials, special effort should be directed toward education of both parent and child regarding target symptoms and potential adverse effects of each medication used.

Primary care physician linkage with trauma center staff

Depending on the resources at a given hospital, a wide variety of physicians may be involved in the care of an injured child. Trauma centers typically possess pediatric intensivists, pediatric surgeons, emergency medicine physicians, general trauma surgeons, and other specialists. As a result, the PCP may find it difficult to establish contact and obtain specific information regarding a patient. Sabin and colleagues [65] found that trauma center staff documented contact with the PCP during hospitalization for only 7.4% of patients with ANY posttraumatic stress symptoms and 0% for patients with high posttraumatic stress symptoms. Because patients may be instructed by trauma center staff to return to their PCP after hospitalization, linkage between the PCP and trauma center is important for seamless follow-up care.

Important needs are also present in day-to-day trauma care. Nearly 40% of adolescents admitted to a trauma center had no identifiable source of primary care [65]. Of those with a PCP, only 37% had at least one office visit during the 6 months after discharge despite high levels of posttraumatic stress symptoms in 30% [65]. It cannot be assumed that a trauma center has provided counseling because no patients in Stallard's study of motor vehicle crashes received any psychological help at hospitalization (one in three had PTSD) [36]. Unfortunately, more than 88% of sampled American Academy of Pediatrics (AAP) practitioners identified barriers to patient access of mental health services, constructed by the managed care environment, and only 49% believed they had skills to detect PTSD [66]. Inadequate training and office time constraints are widely cited as significant barriers [24,33,66].

Assessment of traumatic stress reactions

Although the clinical presentation of PTSD in children can be similar to the presentation in adults, children have consistently displayed a number of differences in symptom manifestation. Therefore, it is essential that practitioners be aware of the variety of symptoms that can be exhibited by children who have been exposed to complex trauma situations [67].

As previously stated, there are three clusters of symptoms that are characteristic of PTSD. The cluster involving intrusive symptoms often is expressed through recurring themes in children's play with toys or with other children [68].

Children tend to demonstrate the symptoms of avoidance and hyperarousal in a cyclical pattern. They often fluctuate between periods of irritability and psychological reactivity and periods of restricted emotionality and numbness [69].

When assessing children for trauma reactions, three areas of functioning must be evaluated. These include using cognitive, academic, and behavioral measures [69]. These areas must be assessed through multiple sources of information and through multiple formats including direct observation; interviews with the child, parents, and teachers; tests; and questionnaires. Specific methods used will vary depending on the age of the child.

In conducting assessments, it is not enough to rely on parental information alone. Shemesh and colleagues [70] found that although the child's report of symptoms statistically correlated with the child's PTSD, the parent's report did not. Parent–child discordance was most pronounced in the adolescent age group [70]. One must also be careful not to reach premature conclusions concerning PTSD in young children because eight of 18 PTSD criteria require a verbal description above their skill levels [47].

Assessing PTSD in preschool-age children poses the greatest level of difficulty. Among this age group, symptoms are almost exclusively expressed through nonverbal behaviors. As a result, assessment measures will rely heavily on the parents and other adults that are in close contact with the child [68]. When children reach school age, assessment becomes clearer. By this time, children show increasing levels of verbal skills and the ability to apply temporal sequencing to traumatic events and symptoms. In both age groups, behavioral representations of symptoms dominate and should be a strong focus of assessment methods. Once children reach preadolescent ages, they are more capable of self-reporting symptoms and events. This is also the time period during which symptom presentations begin to reflect those seen in adults.

Table 2 contains a comprehensive list of PTSD assessment tools for children and adolescents. The table also describes the ages at which each tool should be used, length of time required to administer the assessment, and the psychological domain targeted by the measure. One of the most commonly used measures is the Child Posttraumatic Stress Reaction Index (CPTS-RI). This is a semistructured interview that is designed for both the child and the parents. It can be used for children between the ages of 6 and 17 years. The CPTS-RI consists of 20 questions that target the specific symptoms of PTSD as well as their severity. Research indicates that children who with PTSD score much higher than children without the disorder after exposure to traumatic events [67].

A second frequently used trauma assessment measure for children is the anxiety portion of the Diagnostic Interview Schedule for Children and

Table 1
Pharmacotherapy experience in childhood posttraumatic stress disorder

Agent	Neural pathway	Source	Parameters	Outcome
Carbamazepine	Polysynaptic responses	Looff, et al. [53]	Letter to editor. Open trial. Children and adolescents (aged 8–17 years) victims of sexual abuse, N = 28.	Significant improvement or resolution of all symptoms. No adverse effects seen. Baseline laboratory evaluation and gradual dosage increases important.
Citalopram	Serotonergic	Seedat, et al. [54]	Open trial; media advertisement recruitment. Children and adolescents (aged 10–18 years), N = 24 (compared with adult sample, N = 14). All with current DSM-IV PTSD.	Significant reduction in all symptom clusters. No significant difference between groups. Similar safety profile compared with adults. Two subjects withdrawn (one because of nosebleeds; one because of skin rash).
Citalopram	Serotonergic	Seedat, et al. [55]	Open trial; subjects recruited from outpatient clinics. Adolescents (aged 12–18 years), N = 8. All with current DSM-IV PTSD.	Significant improvement in symptoms compared with baseline. One subject withdrawn because of nosebleeds.
Clonidine	Adrenergic	Harmon, et al. [56]	Open trial of referred patients. Children (aged 3–6 years), N = 7. All with current DSM-IV PTSD.	Moderate to great improvement in target symptoms (aggression, impulsivity, emotional outbursts, hyperarousal, hypervigilance, generalized anxiety, oppositionality, insomnia). Clinical caveats include cardiovascular effects and sedation.

Clozapine	Dopaminergic	Kant, et al. [57]	Retrospective chart review. Mixed group of adolescents (bipolar, IED, and PTSD), N = 39 (19 with DSM-IV PTSD).	Hallucinations, aggression, and flashbacks improved. Significant reductions in polypharmacy. Adverse effects for entire group included agranulocytosis (n = 1), neutropenia (n = 2), weight gain (n = 20), sedation (n = 18), and hypersalivation (n = 6).
Clozapine	Dopaminergic	Wheatley, et al. [58]	Open trial. Adolescents (aged 17–19) from inpatient medium secure unit, N = 6. All with chronic DSM-IV PTSD and psychotic symptoms.	Decreased aggression, self-harm, and intrusive hallucinations. Most troublesome side effects (reported by patients): Excessive salivation, dizziness, weight gain, nausea, sedation, and constipation.
Cyproheptadine	Serotonergic/ histaminergic	Gupta, et al. [59]	Case report. Boy (age 9) with PTSD, ADHD, ODD, and nightmares. Nightmares failed to respond to trazodone and diphenhydramine.	Complete remission of nightmares within 1 month. Patient has experienced no side effects.
Guanfacine	Adrenergic	Horrigan [60]	Case report. Girl (age 7) with chronic PTSD and nightmares. Symptoms resistant to clonidine.	Suppression of nightmares by second evening. Longer half-life believed to provide greater "window of suppression." No side effects reported.
Mirtazapine	Adrenergic/ serotonergic	Good and Petersen [61]	Case report. Girl (age 8) with PTSD.	Improvement in anxiety and sleep.
Nefazodone	Serotonergic/ Adrenergic	Domon and Andersen [62]	Letter to editor. Practice experience in adolescents with PTSD.	Improvements seen in anger, aggression, insomnia, and avoidance. Greater degree of engagement in therapy seen. Most common adverse effects: morning somnolence, nausea, and vomiting.

(continued on next page)

Table 1 (*continued*)

Agent	Neural pathway	Source	Parameters	Outcome
Propanolol	Adrenergic	Famularo and colleagues [63]	Open trial. Children (aged 6-12) in off-on-off design, (N = 11). All with DSM-III PTSD.	Significant improvement in PTSD symptom inventory during treatment compared with before medication, and significant decrement after treatment compared with during medication. No child required discontinuation of medication. Top dosage limited by mild adverse effects in three patients.
Quetiapine	Serotonergic/ dopaminergic/ histaminergic/ adrenergic	Stathis and colleagues [64]	Open trial. Male adolescents (aged 15-17) in juvenile detention center, N = 6. All with DSM-IV PTSD.	Significant reduction in dissociation, anxiety, depression, anger, insomnia, and nightmares. Significant (mean = 3.9 kg.) weight gain. No other significant side effects

Abbreviations: IED, Intermittent explosive disorder; ADHD, attention-deficit/hyperactivity disorder; ODD, oppositional defiant disorder.

Table 2
Trauma assessments for children

Assessment	Age	Duration	Domain	Format
Angie/Andy Child Rating Scale (A/A CRS)	6–11	30–45 min	Complicated PTSD	Structured child report
Child PTSD Symptom Scale	8–18	15 min	PTSD severity	Self-report
Child Posttraumatic Stress Reaction Index (CPTS-RI)	6–17	15–45 min	PTSD severity	Semistructured interview (child and parent)
Child Report of Posttraumatic Symptoms (CROPS)	8–13	5 min	Broad symptoms	Self-report (child and parent)
Child's Reaction to Traumatic Events Scale (CRTES)	NS	3–10 min	Psychological response to stress	Interview self-report
Childhood PTSD Interview (CPTSDI)	>18	30 min	PTSD (DSM-IV)	Semistructured interview
Children's PTSD Inventory	7–18	15–20 min	PTSD (DSM IV)	Structured interview
Diagnostic Interview for Children and Adolescents-Revised PTSD Module	6–17	90 min	PTSD (DSM-IV)	Semistructured interview
Parent Report of Child's Reaction to Stress	>18	30–45 min	PTSD (DSM-IV)	Parent report
Parent Report of Posttraumatic Symptoms	>14	5 min	PTSD symptoms	Parent report
PTSD Checklist	>18	5–7 min	PTSD (DSM-IV)	Parent report
Trauma Symptom Checklist for Children	8–16	10–20 min	Distress level	Self-report
Traumatic Event Screening Inventory Child Version (TESI-C)	4+	10–30 min	Traumatic events	Interview (child and parent)

Data from Cook-Cottone C. Childhood posttraumatic stress disorder: diagnosis, treatment, and school reintegration. School Psychology Review 2004;127–39.

Adolescents from the DSM-IV (ADIS). This measure is also a semistructured interview that can be used with children between the ages of 6 and 17 years. One strength of this measure is that it assesses for acute stress reactions as well as PTSD. Both the CPTS-RI and the ADIS are well researched and have shown effectiveness in assessment with children after trauma.

For older children, self-report measures can be used. These measures are brief, reliable instruments that can indicate if more intensive assessment tools should be sought or if referrals for treatment should be made. The most popular of these assessment tools is the Children's PTSD Symptoms Scale (CPSS). This questionnaire consists of 24 items. The majority of the items assess specific symptoms of PTSD. The CPSS can be used for children between the ages of 8 and 18 years and takes less than 15 minutes to complete.

A final factor that must be taken into account when assessing PTSD symptoms in children is the psychological functioning of the parent or caregiver. Research indicates that children's reactions to trauma and their level of resiliency to these events are directly linked to the responses of their parents [71]. Families that show stable, secure, emotional responses to traumatic events serve as a protective factor for children. These children seem to cope more effectively after exposure to the traumatic event [71].

Evidence-based psychological treatments

Two factors guide the selection of information in this part of the chapter. The first is that although a number of approaches such as trauma-focused cognitive-behavioral therapy (CBT) eye movement desensitization and reprocessing (EMDR), play therapy, art therapy, psychodynamic therapy, and pharmacotherapy exist for the treatment of PTSD in children and adolescents, only trauma-focused CBT and EMDR have empirical validity. The second is that randomized, controlled studies of PTSD in children and adolescents have been conducted primarily in the context of child sexual abuse [72,73]. Only a few controlled studies have examined the treatment of PTSD resulting from natural disasters [74], vehicular accidents [75], and war and refugee experiences [76].

Trauma-focused CBT is theoretically grounded and has been validated empirically in a number of different trauma contexts. Its goal is to address the cognitive, behavioral, and physiological symptoms of PTSD, while incorporating the treatment of other co-occurring problems in a coherent fashion. The characteristic features of trauma-focused CBT are exposure and cognitive restructuring. Treatment usually requires approximately 12 weekly sessions that last 60 to 90 minutes each.

EMDR, as it was originally described, combines exposure with saccadic eye movements. Studies later found that attention to other types of left-to-right movement could be substituted for eye movements. In adapting the protocol for children, hand tapping on the shoulders or on the feet has been substituted successfully. Although questions still remain about exactly how EMDR works, it produces marked improvement in relatively few sessions. However, this level of effectiveness has been shown only with single-event traumas and not with those such as abuse that often include multiple traumatic experiences [77]. Further information may be found at: http://www.emdr.com.

Important elements of psychological treatment

Treatment, irrespective of type, includes a number of essential elements: psycho education about trauma symptoms, exposure to trauma-related cues to bring about habituation of stress reactions, coping skills to manage fear and anxiety, and training parents to play a facilitating role in their child's recovery. The type of trauma, severity of trauma reactions and the child's developmental level determine the content of treatment.

Psycho education

The goal of psycho education is to reassure that trauma reactions are not indications of "craziness" and to provide a rationale for treatment. The symptoms of PTSD should be explained in a way that is understandable to children given their developmental level.

Symptom monitoring

Symptom monitoring is a way of determining the frequency and severity of stress reactions. Children are asked to record the frequency and intensity of trauma symptoms, and typically, a few key symptoms are selected from each cluster.

Exposure

All exposure procedures involve recalling the traumatic event in detail, holding it in consciousness, and tolerating the associated feelings of anxiety until anxiety reduces through the process of habituation. This element of treatment is essential and cannot be dropped from the treatment package. In CBT, exposure may be conducted imaginally or in vivo, although writing or using play or drawings are all effective alternatives.

Children should be informed that when they begin the exposure, they will experience an increase in anxiety, which will peak and then gradually lessen. Exposure is a difficult process and may require many trials before habituation of anxiety to a satisfactory degree is acquired.

In vivo exposure or real-life exposure is usually begun only after habituation to the most stressful level of the graded hierarchy of exposure scenes has been obtained by means of imaginal exposure. In vivo exposure involves making visual, physical, or experiential contact with trauma-related stimuli. This too is often conducted in real life and in a graduated fashion. Parents often are enlisted to act as cotherapists during this part of treatment.

Coping skills

Coping skills are techniques that children can use to regain control over their anxiety. The purpose of coping skills is to enable further contact with trauma-related stimuli rather than to avoid it. Progressive muscle relaxation is a skill in which children learn to recognize the muscle tension associated with anxiety verses being in a calm, relaxed state.

A caveat to the usefulness of coping techniques from the adult anxiety literature is that when they are used to avoid engaging with fear-relevant stimuli during therapy, the treatment gains are significantly lessened [78]. Therefore, the therapist needs to ensure that coping skills are used in the service of engagement rather than avoidance.

Cognitive restructuring

Cognitive restructuring involves identifying maladaptive beliefs that often develop as a result of trauma, challenging them through both dialogue and behavioral experiments, and formulating more adaptive interpretations.

Homework

Homework helps to consolidate the work that is done in session and functions as a reality check as to the effectiveness of the treatment content. Early homework assignments typically involve symptom monitoring and practice of coping skills. Once exposure is begun in session, homework assignments also include exposure-related tasks. Homework assignments should always be jointly agreed on by both the therapist and the client and should be presented in manageable amounts that encourage mastery.

Parent training

Parents provide the support that children need to progress through the stages of therapy. It is important to evaluate the degree to which parents are capable of playing "cotherapist" because some of them may also be experiencing symptoms of psychological distress.

One of the most valuable things that parents need to know is that it is important to talk about the trauma or loss. Children often minimize their suffering because they don't want to upset their parents. Parents are trained to monitor homework; manage problems related to school, sleep, anger and other issues; and to use reinforcement to encourage and reward the child. They also provide the therapist with a second source of feedback regarding the child's difficulties and progress.

Grief work

Grief work is necessary in instances of bereavement or separation from loved ones. It can be conducted in a family setting because the entire family experiences the loss, and it sometimes requires reorganization of the family system.

Reestablishing routines

Returning to a normal routine as soon as possible is important in helping children to regain a sense of normalcy. This includes returning to school, regular sleep and mealtimes, peer interactions, and other activities that used to be a part of their lives before the trauma. To facilitate returning to prior routines, school personnel may also need to be consulted.

Addressing comorbidity and problem behavior

Children may also develop other difficulties besides PTSD as a result of the trauma. Depression and other phobias are common co-occurring disorders. Younger children may refuse to be separated from their parents, some may engage in aggressive behaviors, and older children may use substances as a way of relieving the PTSD symptoms.

Other sources of information

- The National Center for PTSD provides information about PTSD in children and adolescents and types of treatment available and personnel qualified to provide treatment. The website is: http://www.ncptsd.va.gov.
- Cohen [79] and Vernberg and Vogel [80] provide further guidelines for the treatment of PTSD in children and adolescents.
- Cohen and colleagues [81] provide details regarding the treatment of adolescents presenting with PTSD and comorbid substance abuse.
- The International Society for Traumatic Stress Studies has a membership directory with a geographical listing of therapists who treat children and adolescents. The web address is: http://www.istss.org/index.htm.

Summary

Here we have provided an overview of children's experience of trauma and its effects. We have discussed the evidence base regarding dimensions of trauma's short- and long-term effects and its complications given emerging developmental issues and have described intervention procedures that have empirical support as well as (in the case in which empirical science has not yet been developed) selected common practices representing the best judgments of medical clinicians. We have pointed to the need for continuity of care and ongoing consultation among treating professionals. And finally we have provided access routes to additional resources that might assist the PCP in addressing the needs of traumatized children.

References

[1] Giaconia RM, Reinherz HZ, Silverman AB, et al. Traumas and posttraumatic stress disorder in a community population of older adolescents. J Am Acad Child Adolesc Psychiatry 1995;34(10):1369–80.
[2] Cuffe SP, Addy CL, Garrison CZ, et al. Prevalence of PTSD in a community sample of older adolescents. J Am Acad Child Adolesc Psychiatry 1998;37(2):147–54.
[3] American Psychiatric Association. Diagnostic and statistical manual of mental disorders. 4th edition (text revision). Washington, DC: American Psychiatric Association; 2000.
[4] Joshi PT, O'Donnell DA. Consequences of child exposure to war and terrorism. Clin Child Fam Psychol Rev 2003;6:275–92.
[5] Fox L, Long SH, Anglois A. Patterns of language comprehension deficit in abused and neglected children. J Speech Hear Disord 1988;53:239–44.
[6] Perez CM, Widom CS. Childhood victimization and long-term intellectual and academic outcomes. Child Abuse Negl 1994;18:617–24.
[7] Durkin MS, Khan N, Davidson LL, et al. The effect of a natural disaster on child behavior: evidence for posttraumatic stress. Am J Public Health 1993;83:1549–53.
[8] Klimes-Dougan B, Kistner J. Physically abused preschoolers' response to peers' distress. Dev Psychol 1990;26:599–602.
[9] Cicchetti D, Toth SL. A developmental psychopathology perspective on child abuse and neglect. J Am Acad Child Adolesc Psychiatry 1995;34:541–65.
[10] Rogosch FA, Cicchetti D, Shields A, et al. Parenting dysfunction in child maltreatment. In: Bornstein MH, editor. Handbook of parenting (vol. 4). Hillsdale (NJ): Erlbaum; 1995. p. 127–59.
[11] Camras L, Ribordy S, Hill J, et al. Recognition and posing of emotional expressions by abused children and their mothers. Dev Psychol 1988;24:776–81.
[12] Beeghly M, Cicchetti D. Child maltreatment, attachment, and the self-system: emergence of an internal state lexicon in toddlers at high social risk. In: Hertzig ME, Farber EA, editors. Annual progress in child psychiatry and child development. Philadelphia: Brunner/Mazel; 1996. p. 127–66.
[13] Haskett M, Kistner J. Social problem solving skills and young physically abused children. Child Psychiatry Hum Dev 1990;21:109–18.
[14] Smith M, Walden T. Understanding feelings and coping with emotional situations: a comparison of maltreated and nonmaltreated preschoolers. Soc Dev 1999;8:93–116.
[15] Brown GL, Ebert MH, Goyer DC, et al. Aggression, suicide and serotonin: relationships to CSF amine metabolites. Am J Psychiatry 1982;139(6):741–6.
[16] Higley JD, Mehlman PT, Poland RE, et al. CSF testosterone and 5-HIAA correlate with different type of aggressive behaviors. Biol Psychiatry 1996;40:1067–82.
[17] McEwen BS. Early life influence on life-long patterns of behavior and health. Ment Retard Dev Disabil Res Rev 2003;9:149–54.
[18] Swiergiel AH, Takahashi LK, Kalin NH. Attention of stress-induced behavior by antagonism of corticotropin-releasing factor receptors in the central amygdale in the rat. Brain Res 1993;623:229–34.
[19] Wiersma A, Baauw AD, Bohus B, et al. Behavioral activation produced by CRH but not α-helical CRH (CRH-receptor antagonist) when microinfused into the central nucleus of the amygdala under stress-free conditions. Psychoneuroendocrinology 1995;20:423–32.
[20] Richert KA, Carrion VG, Karchemskiy A, et al. Regional differences of the prefrontal cortex in pediatric PTSD: an MRI study. Depress Anxiety 2006;23:17–25.

[21] Roberts AC. Introduction. In: Roberts AC, Robbins TW, Weiskrantz L, editors. The prefrontal cortex: executive and cognitive functions. New York: Oxford University Press; 1998. p. 1–8.
[22] Damasio AR. The somatic marker hypothesis and the possible functions of the prefrontal cortex. In: Roberts AC, Robbins TW, Weiskrantz L, editors. The prefrontal cortex: executive and cognitive functions. New York: Oxford University Press; 1998. p. 36–50.
[23] Hamner MB, Lorberbaum JP, George MS. Potential role of the anterior cingulate cortex in PTSD: review and hypothesis. Depress Anxiety 1999;9(1):1–14.
[24] Cohen JA. Treating traumatized children: current status and future directions. J Trauma Dissociation 2005;6(2):109–21.
[25] National Collaborating Center for Mental Health. Post-traumatic stress disorder: the management of PTSD in adults and children in primary and secondary care. London: The Royal College of Psychiatrists (Gaskell) and the British Psychological Society; 2005. p. 104–32.
[26] Heim C, Wagner D, Maloney E, et al. Early adverse experience and risk for chronic fatigue syndrome: results from a population-based study. Arch Gen Psychiatry 2006;63:1258–66.
[27] Kato K, Sullivan PF, Evengård B, et al. Premorbid predictors of chronic fatigue. Arch Gen Psychiatry 2006;63:1267–72.
[28] Lecrubier Y. Posttraumatic stress disorder in primary care: a hidden diagnosis. J Clin Psychiatry 2004;65(Suppl 1):49–54.
[29] Yehuda R. Post-traumatic stress disorder. N Engl J Med 2002;346(2):108–14.
[30] Geltman PL, Grant-Knight W, Mehta SD, et al. The "lost boys of Sudan": functional and behavioral health of unaccompanied refugee minors re-settled in the United States. Arch Pediatr Adolesc Med 2005;159(6):585–91.
[31] Morgan L, Scourfield J, Williams D, et al. The Aberfan disaster: 33-year follow-up of survivors. Br J Psychiatry 2003;182:532–6.
[32] Yule W, Bolton D, Udwin O, et al. The long-term psychological effects of a disaster experienced in adolescence: I: the incidence and course of PTSD. J Child Psychol Psychiatry 2000; 41(4):503–11.
[33] Augustyn M, Groves BM. Training clinicians to identify the hidden victims: children and adolescents who witness violence. Am J Prev Med 2005;29(5 Suppl 2):272–8.
[34] Bryant B, Mayou R, Wiggs L, et al. Psychological consequences of road traffic accidents for children and their mothers. Psychol Med 2004;34(2):335–46.
[35] Stallard P, Salter E, Velleman R. Posttraumatic stress disorder following road traffic accidents—a second prospective study. Eur Child Adolesc Psychiatry 2004;13(3):172–8.
[36] Stallard P, Velleman R, Baldwin S. Prospective study of post-traumatic stress disorder in children involved in road traffic accidents. BMJ 1998;317(7173):1619–23.
[37] Sturms LM, van der Sluis CK, Stewart RE, et al. A prospective study on paediatric traffic injuries: health-related quality of life and post-traumatic stress. Clin Rehabil 2005;19(3): 312–22.
[38] Peters V, Sottiaux M, Appelboom J, et al. Posttraumatic stress disorder after dog bites in children. J Pediatr 2004;144(1):121–2.
[39] Sanders MB, Starr AJ, Frawley WH, et al. Posttraumatic stress symptoms in children recovering from minor orthopaedic injury and treatment. J Orthop Trauma 2005;19(9):623–8.
[40] Holbrook TL, Hoyt DB, Coimbra R, et al. Long-term posttraumatic stress disorder persists after major trauma in adolescents: new data on risk factors and functional outcome. J Trauma 2005;58(4):764–9.
[41] Rees G, Gledhill J, Garralda ME, et al. Psychiatric outcome following paediatric intensive care unit (PICU) admission: a cohort study. Intensive Care Med 2004;30(8):1607–14.
[42] Mintzer LL, Stuber ML, Seacord D, et al. Traumatic stress symptoms in adolescent organ transplant recipients. Pediatrics 2005;115(6):1640–4.
[43] Stuber ML, Shemesh E, Saxe GN. Posttraumatic stress responses in children with life-threatening illnesses. Child Adolesc Psychiatr Clin North Am 2003;12(2):195–209.

[44] Thienkrua W, Cardozo BL, Chakkraband ML, et al. Symptoms of posttraumatic stress disorder and depression among children in tsunami-affected areas in southern Thailand. JAMA 2006;296(5):549–59.
[45] Schaal S, Elbert T. Ten years after the genocide: trauma confrontation and posttraumatic stress in Rwandan adolescents. J Trauma Stress 2006;19(1):95–105.
[46] Hagan JF Jr. American Academy of Pediatrics Committee on Psychosocial Aspects of Child and Family Health; Task Force on Terrorism. Psychosocial implications of disaster or terrorism on children: a guide for the pediatrician. Pediatrics 2005;116(3):787–95.
[47] Kaminer D, Seedat S, Stein DJ. Post-traumatic stress disorder in children. World Psychiatry 2005;4(2):121–5.
[48] Fairbrother G, Stuber J, Galea S, et al. Posttraumatic stress reactions in New York City children after the September 11, 2001, terrorist attacks. Ambul Pediatr 2003;3(6):304–11.
[49] Montgomery V, Oliver R, Reisner A, et al. The effect of severe traumatic brain injury on the family. J Trauma 2002;52(6):1121–4.
[50] Vieweg WV, Julius DA, Fernandez A, et al. Posttraumatic stress disorder: clinical features, pathophysiology, and treatment. Am J Med 2006;119(5):383–90.
[51] Donnelly CL. Pharmacologic treatment approaches for children and adolescents with posttraumatic stress disorder. Child Adolesc Psychiatr Clin N Am 2003;12(2):251–69.
[52] Cohen JA, Mannarino AP, Rogal S. Treatment practices for childhood posttraumatic stress disorder. Child Abuse Negl 2001;25(1):123–35.
[53] Looff D, Grimley P, Kuller F, et al. Carbamazepine for PTSD. J Am Acad Child Adolesc Psychiatry 1995;34(6):703–4.
[54] Seedat S, Stein DJ, Ziervogel C, et al. Comparison of response to a selective serotonin reuptake inhibitor in children, adolescents, and adults with posttraumatic stress disorder. J Child Adolesc Psychopharmacol 2002;12(1):37–46.
[55] Seedat S, Lockhat R, Kaminer D, et al. An open trial of citalopram in adolescents with posttraumatic stress disorder. Int Clin Psychopharmacol 2001;16(1):21–5.
[56] Harmon RJ, Riggs PD. Clonidine for posttraumatic stress disorder in preschool children. J Am Acad Child Adolesc Psychiatry 1996;35(9):1247–9.
[57] Kant R, Chalansani R, Chengappa KN, et al. The off-label use of clozapine in adolescents with bipolar disorder, intermittent explosive disorder, or posttraumatic stress disorder. J Child Adolesc Psychopharmacol 2004;14(1):57–63.
[58] Wheatley M, Plant J, Reader H, et al. Clozapine treatment of adolescents with posttraumatic stress disorder and psychotic symptoms. J Clin Psychopharmacol 2004;24(2):167–73.
[59] Gupta S, Austin R, Cali LA, et al. Nightmares treated with cyproheptadine. J Am Acad Child Adolesc Psychiatry 1998;37(6):570–2.
[60] Horrigan JP. Guanfacine for PTSD nightmares. J Am Acad Child Adolesc Psychiatry 1996;35(8):975–6.
[61] Good C, Petersen C. SSRI and mirtazapine in PTSD. J Am Acad Child Adolesc Psychiatry 2001;40(3):263–4.
[62] Domon SE, Andersen MS. Nefazodone for PTSD. J Am Acad Child Adolesc Psychiatry 2000;39(8):942–3.
[63] Famularo R, Kinscherff R, Fenton T. Propranolol treatment for childhood posttraumatic stress disorder, acute type. A pilot study. Am J Dis Child 1998;142(11):1244–7.
[64] Stathis S, Martin G, McKenna JG. A preliminary case series on the use of quetiapine for posttraumatic stress disorder in juveniles within a youth detention center. J Clin Psychopharmacol 2005;25(6):539–44.
[65] Sabin JA, Zatzick DF, Jurkovich G, et al. Primary care utilization and detection of emotional distress after adolescent traumatic injury: identifying an unmet need. Pediatrics 2006;117(1):130–8.
[66] Laraque D, Boscarino JA, Battista A, et al. Reactions and needs of tristate-area pediatricians after the events of September 11th: implications for children's mental health services. Pediatrics 2004;113(5):1357–66.

[67] Saxe GN, Stoddard F, Hall E, et al. Pathways to PTSD, part I: children with burns. Am J Psychiatry 2005;162(7):1299–304.
[68] Faust J, Katchen LB. Treatment of children with complicated posttraumatic stress reactions. Psychotherapy: Theory, Research, Practice, Training 2004;41:426–37.
[69] Cook-Cottone C. Childhood posttraumatic stress disorder: diagnosis, treatment, and school reintegration. School Psych Rev 2004;33(1):127–39.
[70] Shemesh E, Newcorn JH, Rockmore L, et al. Comparison of parent and child reports of emotional trauma symptoms in pediatric outpatient settings. Pediatrics 2005;115(5):e582–9.
[71] Fremont WP. Childhood reactions to terrorism-induced trauma: a review of the past 10 years. J Am Acad Child Adolesc Psychiatry 2004;43:381–90.
[72] Cohen JA, Deblinger E, Mannarino AP, et al. A multisite, randomized controlled trial for children with sexual abuse-related PTSD symptoms. J Am Acad Child Adolesc Psychiatry 2004;43(4):393–402.
[73] Deblinger E, Steer RA, Lippmann J. Two-year follow-up study of cognitive behavioral therapy for sexually abused children suffering post-traumatic stress symptoms. Child Abuse Negl 1999;23(12):1371–8.
[74] Goenjian AK, Walling D, Steinberg AM, et al. A prospective study of posttraumatic stress and depressive reactions among treated and untreated adolescents 5 years after a catastrophic disaster. Am J Psychiatry 2005;162(12):2302–8.
[75] Stallard P, Velleman R, Salter E, et al. A randomised controlled trial to determine the effectiveness of an early psychological intervention with children involved in road traffic accidents. J Child Psychol Psychiatry 2006;47(2):127–34.
[76] Ehntholt KA, Smith PA, Yule W. School-based cognitive-behavioural therapy group intervention for refugee children who have experienced war-related trauma. Clin Child Psychol Psychiatry 2005;10(2):235–50.
[77] Tufnell G. Eye movement desensitization and reprocessing in the treatment of pre-adolescent children with post-traumatic symptoms. Clin Child Psychol Psychiatry 2005;10(4): 587–600.
[78] Powers MB, Smits JA, Telch MJ. Disentangling the effects of safety-behavior utilization and safety-behavior availability during exposure-based treatment: a placebo-controlled trial. J Consult Clin Psychol 2004;72(3):448–54.
[79] Cohen JA. Practice parameters for the assessment and treatment of children and adolescents with posttraumatic stress disorder. J Am Acad Child Adolesc Psychiatry Special Issue: Practice parameters 1998;37(10 Suppl):4S–26S.
[80] Vernberg EM, Vogel JM. Psychological responses of children to natural and human-made disasters: II. Interventions with children after disasters. J Clin Child Psychol 1993;22(4): 485–98.
[81] Cohen JA, Mannarino AP, Zhitova AC, et al. Treating child abuse-related posttraumatic stress and comorbid substance abuse in adolescents. Child Abuse Negl 2003;27(12):1345–65.

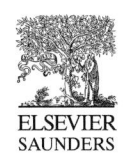

Psychologic Impact of Deafness on the Child and Adolescent

Asiah Mason, PhD[a],*, Matthew Mason, PhD[b]

[a]National Mission Initiatives, Laurent Clerc National Deaf Education Center, Gallaudet University, 800 Florida Avenue NE, Washington, DC 20002, USA
[b]Norbel School, 12007 Yellow Bell Lane, Columbia, MD 21044, USA

"The only thing that a deaf person cannot do is hear."
—I. King Jordan (1988)

Deaf and hard-of-hearing children and adolescents comprise a heterogeneous population. They come from every region and state; from farms, inner cities, and suburbs; and from every racial, ethnic, and socioeconomic group. They may be adopted or fostered, have many siblings or none, and live in large or small extended families in which parents speak English or one of many other languages. Those parents may be hearing, deaf, or hard of hearing and married or single, living with a partner, divorced, or separated. The children themselves may be deaf or hard of hearing, may or may not have additional conditions, and may or may not be developing at age level [1]. All these characteristics have an impact on the development and well-being of deaf and hard-of-hearing children and adolescents.

Within this heterogeneous background, in more than 90% of families with deaf children, the parents are hearing and usually have no knowledge of or experience with deafness [2]. Deafness has an impact on the family as well as on the deaf child [3]. The families of newly diagnosed deaf children experience a changed world as a result of the diagnosis. This world involves more than just the absence of hearing. Hearing parents who are not familiar with deafness often view their deaf child with uncertainty [4]. They may not know what to expect in terms of goals and expectations for their deaf child's future. They also may wonder about their role and how to be effective parents in this unfamiliar situation. They may experience feelings of guilt, confusion, and helplessness, all of which are understandable [5].

---

* Corresponding author.
  E-mail address: asiah.mason@gallaudet.edu (A. Mason).

The purpose of this article is to provide a brief overview of the psychologic impact (stimuli and events that influence cognitive, social, and emotional development) of deafness on children and adolescents. In addition, methods for connecting with families to provide information, support, and resources to enhance deaf children's development are described. In this context, cognitive development refers to changes in a person's intellectual abilities, including attention, memory, academic and everyday knowledge, problem solving, imagination, creativity, and language. Social-emotional development refers to changes in attachment, emotional communication, self-understanding, knowledge about other people, interpersonal skills, friendships, intimate relationships, and moral reasoning and behavior [6]. To understand the psychologic impact of deafness on children and adolescents, it is necessary to take a look at the contextual experience of deafness from infancy, early childhood, and middle childhood to adolescence.

Today, families are looking more to the growing body of research on human development for answers to the age-old question of how best to support the needs of their children [7]. For some 5000 American families experiencing the birth of a deaf infant each year [8], this question comes to the forefront as the developmental issues become more complex and uncertain. Research on so-called "protective" factors surrounding children who demonstrate successful adaptation to deafness represents an important aspect of support to these families in their search for answers [9–11]. Concerns still exist regarding how deafness affects the developing child, how the child affects the family's functioning, and how the family's decisions and actions can support the child in the short term and across his or her life span.

This article incorporates what has been learned from research on childhood disabilities, child development, developmental psychopathology, and life span development using a framework of "person-environment interaction" or "transactional adaptation" [12,13]. The continuous interplay between individual child characteristics and environmental factors (including setting and family variables) is crucial to demystifying and predicting the deaf child's development. Commonly, the diagnosis of deafness is so shocking that for many families, it can become a singular focus [14] that can distract them from considering other influences affecting developmental trajectories, such as early socioemotional development, including communication, self-regulation, emotional expressiveness, and self-recognition.

Impact of deafness during infancy and toddlerhood: attachment and language development

The emotional bond that develops between the infant and caregivers during the first year of life is called attachment. Attachment is the strong affectional tie we feel for special people in our lives that leads us to experience pleasure and joy when we interact with them and to be comforted by their nearness during times of stress. By the end of the first year, infants have become attached to familiar people who have responded to their needs for physical care and stimulation [15]. The infant's ability to thrive physically and psychologically depends on the quality of this attachment [16]. When caregivers are consistently warm and responsive to their infant's needs, the infant develops a secure attachment. Conversely, insecure attachment may develop when the caregivers are neglectful, inconsistent, or insensitive to their infant's moods or behaviors. The quality of attachment during infancy is associated with a variety of long-term effects [17]. Studies have shown that hearing preschoolers with a history of secure attachment tend to be more prosocial, empathic, and socially competent than are preschoolers with a history of insecure attachment [18,19]. Hearing adolescents with secure attachment histories demonstrate fewer problems, do better in school, and have more successful relationships with peers than do adolescents with insecure attachment in infancy [20].

Normal linguistic development emerges out of the typical and almost universal interactions between mothers and their infants, and this forms the basis for attachment. During this socialization process, secure attachment is reinforced by the mother touching and caressing the child, talking to the child, or picking up the child when, for example, the infant cries. The infant usually ceases fussing and looks at the mother, who is smiling or speaking, and the infant responds by vocalizing. Such interactions continue back and forth as the dyad gives each other cues. Over time, this procedure increases in complexity [5]. Hearing newborns are exposed to almost continuous auditory information. They recognize their mother's voice early and become familiar with noises. Vision and voice enter reciprocally into play and become part of the early communication constantly surrounding the infants [21]. When the mother leaves physically, infants can still hear her even if they cannot see her.

Developing social attachments, developing an awareness of self, being able to interpret cues from others through social referencing, and learning to regulate one's own emotional responses are important accomplishments during the first few years. The implications of these developments for deaf infants are somewhat different than for hearing babies. In the case of children whose diagnosis of deafness is delayed, hearing parents do not know that their deaf infant cannot hear. They unknowingly deprive the infant of their presence every time they exit the infant's visual field [21]. Deaf infants depend on tactile sensations, direct contact, and visual input for communication. They are incapable of foreseeing an arrival by means of noise, the sound of approaching steps, or a voice calling from the other room. If lack of hearing is not compensated for by visual and tactile stimulation on an ongoing basis, the deaf child's sense of isolation can be exacerbated [5].

The degree to which attachment is affected by deafness may also be influenced by such factors as communication proficiency. It has been shown, for example, that deaf preschoolers with poor communications skills were often insecurely attached, whereas those able to communicate more easily developed secure attachments [22]. Other researchers have found that deaf children with deaf parents (presumably dyads with high communicative competence) develop attachment patterns similar to those observed in hearing children with hearing parents [23]. These studies conclude there is currently little evidence that deafness itself contributes directly to insecure attachment; it is more likely the case that the other contextual influences discussed previously have a far greater impact on the attachment process.

Marschark [24] posited that early researchers described deaf children with hearing parents as less likely to be securely attached to their mothers based on anecdotal or observational rather than empiric studies. They reasoned that the apparent role of hearing and speech enables the development of normal reciprocal mother-child relationships. Without this communication, reciprocity cannot transfer from nonverbal to verbal processes. Researchers theorized that the stress of waiting to confirm a child's hearing loss may lead to the mothers making incorrect interpretations of infant or child behaviors during the attachment process, such as thinking that the child may be mentally retarded. The hearing mother–deaf child dyad may develop reciprocal behavior patterns that differ from those typically seen in hearing mother–hearing child dyads [5].

Two studies that tried to understand the interactions between mothers' communication effectiveness and attachment in hearing-deaf dyads [22,25] compared the relationships of deaf toddlers and their hearing mothers with those of a matched group of hearing toddlers and their mothers. They found that deaf toddlers and their mothers did not communicate with each other as well as hearing toddlers and their mothers. Mothers would talk and gesture when their children were not looking at them, and this frequently led to termination of the interaction. The mothers had not yet learned to coordinate communication with the children's visual attention. Also, deaf toddlers and their hearing mothers spent less of the free-play session interacting with each other than hearing toddlers and their mothers, perhaps in part because deaf children must divide their attention between mother and toys.

The deaf infants themselves typically responded by mirroring their parents' signs [26]. Specifically, these infants frequently moved their own hands and arms, with parental praise and encouragement reinforcing these movements. These responses represent the precursor to the early gestures and signed communications produced by deaf infants and are part of the attachment process.

Eye gaze and maintaining eye contact during interaction are of particular importance. Koester and colleagues [26] report findings concluding that deaf infants alternate their gaze between their deaf mothers and the surroundings more frequently. The length of time the deaf infants gazed at their deaf mothers tended to be longer in comparison to deaf infants with hearing mothers, who spent more time looking at the surroundings [5].

Some research suggests that early dyadic communication can easily be disturbed by difficult-to-read infant signals [27] or by lack of infant responsiveness to caregivers' bids [28]. These patterns may be important predictors of later interactional emotional difficulties between parent and child [29]. In either case, having a child diagnosed with a hearing loss can easily alter the typical flow of reciprocal interactions, and thus change parent-infant dynamics, at least temporarily, until mutuality is re-established and each partner's signals become more easily interpreted by the other partner. As in the case of temperament, however, the initial fit between parental expressive communication styles and the infant's receptive abilities and preferences plays an important role in determining the outcome for the deaf infant's early social, emotional, and linguistic development. When a deaf child does not orient or calm to a parent's voice, parents may gradually perceive this as a rejection or cause for concern about their caregiving abilities [30].

Impact on development of self-regulation and emotional expressiveness

Emotional self-regulation refers to the strategies we use to adjust our emotional state to a comfortable level of intensity so that we can accomplish our goals [15]. If one drinks a cup of coffee to wake up in the morning, reminds oneself that an anxiety-provoking event is going to be over soon, or decides not to see a scary horror film, one is engaging in emotional self-regulation. In the early months of life, infants have only a limited capacity to regulate their emotional states. Although they can turn away from unpleasant stimulation and mouth and suck when their feelings get too intense, they are easily overwhelmed. They depend on the soothing interventions of caregivers: lifting the distressed baby to the shoulder, rocking, and talking softly. Rapid development of the cortex gradually increases the baby's tolerance for stimulation. When infants are between 2 and 4 months of age, caregivers start to build on this capacity through engaging in verbal and face-to-face play and verbally encouraging attention to objects. In these interactions, parents arouse pleasure in the baby while adjusting the pace of their own behavior so that the infant does not become overwhelmed and distressed. As a result, the baby's tolerance for stimulation increases further. By the end of the first year, infants' ability to move about permits them to regulate feelings more effectively by approaching or retreating from various situations.

In deaf infants, these self-regulatory behaviors are reinforced when caregivers use facial and body expressions that the infants can imitate. Deaf mothers tend to be highly active and animated with their infants. This tends to elicit positive responses from the infants. When parents of deaf infants omit the use of eye contact or facial expressions, deaf infants are more likely to respond with protestations [31]. Deaf infants do vocalize, but they do so more for protesting or stimulation. Without amplification that conveys speech sounds, the ability to learn conversational skills like hearing infants is not reinforced. Visual stimuli, such as exaggerated facial expressions and visual language, as well as increased use of tactile contact and auditory amplification facilitate interactive communication and set the foundation for language development [5].

It is tremendously helpful when hearing parents understand that deafness is a visual experience, even when auditory amplification is provided. They may require special help in learning to respond to and foster their deaf child's understanding of visual stimuli and signals, because this is a different communicative style for them [32]. Parents may need to be taught the importance of responding to the deaf child's early gestures using visual-gestural modes in addition to auditory stimuli. This entails awareness of eye contact and shifts in eye gaze, which indicate the infant's interests, level of attention, and receptiveness to environmental input [5]. Early interventionists and hearing caregivers have much to learn from how deaf parents use visual strategies, such as those already described, for interactive communication and for reinforcing self-regulatory behaviors [26,32].

As caregivers help infants to regulate their emotional states, they also provide lessons in socially approved ways of expressing feelings. As von Salisch [33] noted, "...Parents talk to their children about verbal labels for their inner experiences, about antecedents of other people's emotional expressions, and about the consequences of their own expressive displays." Most hearing infants in North American cultures are frequently exposed to conversations about feelings, internal states, and subjective experiences. By the second year of life, growth in representation and language leads to new ways of regulating emotions. A vocabulary for talking about feelings, such as happy, love, surprised, scary, yucky, and mad, develops rapidly after 18 months [15]. In infants, the result is an accumulation of practice labeling and articulating their own emotions and developing strategies for modulating their emotional responses to affectively laden experiences. How does this process occur before the establishment of a shared and effective system of communication when the infant is deaf and the primary caregiver is hearing? What is the long-term effect of having missed so many of these early opportunities for learning to express one's feeling through language, making one's needs known to others through spoken communication, and receiving the linguistic feedback that validates one's emotional responses?

When a deaf child has hearing parents, creating shared meaning and relatedness through language is a greater challenge. The absence of an available symbolic system in which to share personal knowledge or create a linguistic construct for an affective or emotional inner experience makes the possibility of developmental arrest or delay more likely. Without words, signs, gestures, or communicative silence, there is no ability to express experiences, thoughts, or feelings [34].

The concept of "goodness of fit" is frequently mentioned in literature describing temperament studies. Temperament refers to stable individual differences in quality and intensity of emotional reaction, activity level, attention, and emotional self-regulation [15]. Children with different temperaments have unique child-rearing needs. Chess and Thomas [35] proposed a goodness-of-fit model to explain how temperament and environment can work together to produce favorable outcomes. Goodness of fit involves creating child-rearing environments that recognize each child's temperament while helping the youngster to achieve more adaptive functioning. The goodness-of-fit model applies to the child-rearing practice of deaf children and adolescents. The concept is also applicable when considering the development of emotional regulation in a deaf child who, in most instances, has hearing parents. The importance of shared meanings cannot be overemphasized and is critical in facilitating the emergence of flexible and adaptive self-regulatory behaviors on the part of the deaf child.

Impact of deafness on social and emotional development

Effective social-emotional development requires not only the prevention of social or personal ills but the promotion of healthy growth and development (ie, having healthy relationships, managing stress effectively, self-efficacy). Healthy social-emotional development is a critical foundation for life success. Competencies that are generally accepted as defining healthy social-emotional development are also applicable to helping individuals realize their academic and vocational potential [36]. Unfortunately, as a group, deaf children and adolescents demonstrate reduced mastery in many of these areas of competence, and thus are at risk for several adverse outcomes [37–39]. These outcomes include low academic achievement, underemployment, and higher rates of social maladaption (eg, violence, drug and alcohol problems) and psychologic distress and disorder [24,37]. Not all deaf children develop adjustment problems, however, and the impact of deafness on the child's overall development is influenced by several factors, including the quality of the family environment, parental adaptation to deafness, family coping, the nature of school and community resources, and the child's characteristics and transactions with his or her ecology [21,40–42].

Previous reviews of social-cognition in childhood (eg, the study by Greenberg and Kusche [37]) noted that deaf children are often delayed in language development, tend to show greater impulsivity and poorer emotional regulation, and often have an impoverished vocabulary of emotion language. Thus, for some deaf children as well as for other individuals who have experienced delays in language or who have been deprived of sufficient language-mediated experience, the inability to mediate experience with linguistic symbols and label aspects of inner emotional states spontaneously may be one important factor leading to serious gaps in social-emotional development. For example, young children generally act on their own curiosity with impulsive behavior, such as touching or exploring an object that may not be safe, or experience a feeling but have no linguistic label for it. After numerous warnings or feeling identification from caregivers, children can develop their own internal linguistic dialog to temper the impulsive desire to touch and explore or understand their own feeling states by telling themselves, "It's not safe," "It doesn't belong to me," "Don't touch," "I am sad," or "I feel angry." This process is interrupted (or never begins) when children do not or cannot perceive their caregivers' language, however [43].

Furthermore, there are other important factors to be considered in understanding obstacles faced by deaf children in developing social and emotional competence that have direct implications for educational interventions. Meadow and Dyssegaard [44] hypothesized that the deficits in motivation and initiative, important factors for social maturity, may be attributable to hearing parents and teachers being highly directive and not providing deaf children with rich opportunities for taking independent action and responsibility.

When parents find out that their child is deaf, they often experience an emotional crisis and loss of confidence in their ability to know what is best for their child. Parents turn to professionals for support and guidance with respect to intervention approaches. This can be a confusing time for parents, given the disparate approaches advised by some professionals. Despite this initial stress, the implementation of universal screening for hearing loss in newborns, early identification, and early intervention have demonstrated significant gains in the language and communication skills for deaf children. These gains have shown lasting effects into early childhood for better success in language, academic, and social-emotional outcomes for deaf children [11,45]. Koester [12] and Sass-Lehrer and Bodner-Johnson [9] provide an in-depth review of the importance of this initial phase in deaf children's lives to their overall development and their families' adjustment.

After the initial impact of diagnosis and early intervention, a variety of obstacles in parenting can accompany the significant communication problems that are often found between deaf children and their hearing parents [46–48]. Parents frequently report that because their deaf children do not understand them, they have limited options available for socializing their children. As a result, some deaf children have fewer opportunities to learn what they did wrong and why it was wrong, how their behavior affected others, and what alternatives they could have chosen instead. Moreover, their parents are more likely to model avoidance and physical action as methods for solving problems. Similarly, parental frustration attributable to communication barriers often leads parents to "take on" their children's problems. When this happens, deaf children are then afforded little opportunity to learn from and resolve their own difficulties. The impact of limited explanations and restricted experiences denies to many deaf children their rightful opportunity to learn to understand others.

Impact of deafness within a family system: stress, overprotection, and acceptance

It has been reported that the stress of the child's hearing loss negatively affects family functioning and, consequently, the development of the child [43]. Protective factors thought to ameliorate negative relationships between familial stress and healthy child development include parental attitudes [49], beliefs [10], attributions [50], internal and external family resources [51], and the quality of social support [52]. These factors can support parents' abilities to adapt successfully to stressors (eg, the results of the questionnaire developed by Minnes and Nachsen [53]), facilitating their parenting effectiveness, and hence child outcomes.

For families with deaf infants, a unique source of stress stems from conflicting professional opinions regarding different intervention and communication options [54]. The existence of social networks of families with deaf children also corresponds to positive mother-child interactions [1], however, perhaps effectively buffering negative effects of familial stress on children's development.

Plasticity is another related concept of particular interest. According to this approach, certain skills or attributes may still be developed at some later point even if the typical time of emergence has been missed, and this approach is applicable to deaf and hearing infants. Although there may be sensitive periods during which a given skill, such as language, develops most readily and perhaps most fully [55], the possibility remains for personal and contextual modifications to facilitate this development later. In the primarily auditory linguistic contexts provided by most hearing families, the mode of language input may not be the best fit for the communication needs of a deaf child. It seems plausible then that the language delays with which most deaf children of hearing parents enter formal educational settings may be partially explained by the concept of goodness of fit during the preschool years [56] instead of putting the blame or causal factor on the child's deafness.

In addition to the other factors already discussed, more subtle factors are involved in the constellation of immature behaviors that are frequently noted with deaf children. For example, for many (if not most) adults living and working with deaf children, manual-sign communication is a second language that has been acquired late in life and is never as natural as their native spoken language. Nor is it natural for hearing people to remain acutely attuned to the needs of a deaf person who relies on lip reading or on residual hearing. Therefore, in addition to the deaf child's communication difficulties, there is an issue of lack of communication skill, which can be insecurity on the part of many adults. This combination of fear of misunderstanding or being misunderstood and communication deficiencies in adult role models results in an insidious form of "linguistic overprotection." This often unconscious fear leads adults to "talk down" to or reduce the linguistic and cognitive complexity of communications to deaf children [57]. This phenomenon, in turn, limits the children's opportunities to learn about social and emotional states and characteristics as well as limiting their opportunities to learn more advanced language.

Bat-Chava [58,59] found that those deaf people and their families who embraced values of the hearing world and the deaf world seemed to have the highest level of self-esteem. They were able to reap professional and academic success while also being able to advocate for social change in the majority's view of their minority culture. They did not accept the differential (lower) expectations by the majority culture, which can result in deaf individuals limiting their own personal goals; developing negative self-concepts; or internalizing cognitive attributions of helplessness, failure, and inferiority.

Stinson and Foster [42] wrote about the impact on the identity and social adjustment of deaf children as a result of the availability of hearing or deaf peers to socialize with in their respective educational placements. The most common placements are inclusion in the child's neighborhood school, self-contained classrooms, regular hearing schools, or deaf residential programs. Each of these placements and respective peer groups promotes different aspects of social competence and sense of identity in deaf or hard-of-hearing children. When combined with the family environment and parent-child communication strategies investigated by Sheridan [60] and Steinberg [34], the complex set of influences that affect the achievement of positive self-acceptance and secure identity for deaf individuals is evident.

Osofsky and Thompson [61] posed two important questions regarding ways in which less than optimal situations might be improved for families, and thus lead to better outcomes: (1) how can adaptive parenting be supported and fostered, and (2) what are the conditions most likely to enhance resilience in families at risk for parent-child difficulties? Finding the most appropriate and supportive context for a deaf child (facilitating this particularly within the family during the early years) may be one of the most pressing tasks for early interventionists, deaf education specialists, parents, and researchers.

Impact of deafness on incidental learning

Understanding ourselves, our culture, and rules for how people and families communicate is strongly influenced by incidental learning. Incidental learning is the process by which information is learned by virtue of passive exposure to events witnessed or overheard [43]. The meaning of such information is not directly taught or necessarily intended for instruction; yet, important information and nuances for behavior or beliefs are transmitted and absorbed consciously or unconsciously. Because the constant use of sign language by hearing people is rare and deaf children cannot overhear spoken conversations, there are many types of messages that are not readily available to deaf children (eg, parent or teacher discussions, problem solving, arguments when children are out of sight but not out of hearing range, television and radio in the background environment, telephone calls with relatives or friends, praise or disciplinary procedures directed toward another child). In the case of deaf children, all communications must be directed specifically to them, and they, in turn, must also pay close visual attention. This can be a tiring process for these children as well as for others communicating with them and may sometimes interfere with ongoing activities.

Thus, deafness itself may limit some avenues of incidental learning commonly experienced by hearing children. As a result, programs to promote parent-child communication and social and emotional competence should be used with all deaf children (not only with those who are manifesting problems) to help remediate understanding that may be missed or distorted through gaps in incidental learning [43].

Impact of deafness during adolescent years: competence, social independence, and identity development

In his seminal work, Marschark [30] wrote that as young children develop into more social organisms, the variety of their relationships with family, peers, and other adults (eg, teachers) increases far beyond that established with the mother and other caregivers within the home. Most children exhibit an affinity toward others, displaying instrumental and emotional (or person-oriented) dependence. Instrumental dependence refers to seeking attention from others to satisfy needs or wants, whereas emotional dependence refers to the extension of attachment-like bonds as children strive for proximity, approval, and affection from others. The child who is independent still displays appropriate instrumental and emotional dependence but blends such behavior with self-reliance, assertiveness, and a need for achievement.

In general, children and adolescents with disabilities are likely to encounter difficulty in establishing their independence. In part, the relatively greater need for instrumental assistance is a real one, the qualities and extent of which vary with the nature of the child's handicap. The frequent overprotection of children and adolescents with disabilities by their parents creates further impediments to social independence, however, because those children are often able to perform a variety of tasks that others typically do for them. As Meadow [62] noted:

> ... parents generalize from the narrow range of tasks that the handicapped child actually cannot do, and assume that there is a much larger spectrum of tasks of which he is incapable. Eventually, the assumed inability becomes a real inability because the child does not have the opportunity to practice

tasks and develop new levels of expertise. In addition, it takes more patience and time for handicapped children to perform the trial-and-error process of skill acquisition-time and patience that parents may not have or be unwilling to give. For deaf children with deficient communication skills, it takes additional time and patience merely to communicate what is expected, required, and necessary for the performance of even a simple task.

Intimate attachments to parents and peers as a feeling of belonging to a social network are important in healthy identity development in adolescence. One's social network might include a variety of individuals, including relatively close friends, members of one's extended family, coworkers or classmates, neighbors, casual acquaintances, and members of organizations or groups in which the adolescent actively participates. Intimate attachments and one's social group can be invaluable resources for coping with stress by providing a variety of functions, including emotional support, validation, information, advice, feelings of solidarity, and actual physical or financial assistance. For these reasons, it is important for deaf adolescents to feel connected with other deaf peers or adults through school programs, recreational programs, deaf clubs, or other organized activities [43].

Impact of deafness personality development

Marschark [30] emphasized it is important to recognize that in the case of deaf children, and particularly for those of hearing parents, the rules, customs, and social behaviors learned in the home may not generalize to social situations outside the home. In part, this situation results from deaf children's emerging from hearing homes having had a relatively more restricted range of interpersonal interactions than hearing peers or deaf peers who have deaf parents. Furthermore, the interaction patterns that such children acquire at home frequently differ from those of children raised in homes in which children and parents share a common hearing status and a common mode of communication. For deaf children with deaf parents, the transfer of social processes to a broader audience is likely to be easier. Social interactions with individuals outside the immediate family are thus more likely to be similar to those within the family.

Deaf children of deaf parents are more likely than those with hearing parents to have experienced consistent parenting behaviors, effective communication, and more tolerant social environments [37]. Deaf children of deaf parents also are at an advantage in that they have better linguistic means with which to deal with new social settings. Regardless of parental hearing status, social interactions and communication fluency at home form the bases for deaf children's social development. Often, deaf children reared by hearing parents and surrounded by hearing peers have fewer opportunities or reduced capacity to learn from social interactions, stemming from inadequately developed communication skills. A decreased sense of independence, poorer self-esteem, and lower quality of relationships may arise. Many of these children are labeled as impulsive, egocentric, and overly dependent; it is important to recognize that these traits may be a strong reflection of the differences deaf children experience vis-à-vis their child-parent relationship compared with hearing children. It is fascinating to consider that deaf children and adolescents have an unusual but necessary overdependency on their family members for social modeling and role identification. The breadth of their social sphere is restricted depending on whether persons in their community can competently communicate with them.

Deaf children and adolescents are often described as emotionally immature compared with their hearing peers [37]. In the case of deaf children of hearing parents, one could argue that lags in social and emotional development result, in part, from the lack of appropriate social models with whom they can identify and communicate. Clearly, the lack of communication between parents and children leaves both sides unclear about the needs, wants, and capabilities of the other [63–65].

Theories of moral development recognize that conscience begins to take shape in early childhood. Most agree that at first, the child's morality is externally controlled by adults' verbalization and nonverbal expression of right and wrong. Gradually, it becomes regulated by inner standards. Truly moral individuals do not just do the right thing when authority figures are around. Instead, they have developed principles of good conduct and compassion that they follow in a wide variety of situations [20]. Many environmental factors promote moral stage change, including child-rearing practices, schooling, peer interaction, and aspects of culture. Growing evidence suggests that the way these experiences work is to present young people with cognitive challenges that stimulate them to think about moral problems in more complex ways. When linguistic and experiential confounds are removed, deaf children, as a group, show evidence of sophisticated moral reasoning [24].

Any interpretation of findings concerning moral reasoning in deaf children must keep in mind the sociocultural context of their social development. At one level, it would not be at all surprising if deaf children perform at more concrete or superficial levels in moral reasoning tasks if they have been raised in situations in which their parents and other adult figures have not communicated affective responses, goals, and desires [63] and have provided immediate gratification rather than rational explanations for behavior. Moreover, for deaf children with hearing parents, the inconsistency of social feedback and alternating permissiveness and physical punishment frequently have led to a resistance to parental values as early as the middle school years. In the case of deaf children with deaf parents, one would expect that the consistency of early social interaction and moral training would lead to higher levels of moral reasoning in context-appropriate settings, but comparisons of the moral reasoning abilities of deaf children with deaf versus hearing parents apparently have not been made.

Deaf children and adolescents may be able to infer moral values by observing the consequences of their own and others' behavior to a limited extent. This process is far slower and less efficient for the communication of moral values than is the use of language, however. For those deaf children who lack effective abstract communication within the home, the major portion of moral training does not begin until they enter a special deaf preschool or classroom. In those contexts, morality is learned, in part, from teachers and other adults who also have a variety of more explicit responsibilities. Most moral training, one suspects, comes from peers who may have been raised in similar circumstances, and thus also have relatively limited exposure to alternative bases for moral reasoning [24].

Impact of deafness on education of deaf children

One of the biggest controversies in the field of deafness is the issue of education for deaf children. It is not the intention of this article to discuss or debate the opposing viewpoints of this issue. It is the authors' intention to reflect the belief that deaf education and the experiences of deaf children must be made as normal as possible. This conclusion is not a call for mainstreaming deaf children into regular classrooms [2]. Public Law 94-142 (Education for All Handicapped Children Act) mandates that deaf and other children with disabilities should be placed with children without disabilities "to the greatest appropriate degree." It also recognizes, however, that regular classrooms may be inappropriate. In practice, the mainstreaming of deaf students frequently consists of integration in nonacademic or vocational domains but not in academics. Being in a normal school or normal classroom does not necessarily provide deaf children with the same education as hearing peers.

In the absence of comparable early environments, many deaf children are ill equipped to deal with the content or the context of the hearing public school classroom. Such a setting would be neither "normal" nor facilitative [24]. The problems facing deaf education go far beyond children's inability to hear, speak, and read. Most of those problems did not develop during the school years, and it is unlikely that they can be resolved then [43].

In addition to all the variables presented herein, a most significant factor affecting deaf children's mental health is their vulnerability to multiple risk factors. Deaf children are especially at risk for mental health issues because of family dysfunction, lack of access to equal opportunities in access to services, and increased vulnerability for childhood physical and sexual abuse [66,67]. The limited focus of this article does not allow for full coverage of this topic. Nevertheless, it is especially important to understand that any developing child is at risk for developing mental health conditions and that the development of such conditions depends on genetic, physiologic, environmental, and social risk factors. Because deaf children are at a higher risk for increased family or relationship problems and language development difficulties as a result of the nature of their physiologic difference compared with hearing peers, these risk factors must be considered when evaluating a deaf child. When the family of the deaf child provides a nurturing and appropriate support for communication development, such deaf children pose no more risk for developing a mental health disorder compared with their hearing peers [3,5,21].

Summary

Sacks [68] states that infants who are congenitally and profoundly deaf begin their lives lacking what is perhaps the most universal of parent-child communications devices not only in humans but across a variety mammalian and other species: the oral-aural channel. Surely, there is compensation and accommodation in that situation that serve to provide a reciprocal relationship between the parent and child in a somewhat different manner than that of hearing children. It is only by understanding those differences, however, that one can hope to understand the psychologic functioning of deaf individuals [43].

A growing body of research documents the positive effects of early comprehensive intervention for the social and cognitive development of children born at risk for developmental delay [69]. For children who are deaf or hard of hearing, positive results of early intervention are shown for social and communicative competence, and support networks relate to positive mother-child interaction and better language development [40,70]. Children and adolescents in responsive and supportive families demonstrate better socioemotional, communicative, and cognitive development compared with others [1].

Families identify communication choice as one of the most stressful decisions they have to make. Lack of information and resources or biased, incomplete, and inaccurate information from professionals makes the decision even more difficult. Although a decision about the best mode of communication may take time, parent-child relationships and language acquisition cannot be sacrificed or put on hold. Effective communication—signed, spoken, cued, or a combination—is vital to the quality of family life and to the child's emotional adjustment, language development, and future academic achievement. Many parents do not achieve the sign fluency they would like but use signs nevertheless to clarify messages and reduce communication frustration. Because parents want their children to have every opportunity, they do whatever they can to achieve this goal [1].

There are qualitative differences in various aspects of the development of deaf versus hearing children [43]. Nevertheless, it is important not to view developmental differences as deficiencies [24]. Certainly, deaf children bring different personal attributes to environmental challenges or developmental demands than do hearing children.

Researchers in the field of deafness have presented evidence indicating that deaf children, on average, are relatively more restricted in their range of experience; they tend to have more concrete and informationally deficient linguistic interchanges with others and do not have as many available sources of content and social knowledge as hearing age-mates [24]. In a real sense, then, many of the interactions observed between deaf children and their early environments seemed to orient them toward the concrete, the superficial, and the immediate. Such patterns held primarily for deaf children of hearing parents, especially the children of parents who, for whatever reason, had minimal or only later communication with their children. Deaf parents, on average, are found to have greater expectations for and involvement in their children's education, in addition to having more consistent child-rearing practices. It is therefore difficult to separate child-related from parent-related factors in deaf children's successes and failures. We can be sure only that the two interact in a variety of ways, and we can then try to identify the dimensions that seem to be most salient in determining the course of psychologic development in deaf children. Marschark [43], in his ground-breaking work, indicated that three such factors now seem to stand out as having central implications for deaf children's normal development and competence in dealing with the world.

Early language experience

Regardless of its mode, all evidence from deaf and hearing children points to the need for effective early communication between children and those around them. Obvious in some sense, the need for symbolic linguistic interaction goes beyond day-to-day practicalities and academic instruction. The deaf children who seem most likely to be the most competent in all domains of childhood endeavor are those who actively participate in linguistic interactions with their parents from an early age. From those interactions, they not only gain facts but gain cognitive and social strategies, knowledge of self and others, and a sense of being part of the world. In social as well as academic domains, lack of the ability to communicate about the abstract and the absent prevents children from reaching their potential.

Diversity of experience

It is through active exploration of the environment and through experience with people, things, and language that children acquire knowledge, including learning to learn. The operating principles for development outlined previously in this article are unlikely to be innate. They derive from the application of basic perceptual, learning, and memory processes (which are more likely to have innate components) as a result of experience. With sufficient resources, learning becomes a self-motivating and self-sustaining pursuit. In the absence of diversity, there are no problems to solve, and thus no need for flexibility. When attempting to ensure that deaf children have the necessities for academic and practical pursuits, we sometimes forget that the basic elements must fit the larger puzzle if they are to make sense, be retained, and be appropriately implemented.

Social interaction

Deaf children's relationships with others frequently have been characterized as impulsive, remote, and superficial. Deaf children with deaf parents and those whose hearing parents are involved in early intervention programs, however, showed relatively normal patterns of social development. Beyond the biologic and cognitive functions of social interaction, children use such relationships to develop secure bases for exploration and to identify with others who are like them; moreover, they use others for instrumental and emotional support. Social relationships make children part of peer and cultural groups, and they lead to self-esteem, achievement motivation, and moral development. Children who are denied such opportunities early in life because of child-related, familial, or societal factors cannot fully benefit from other aspects of experience.

Deaf children with deaf parents and those whose hearing parents are involved in early intervention programs show relatively normal patterns of communication, emotional, and social development. It is the consequent development of positive supportive social relationships that predicts the deaf child's future mental and cognitive strength over his or her life span.

References

[1] Meadow-Orlans K, Mertens D, Sass-Lehrer M. Parents and their deaf children: the early years. Washington, DC: Gallaudet University Press; 2003.
[2] Moores D. Educating the deaf: psychology, principles, and practices. 5th edition. Boston: Houghton Mifflin; 2001.
[3] Koester L, Meadow-Orlans K. Parenting a deaf child: stress, strength, and support. In: Moores DF, Meadow-Orlans K, editors. Educational and developmental aspects of deafness. Washington, DC: Gallaudet University Press; 1990.
[4] Christiansen J, Leigh I. Cochlear implants in children: ethics and choices. Washington, DC: Gallaudet University Press; 2002.
[5] Andrews JF, Leigh IW, Weiner MT. Psychological issues in childhood. In: Deaf people: evolving perspectives from psychology, education and sociology. Boston: Allyn and Bacon; 2004. p. 157–79.
[6] Berk L. Theory and research in human development. In: Development through the lifespan. 2nd edition. Needham Heights (MA): Allyn & Bacon; 2001. p. 2–43.
[7] Horowitz F. Child development and the PITS: simple questions, complex answers, and developmental theory. Child Dev 2000;71:1–10.
[8] Thompson D, McPhillips H, Davis R, et al. Universal newborn hearing screening: summary of evidence. JAMA 2001;286:2000–10.

[9] Sass-Lehrer M, Bodner-Johnson B. Early intervention: current approaches to family-centered programming. In: Marschark M, Spencer P, editors. Deaf studies, language, and education. New York: Oxford University Press; 2003. p. 65–81.
[10] Erting C, Thumann-Prezioso C, Benedict B. Bilingualism in a deaf family: finger-spelling in early childhood. In: Spencer P, Erting C, Marschark M, editors. The deaf child in the family and at school. Mahwah (NJ): Lawrence Erlbaum Associates; 2000. p. 41–54.
[11] Yoshnaga-Itano C, Sedey A, Coulter D, et al. Language of early and later identified children with hearing loss. Pediatrics 1998;102:1161–71.
[12] Traci M, Koester L. Parent-infant interactions: a transactional approach to understanding the development of deaf infants. In: Marschark M, Spencer P, editors. Deaf studies, language, and education. New York: Oxford University Press; 2003. p. 190–202.
[13] Fougeyrollas P, Beauregard L. Disability: an interactive person-environment social creation. In: Albrecht G, Seelman K, Bury M, editors. Handbook of disability studies. Thousand Oaks (CA): Sage; 2001. p. 171–94.
[14] Sameroff AJ, Fiese BH. Transactional regulation and early intervention. In: Meisels SJ, Shonkoff JP, editors. Handbook of early childhood intervention. Cambridge: Cambridge University Press; 1990. p. 119–49.
[15] Berk L. Emotional and social development in infancy and toddlerhood. In: Development through the lifespan. 2nd edition. Needham Heights (MA): Allyn & Bacon; 2001. p. 176–205.
[16] Bowlby J. The nature of the child's tie to his mother. Int J Psychoanal 1958;39:350–73.
[17] Goldsmith H, Harman C. Temperament and attachment: individuals and relationships. Current Directions in Psychological Science 1994;3:53–61.
[18] Collins WA, Gunnar M. Social and personality development. Annu Rev Psychol 1990;41: 387–416.
[19] Kestenbaum R, Farber EA, Sroufe LA. Individual differences in empathy among pre-schoolers: relation to attachment history. In: Eisenberg N, editor. Empathy and related emotional responses (new directions for child development), 33. San Francisco (CA): Jossey-Bass; 1989. p. 51–64.
[20] Berk L. Emotional and social development in adolescence. In: Development through the lifespan. 2nd edition. Needham Heights (MA): Allyn & Bacon; 2001. p. 388–417.
[21] Montanini Manfredi M. The emotional development of deaf children. In: Marschark M, Clark MD, editors. Psychological perspectives on deafness. Hillsdale (NJ): Erlbaum; 1993. p. 49–63.
[22] Greenberg MT, Marvin RS. Attachment patterns in profoundly deaf preschool children. Merrill Palmer Q 1979;25:265–79.
[23] Meadow KP, Greenberg MT, Erting CJ. Attachment behavior of deaf children with deaf parents. J Am Acad Child Psychiatry 1983;22:23–8.
[24] Marschark M. Social and personality development during the school years. In: Psychological development of deaf children. New York: Oxford University Press; 1993. p. 55–72.
[25] Lederberg AR, Mobley CE. The effect of hearing impairment on the quality of attachment and mother-toddler interaction. Child Dev 1990;61:1596–604.
[26] Koester LS, Papousek H, Smith-Gray S. Intuitive parenting, communication, and interaction with deaf infants. In: Spencer PE, Erting CJ, Marschark M, editors. The deaf child in the family and at school. Mahwah (NJ): Erlbaum; 2000. p. 57–71.
[27] Handler MK, Oster H. Mothers' spontaneous attributions of emotion to infant's expressions: effects of craniofacial anomalies and maternal depression. Paper presented at the Biennial Meetings of the Society for Research in Child Development. Minneapolis (MN), 2001.
[28] Papousek H, von Hofacker N. Persistent crying in early infancy: a nontrivial condition for the developing mother-infant relationship. Child Care Health Dev 1998;24:395–424.
[29] Mundy P, Willoughby J. Nonverbal communication, joint attention, and early socioemotional development. In: Lewis M, Sullivan MW, editors. Emotional development in atypical children. Mahwah (NJ): Lawrence Erlbaum Associates; 1996. p. 65–86.

[30] Marschark M. The early years: the social-emotional context of development. In: Psychological development of deaf children. New York: Oxford University Press; 1993. p. 38–54.
[31] Terwilliger L, Kamman T, Koester LS. Self-regulation by deaf and hearing infants at 9 months. Poster session presented at the Annual Meeting of the Rocky Mountain Psychological Association, Reno (NV), 1997.
[32] Swisher V. Learning to converse: how deaf mothers support the development of attention and conversation skills in their young deaf children. In: Spencer T, Erting C, Marschark M, editors. The deaf child in the family and at school. Mahwah (NJ): Erlbaum; 2000. p. 21–39.
[33] von Salisch M. Children's emotional development: challenges in their relationships to parents, peers, and friends. International Journal of Behavioural Development 2001;25: 310–9.
[34] Steinberg A. Autobiographical narrative on growing up deaf. In: Spencer PE, Erting CJ, Marschark M, editors. The deaf child in the family and at school. Essays in honor of Kathryn P. Meadow-Orlans. Mahwah (NJ): Lawrence Erlbaum Associates; 2000. p. 93–108.
[35] Chess S, Thomas A. Temperament: theory and practice. New York: Brunner-Mazel; 1996.
[36] Goleman D. Emotional intelligence. New York: Bantam Books; 1995.
[37] Greenberg M, Kusche C. Cognitive, personal and social development of deaf children and adolescents. In: Wang MC, Reynolds M, Walberg HJ, editors. Handbook of special education: research and practice, 1. Oxford (UK): Pergamon Press; 1989. p. 95–129.
[38] Marschark M. Raising and educating a deaf child: a comprehensive guide to the choices, controversies, and decisions faced by parents and educators. New York: Oxford University Press; 1997.
[39] Meadow KP, Greenberg MT, Erting C, et al. Interactions of deaf mothers and deaf preschool children: comparisons with three other groups of deaf and hearing dyads. Am Ann Deaf 1981;126:454–68.
[40] Calderon R. Parent involvement in deaf children's education programs as a predictor of child's language, reading, and social-emotional development. J Deaf Stud Deaf Educ 2000;5:140–55.
[41] Calderon R, Greenberg MT. The effectiveness of early intervention for deaf children and children with hearing loss. In: Guralnick MJ, editor. The effectiveness of early intervention. Baltimore (MD): Paul H. Brookes; 1997. p. 455–82.
[42] Stinson MS, Foster S. Socialization of deaf children and youths in school. In: Spencer PE, Erting CJ, Marschark M, editors. The deaf child in the family and at school: essays in honor of Kathryn P. Meadow-Orlan. Hillsdale (NJ): Lawrence Erlbaum Associates; 2000. p. 191–209.
[43] Calderon R, Greenberg M. Social and emotional development of deaf children: family, school, and program effects. In: Marschark M, Spencer P, editors. Deaf studies, language, and education. New York: Oxford University Press; 2003. p. 177–89.
[44] Meadow KP, Dyssegaard B. Social-emotional adjustment of deaf students: teacher's ratings of deaf children: an American-Danish comparison. Int J Rehabil Res 1983;6(3):345–8.
[45] Calderon R, Naidu S. Further support of the benefits of early identification and intervention with children with hearing gloss. In: Yoshinaga-Itano C, editor. Language, speech and social-emotional development of deaf and hard of hearing children: the early years [monograph]. Volta Rev 2000;100(5):53–84.
[46] Schlesinger HS. The antecedents of achievement and adjustment: a longitudinal study of deaf children. In: Anderson G, Watson D, editors. The habilitation and rehabilitation of deaf adolescents. Washington, DC: The National Academy of Gallaudet College; 1984. p. 48–61.
[47] Schlesinger HS, Meadow KP. Sound and sign: childhood deafness and mental health. Berkeley (CA): University of California Press; 1972.
[48] Vaccari C, Marschark M. Communication between parents and deaf children: implications for social-emotional development. J Child Psychol Psychiatry 1997;38:793–802.

[49] Hadadian A. Attitudes toward deafness and security of attachment relationships among young deaf children and their parents. Early Educ Dev 1995;6:181–91.
[50] Miller CL. Parent's perceptions and attributions of infant-vocal behaviour and development. First Language 1988;8:125–42.
[51] Pelchat D, Richard N, Bouchard JM, et al. Adaptation of parents in relation to their 6-month old infant's type of disability. Child Care Health Dev 1999;25:377–97.
[52] Meadow-Orlans KP, Steinberg A. Effects of infant hearing loss and maternal support on mother-infant interactions at 18 months. J Appl Dev Psychol 1993;14:407–26.
[53] Minnes P, Nachsen JS. The family and support questionnaire: focusing on the needs of parents. Journal of Developmental Disabilities 1997;5:67–76.
[54] Meadow-Orlans KP, Sass-Lehrer M. Support services for families with children who are deaf: challenges for professionals. Topics in Early Childhood Special Education 1995;15:314–34.
[55] Newman AJ, Bavelier D, Corina D, et al. A critical period for right hemisphere recruitment in American Sign Language processing. Nat Neurosci 2002;5:76–80.
[56] Clark MD. A contextual/interactionist model and its relationship to deafness research. In: Marschark M, Clark MD, editors. Psychological perspectives on deafness. Mahwah (NJ): Lawrence Erlbaum Associates; 1993. p. 353–62.
[57] Schlesinger HS. Effects of powerlessness on dialogue and development: disability, poverty and the human condition. In: Heller B, Flohr L, Zegans L, editors. Expanding horizons: psychosocial interventions with sensorily-disabled persons. New York: Grune and Stratton; 1987. p. 1–27.
[58] Bat-Chava Y. Group identification and self-esteem of deaf adults. Pers Soc Psychol Bull 1994;20:494–502.
[59] Bat-Chava Y. Diversity of deaf identities. Am Ann Deaf 2000;145:420–8.
[60] Sheridan MA. Images of self and others: stories from the children. In: Spencer PE, Erting CJ, Marschark M, editors. The deaf child in the family and at school: essays in honor of Kathryn P. Meadow-Orlans. Hillsdale (NJ): Lawrence Erlbaum Associates; 2000. p. 5–19.
[61] Osofsky JD, Thompson MD. Adaptive and maladaptive parenting: perspectives on risk and protective factors. In: Shonkoff JP, Meisels SJ, editors. Handbook of early childhood intervention. 2nd edition. New York: Cambridge University Press; 2000. p. 54–75.
[62] Meadow KP. Personality and social development of deaf people. Journal of Rehabilitation of the Deaf 1976;9:1–12.
[63] Harris AE. The development of the deaf individual and the deaf community. In: Liben L, editor. Deaf children: developmental perspectives. New York: Academic Press; 1978. p. 217–34.
[64] Kusche CA, Greenberg MT. Evaluative understanding and role-taking ability. A comparison of deaf and hearing children. Child Dev 1983;54:141–7.
[65] Young EP, Brown SL. The development of social-cognition in deaf preschool children. A pilot study. Paper presented at meetings of the Southeastern Psychological Association, Atlanta, 1981.
[66] Vernon M. Deaf people and the criminal justice system. A deaf American monograph 1996;46:149–53.
[67] Burke F, Gutman V, Dobosh P. Treatment of survivors of sexual abuse: a process of healing. In: Leigh IW, editor. Psychotherapy with deaf clients from diverse groups. Washington, DC: Gallaudet University Press; 1999. p. 279–305.
[68] Sacks O. Seeing voices: a journey into the world of the deaf. New York: Harper Collins; 1990.
[69] Hauser-Cram P, Warfield ME, Shonkoff JP, et al. Children with disabilities: a longitudinal study of child development and parent well-being. Monogr Soc Res Child Dev 2001;66(3).
[70] Yoshinaga-Itano C. Development of audition and speech: implications for early intervention with infants who are deaf and hard of hearing. Volta Rev 2000;100:213–34.

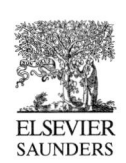

Pediatric Insomnia: A Behavioral Approach

Mark G. Goetting, MD*, Jori Reijonen, PhD

Sleep Health: Comprehensive Sleep Medicine, 3200 West Centre Avenue, Suite 203, Portage, MI 49024, USA

A child who experiences insomnia suffers, as does the child's family and society at large. The ripples from a child's bad night of sleep often cause marital tension, diminished care of siblings, and daytime sleepiness of all involved and can also reduce parental employment productivity and increase the potential for physical abuse of the insomniac, especially during the sleepless nights. The family's quality of life is the most common casualty. It is essential to consider all these consequences while assessing and treating pediatric sleep disorders.

Sleeplessness in infants, children, and adolescents is common. These problems are underreported to health care providers. Reasons for underreporting include an unclear understanding of what is normal sleep and a parent's belief that the physician does not take the complaint seriously, has no useful advice, or may prescribe a potentially harmful medication.

Value of sleep

Poets, philosophers, theologians, and physicians have long puzzled over the meaning of sleep. No one can answer why we sleep any more than why we are awake. It is clear that it is an essential biologic drive like eating and drinking. It is unique among these drives in that by the time a person senses the need for sleep, deterioration in cognitive function has already begun and worsens until sleep is attained.

When viewed from the wake perspective, sleep is a necessary hiatus in activity. Technology advances in lighting, entertainment, and communication have led to a marked reduction in sleep time over the past century. This

---

* Corresponding author.
  E-mail address: mgoetting@gmail.com (M.G. Goetting).

reflects a fundamental attitude that sleep is "down time" and has led modern society to a widespread sleep-deprived state. It may be surprising to know that other societies view sleep as an equally important state or even the primary state of existence. For example, Tibetan dream yoga is an ancient practice involving spiritual teaching and transformation that can only occur during sleep. Western mystics, the Rosicrucian movement in particular, write that since the Middle Ages, they have mastered what is likely non-rapid eye movement (REM) sleep to do the work of healing others. More recently, dream exploration, lucid dreaming, and sleep paralysis with out of body experiences are gaining popularity.

Science is limited to describing what happens during normal sleep and what the consequences are of various perturbations to this sleep. Various theories on the function of sleep include memory consolidation, energy conservation, and avoidance of nocturnal predators by becoming silent and still. The following five statements are known about sleep:

1. At 5 years of age, more than half of a child's life has been spent asleep; it is projected to be approximately a third at the end of a lifetime.
2. We cannot work, eat, drink, or procreate during this state of sleep.
3. Muscle tone is decreased in non-REM sleep and lost in REM sleep. Thus, we cannot maintain an antigravity posture and are susceptible to injury.
4. We are unconscious during sleep. We can neither act on danger nor even detect it.
5. Sleep deprivation compromises cognitive, emotional, neurologic, metabolic, and immune function.

Intervention in pediatric sleep disorders

Although sleep disorders are common in all stages of life, the following principles are more applicable when addressing children's problems:

1. Durability of repair: a child with a remedied disability is likely to benefit from normal function for many more years than the same in an adult, especially one who is elderly.
2. Trajectory: a minor adjustment in function at an early age is amplified by developmental processes into adulthood. The analogy is that raising a rifle a few degrees can have a large effect on the bullet's striking point.
3. Window of opportunity: growth and development create vulnerable transient situations in which conditions can induce aggravated or special morbidity and disability. Early intervention would then be preventative.
4. Influence through dependency: children are high-maintenance humans and tax a family's physical, emotional, and financial resources. A chronically ill or misbehaving child can easily overburden the capabilities of a family and adversely affect all its members and their responsibilities.

Thus far, we have no conclusive evidence that treating pediatric sleep disorders supplies these added values; however, experience and reason are supportive of a positive outcome in this regard. The purpose of this article is to discuss the two common causes of insomnia in children, behavioral insomnia of childhood and delayed sleep phase syndrome. Both of these conditions are primarily treated with behavioral interventions that can be initiated and managed by the primary care provider.

Behavioral sleep medicine

Behavioral sleep medicine (BSM) refers to the psychologic treatment of sleep disorders as a discipline. BSM interventions are based on behavioral and cognitive science research, and they are based on several well-established theories of human behavior and cognition [1]. These theories are briefly described here.

In classic conditioning, previously neutral environmental events automatically elicit behaviors, thoughts, and emotions through a learning history of being associated with involuntary unlearned stimuli and responses (unconditioned stimuli [US] and unconditioned responses [URs]) [1]. In this process, those neutral stimuli become conditioned stimuli (CS) and elicit a conditioned response (CR). For example, states of relaxation and sleepiness are US for falling asleep, which is a UR. If this state of relaxation and sleepiness (US) is consistently paired with nursing and the infant frequently falls asleep while nursing, nursing may become a conditioned stimulus for falling asleep (CR). Extinction occurs over time when the US and CS are no longer paired. In this example, if nursing now stops before the infant falls asleep, over time, nursing no longer functions as a conditional stimulus for falling asleep. The process of classic conditioning can lead people to develop maladaptive beliefs, emotions, and behaviors over time.

Operant conditioning focuses on behaviors generally considered voluntary (with the exception of biofeedback) [1]. Environmental events, called consequences, occur immediately after a behavior and may affect the future probability of similar behavior, causing that behavior to be more or less likely to occur in similar situations. If the consequence makes similar behavior more likely to occur in the future, that behavior has been reinforced. If the consequence decreases the probability of that behavior occurring in the future, that behavior has been punished. Consequences can have an effect on behavior whether the consequence is deliberate or accidental and may not always have the intended effect. For example, a 6-year-old child protests going to bed in the evening and is often allowed to fall asleep on the couch watching television with his or her parents rather than falling asleep in his or her room. If this behavior becomes more likely to happen in the future, the protest behavior has been reinforced.

In operant extinction, a behavior that has previously been followed by a positive consequence (reinforced) is no longer followed by that reinforcer.

For example, the child in the previous example is no longer allowed to fall asleep on the couch and is instead required to go to his or her bed before falling asleep. That child may protest through such actions as crying or having temper tantrums for several nights. If the parents are consistent, over the course of a few nights, the child should cease protesting and go to bed more easily (extinction). Before the protest behavior improves, however, it is likely to increase, which is a predictable phenomenon called the extinction burst.

There are several other important concepts in operant theory. To build new complex behavior, it may be ineffective to wait until the desired behavior occurs before providing reinforcement. Through the process of shaping, successive approximations of the desired behavior are reinforced. For example, although parents would like their child to go to bed when asked, at first, the parents need to ask the child to go to bed, then lead the child to bed, and then provide reinforcement until the child goes to bed when told and waits quietly in bed until being tucked in by the parents.

Long sequences of behavior, such as the prebedtime routine, can be built through the process of chaining. In chaining, a sequence of behaviors is learned, with each step of the sequence being reinforced by the next step in the chain. For example, over time, a child learns a sequence of prebedtime behaviors, including getting into his or her pajamas, brushing his or her teeth, listening to a story, and then getting into bed. The final reinforcer is being tucked into bed by the parent.

In operant conditioning, the frequency and scheduling of reinforcement influence the strength of learned behavior and the ease with which a behavior can be extinguished. Continuous reinforcement, occurring after each instance of the desired behavior, quickly strengthens behavior. That behavior is quickly extinguished if the reinforcement ceases, however. Reinforcement provided on an intermittent schedule builds behaviors that become resistant to extinction. For example, when the child was allowed to fall asleep on the couch, his or her behavior was reinforced, but on other occasions, the child was required to go to bed. The child's protest behavior is more likely to persist if he or she is allowed to fall asleep on the couch after every protest. Parents need to be persistent over several nights before their child's protest behavior diminishes.

Finally, although these concepts may seem to be simple at first, in practice, they can become quite complicated. A child's behavior also influences the parents. The protest behavior is likely to be aversive (punishing) to the parents. Any behavior that stops the protest is reinforced, making the parents more likely to "give in" in the future. Furthermore, both parents may work long hours and enjoy having the extra time with their child when he or she falls asleep on the couch. If an extinction procedure is to be effective, these factors must be addressed.

Social cognitive theory, developed by Albert Bandura, focuses on the reciprocity between environmental events and personal factors, such as behavior and cognition [1]. The importance of observational learning, social reinforcement, and self-efficacy regarding one's own abilities is stressed. Cognitive science, although not providing a unified theory, contributes to BSM through focusing on the cognitive processes that contribute to psychopathology [1]. Distortions in information processing, for example, can fuel the performance anxiety and worry that can contribute to insomnia.

Behavioral insomnia of childhood

Defining insomnia in childhood becomes complicated by the normal developmental changes that occur throughout childhood and by the interactive nature of relationships between children and their parents. Nonetheless, sleep problems seem to be highly prevalent in young children, with prevalence estimates ranging from 20% to 30% [2–4]. Sleep complaints have been found to be highly prevalent among children with psychiatric disturbances, including children diagnosed with attention-deficit hyperactivity disorder (ADHD), mood disorder, or anxiety [5].

In the current diagnostic and coding manual, the International Classification of Sleep Disorders (ICSD) [6], children diagnosed with behavioral insomnia of childhood show a pattern consistent with the sleep-onset association type or the limit-setting type. Diagnosis for both types is based on caregiver reports and requires that other sleep, medical, neurologic, and mental disorders are ruled out and that sleep difficulties are not related to medication use.

In the sleep-onset association type, falling asleep and returning to sleep after nighttime awakenings require special conditions, which can become a problem, necessitating caregiver intervention before the child returns to sleep at night [6]. In the first example, the infant, through classic conditioning, has come to associate nursing with falling asleep. If the infant wakes during the night, he or she is unlikely to fall back to sleep without being nursed.

In the limit-setting type, a child has difficulty in initiating or maintaining sleep or stalls or refuses to go to bed or to return to bed and the caregiver demonstrates inadequate limit-setting behaviors regarding establishing appropriate sleep patterns for the child [6]. In the second example, the parents have not set appropriate limits regarding their child's bedtime and have given in to his or her protests.

It should be noted that elements of both subtypes might be apparent in the same child in clinical practice. For example, over time, the 6-year-old child may come to associate his or her parents' presence with falling asleep. If the child wakes in the middle of the night, he or she may call out to the parents and require that a parent remain in the room until he or she returns to sleep.

Several behavioral interventions have been developed for treating behavioral insomnia of childhood [2–4,7,8]. Research regarding these interventions has been reviewed, and interventions have been rated for efficacy using the Chambless criteria [2,9]. Practice parameters have been developed regarding the use of these interventions by a committee appointed by the American Academy of Sleep Medicine [3]. Overall, research indicates that behavioral therapy for behavioral insomnia of childhood is effective in producing improvements, with more than 80% of the children involved in these studies demonstrating durable clinically significant improvements [2]. Interventions are briefly reviewed here.

Parent education and prevention programs have been found to be effective strategies for preventing the development of sleeping difficulties. Such programs are generally administered during the prenatal period or in the first 6 months of life and focus on the development of healthy sleep habits in infants. Information regarding bedtime routines, sleeping schedules, and promoting self-soothing skills is typically provided. These programs seem to be cost-effective as well as beneficial [2–4,9].

Extinction procedures have also been found to be effective in improving bedtime and night waking behaviors [2–4,8,9]. Traditionally, the extinction procedure involved putting the child to bed and ignoring inappropriate behavior until morning. In practice, many parents have found this procedure to be difficult to administer, and behavior often worsens (the extinction burst) before improving. Modified extinction procedures include graduated extinction, which allows for scheduled parental checks, and extinction with parental presence, which allows the parent to remain in the child's bedroom while ignoring inappropriate behavior.

Scheduled awakenings involve the parent deliberately waking the child shortly before the child's usual time for spontaneous nighttime awakening [2–4,9]. This treatment is appropriate for sleep maintenance difficulties rather than sleep-onset problems. In practice, parents may find this procedure difficult to use because it requires a parent to awaken in time to wake up the child. Further, results may take longer than with extinction procedures.

Other procedures have also been found to be effective [2–4,8,9]. In practice, these procedures are often combined. Faded bedtime with response cost involves delaying the child's bedtime to approximate the usual time of sleep onset. Further, the parent removes the child from bed for a short time if the child does not fall asleep within a certain amount of time. Positive routines involve setting a predictable bedtime routine made up of relaxing and enjoyable activities. These activities form a behavioral chain leading to bedtime.

At the current time, there is not adequate research evidence to recommend one procedure over another [2,3]. Although, in practice, interventions are often combined, research evidence supporting the utility of this practice is not yet available [2,3], leaving the clinician to use his or her own clinical judgment when forming an intervention plan for an individual child and family.

Sleep hygiene recommendations generally include suggestions regarding making the sleep environment conducive to sleep; developing consistent routines; avoiding stimulating activities, foods, and beverages before bedtime; and incorporating developmentally appropriate naps. These recommendations combine several elements consistent with the interventions mentioned previously.

Delayed sleep phase disorder

In delayed sleep phase disorder (DSPD), a child or adolescent's sleep onset is delayed in comparison to the desired time of sleep onset. This can result in bedtime struggles, and waking up at the desired time may become difficult. Daytime sleepiness may result, and school functioning may be impaired. Symptoms suggestive of behavioral problems, ADHD, or mood disorder may develop [10]. The phase delay may initially present as sleep-onset insomnia [11].

According to the ICSD [12], a diagnosis of circadian rhythm disorder, delayed sleep phase type (DSPD), requires that there be a delay in the major sleep period when compared with the desired sleeping and waking times. Evidence for the delay includes an inability to fall asleep and awaken at desired and socially acceptable times. When allowed to be on the preferred schedule, however, sleep is normal in quality and duration and follows a 24-hour pattern. Evidence for the delay should be provided by a sleep log or actigraphic monitoring and sleep diary for at least 7 days. Furthermore, the problem with sleep cannot be explained by other factors, such as another sleep, medical, or neurologic disorder, or by use of medication or other substance.

Although onset of DSPS often occurs in adolescence [13], there is little research evidence supporting use of behavioral treatments commonly used for adults in pediatric populations [9]. Chronotherapy involves delaying bedtime and waking times by 3 hours daily. The delay is repeated until the individual has reached the desired sleeping and waking schedule. Once the desired schedule is reached, it should be maintained by strict adherence to the schedule during weekdays and weekends [9,10,13]. This treatment may be difficult to adhere to and is likely to require parental supervision [10].

Alternatively, advancing sleep phase in small increments has also sometimes been recommended [9,10]. This involves first advancing the waking time, and then bedtime, over subsequent nights until the appropriate bedtime and waking time have been reached. Unfortunately, research on this technique has not supported its use for children and adolescents with DSPS [9].

Phototherapy involves the administration of bright light during the appropriate time of day, corresponding to the early morning hours [10,13]. In addition, light exposure in the late part of the afternoon corresponding to after sunset should be avoided [10]. Although phototherapy has been effective in laboratory settings, appropriate timing of bright light exposure can be difficult in clinical settings. In research settings, appropriate timing in relation to circadian phase was assisted by measurement of body temperature or melatonin levels [13].

In clinical practice, an element of lesser phase delay often occurs in children who have difficulty with sleep onset. For example, many children and adolescents find it difficult to return to their normal school-night sleeping schedule after holiday breaks or extended summer vacations. Anticipating changes in schedule and slowly advancing bedtimes and waking times before the beginning of the new schedule can assist in the adjustment to the new schedule.

Teaching sleep

Can you teach a child to sleep? No. Falling to sleep is a two-phase process. The first involves appropriate sleep pressure (deprivation), sleep hygiene, settling, a conducive bedroom environment, and relaxation. This can be modeled and taught. Ultimately, however, parents can only prepare the child and then hope for sleep. Sleep must come to the child and take him or her away. This second phase is the passive phase and cannot be taught; the more effort and desire at this point, the less is the likelihood of success.

Most children have the capacity of being good sleepers, and this explains why behavioral therapy usually works. The elimination of rewards for waking activity at bedtime prompts the development of settling and self-soothing skills in most cases. Sleep usually soon follows. In some cases, however, sleep does not occur. Common examples include children with neurodevelopmental disorders, depression, and anxiety. We may teach children not to disturb us, which has value, but they may remain awake during much of the night. For these children, treatment of the comorbid condition and the use of a hypnotic agent should be considered.

References

[1] Lichstein KL, Nau SD. Behavioral cognitive science: the foundation of behavioral sleep medicine. In: Perlis ML, Lichstein KL, editors. Treating sleep disorders: principles and practice of behavioral sleep medicine. Hoboken (NJ): John Wiley & Sons, Inc.; 2003. p. 169–89.
[2] Mindell J, Kuhn B, Lewin DS, et al. Behavioral treatment of bedtime problems and night wakings in infants and young children. Sleep 2006;29:1263–76.
[3] Morgenthaler TI, Owens J, Alessi C, et al. Practice parameters for behavioral treatment of bedtime problems and night waking in infants and young children. Sleep 2006;29: 1277–81.
[4] Owens J. Insomnia in children and adolescents. J Clin Sleep Med 2004;1:e454–8.
[5] Ivanenko A, Crabtree VM, O'Brien LM, et al. Sleep complaints and psychiatric symptoms in children evaluated at a pediatric mental health clinic. J Clin Sleep Med 2006;2:42–8.
[6] American Academy of Sleep Medicine. Behavioral insomnia of childhood. In: International classification of sleep disordersDiagnostic and coding manual. 2nd edition. Westchester, IL: American Academy of Sleep Medicine; 2005. p. 21–4.
[7] Lewin DS. Behavioral insomnias of childhood—limit setting and sleep onset association disorder: diagnostic issues, behavioral treatment, and future directions. In: Perlis ML,

Lichstein KL, editors. Treating sleep disorders: principles and practice of behavioral sleep medicine. Hoboken (NJ): John Wiley & Sons, Inc; 2003. p. 365–93.
[8] Sheldon SH. Disorders of initiating and maintaining sleep. In: Sheldon SH, Ferber R, Kryger MH, editors. Principles and practice of pediatric sleep medicine. USA: Elsevier Saunders; 2005. p. 127–60.
[9] Kuhn BR, Amy Elliott. Efficacy of behavioral interventions for pediatric sleep disturbance. In: Perlis ML, Lichstein KL, editors. Treating sleep disorders: principles and practice of behavioral sleep medicine. Hoboken (NJ): John Wiley & Sons, Inc.; 2003. p. 415–51.
[10] Herman JH. Circadian rhythm disorders: diagnosis and treatment. In: Sheldon SH, Ferber R, Kryger MH, editors. Principles and practice of pediatric sleep medicine. USA: Elsevier Saunders; 2005. p. 101–12.
[11] Lack LC, Bootzin RR. Circadian rhythm factors in insomnia and their treatment. In: Perlis ML, Lichstein KL, editors. Treating sleep disorders: principles and practice of behavioral sleep medicine. Hoboken (NJ): John Wiley & Sons, Inc; 2003. p. 305–43.
[12] American Academy of Sleep Medicine. Circadian rhythm disorder, delayed sleep phase type (delayed sleep phase disorder). In: International classification of sleep disorders, 2nd edition. Diagnostic and coding manual. Westchester, IL: American Academy of Sleep Medicine; 2005. p. 118–20.
[13] Wyatt JK. Delayed sleep phase syndrome: pathophysiology and treatment options. Sleep 2004;27:1195–203.

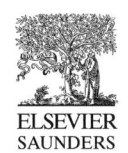

Index

Note: Page numbers of article titles are in **boldface** type.

A

Abuse, sexual, by adolescents. *See* Sexual offenders.

Acute stress disorder, 388

Adaptive skills, assessment of, in intellectual disability, 384

ADHD. *See* Attention-deficit–hyperactivity disorder.

Adolescents. *See* Pediatric patients.

Adult disease prevention, childhood interventions for, **203–217**
  cancer, 206–208
  cardiovascular, 205–206
  diabetes mellitus, 207
  dietary, 209
  exercise programs, 210
  for adolescents, 213–214
  for infants and toddlers, 212
  for school-aged children, 212–213
  multiple chronic diseases and, 208
  osteoporosis, 207–208
  polycystic ovary syndrome, 208
  sexual disease prevention, 210–211
  smoking cessation, 209
  substance abuse, 211
  weight control, 204–208

Ages and Stages Questionnaire, 187–189, 192–193

Alcohol abuse, prevention of, 211

Altruism, as survival skill, 220–221

Amitriptyline, for depression, 253

Amphetamine mixtures, for ADHD
  clinical trials of, 329–330
  formulations for, 330
  side effects of, 330–334
  titration of, 330–331

Antidepressants
  for ADHD, 335
  for depression, 251–253

Anxiety disorders
  ADHD with, 325–326
  depression with, 246

Arithmetic disorder, 367

Asperger's disorder, diagnostic criteria for, 345

Asthma, depression with, 248

Atomoxetine, for ADHD, 334

Attachment, deafness impact on, 408–411

Attention, normal development of, 363

Attention-deficit–hyperactivity disorder, **317–341**
  clinical features of, 322–324
  comorbidity in, 325–326
  depression with, 246
  diagnosis of, 320–322
  epidemiology of, 317–318
  etiology of, 318–319
  impact of, 324–325
  pathophysiology of, 319–320
  risk factors for, 318–319
  treatment of, 326–335
    nonstimulant medications in, 324–325
    patient education on, 327
    psychosocial interventions in, 327–328
    stimulants in, 328–334
  versus learning disorders, 368–369

Auditory development, normal, 363

Autism spectrum disorder, **343–359**
  course of, 343–345
  diagnostic criteria for, 343–345
  medical problems associated with, 352–354
  prevalence of, 345–346
  referral in, 346–347
  screening for, 346–347
  treatment of, 347–352
    biomedical, 349–352
    psychoeducational, 348–349

B

Battelle Developmental Inventory Screening, 196–197

Bayley Infant Neurodevelopmental Screen, 196

Bayley Scales of Infant and Toddler Development, for intellectual disability, 377

Behavioral problems, developmental. *See* Developmental behavioral problems.

Behavioral sleep medicine, 429–431

Behavioral therapy
 for ADHD, 327–328
 for autism spectrum disorders, 347

Biomedical techniques, versus nonbiomedical techniques, 234–235

Birth weight, adult health impact of, 204–205

Bisexual youth. *See* Gay, lesbian, bisexual, transgender, and questioning youth.

Blood pressure, control of, 204–206

Brief-Infant-Toddler Social-Emotional Assessment, 193

Brigance Screens, for developmental behavior, 187, 195

Bupropion
 for ADHD, 335
 for depression, 253

C

Cancer, prevention of, 206–207

Carbamazepine, for posttraumatic stress disorder, 394

Cardiovascular disease, prevention of, 205–206, 208

Casein-free diet, for autism spectrum disorders, 349–350

Checklist for Autism in Toddlers (CHAT), 346–347

Chelation therapy, for autism spectrum disorders, 351

Child abuse, cognitive development and, 388–389

Child Behavioral Checklist, 182, 320–321

Child Posttraumatic Stress Reaction Index, 393

Child sexual abuse, by adolescents. *See* Sexual offenders.

Children. *See* Pediatric patients.

Children's PTSD Symptoms Scale, 398

Cholesterol, high levels of, health impact of, 205

Citalopram
 for depression, 252–253
 for posttraumatic stress disorder, 394

Clonidine
 for ADHD, 335
 for posttraumatic stress disorder, 394

Clozapine, for posttraumatic stress disorder, 395

Cognitive development
 normal, 362
 trauma impact on, 388–389

Cognitive function, assessment of, in intellectual disability, 381–383

Cognitive restructuring, for posttraumatic stress disorder, 400

Cognitive-behavioral therapy
 for ADHD, 327–328
 for posttraumatic stress disorder, 398–399

Communication
 between deaf children and parents, 410–411
 deficits of
  in autism, 344
  in deafness, 416–417

Competence
 as protective factor, in depression, 251
 development of, deafness impact on, 417–418

Complementary and alternative medicine, for depression, 253

Comprehensive Inventory of Basic Skills-Revised Screener, 197

Conduct disorder
 ADHD with, 325–326
 depression with, 247

Confidentiality
 for gay, lesbian, bisexual, transgender, and questioning youth, 297
 for sexual offenders, 312–313

Connors Rating Scale-Revised, 182, 199

Coping skills, teaching of, for posttraumatic stress disorder, 400

Cross-cultural assessment, **227–242**
 awareness in, 235–236
 biomedical and nonbiomedical differences and, 234–235
 factors to address in, 239
 importance of, 227
 management based on, 237–240
 process of, 233–237
 resources for, 228
 terminology of, 227–333

Cross-cultural relationship, definition of, 233

Culture, 229–233
 definition of, 229–230
 Western versus non-Western, 231

Cyproheptadine, for posttraumatic stress disorder, 395

D

Deafness, psychologic impact of, **407–426**
 on attachment, 408–411
 on competence development, 417–418
 on education, 420–421
 on emotional development, 413–414
 on emotional expressiveness, 411–413
 on family functioning, 415–416
 on identity development, 417–418
 on incidental learning, 416–417
 on language development, 408–411
 on personality development, 418–420
 on self-regulation, 411–413
 on social development, 413–414
 on social independence, 417–418

Delayed sleep phase disorder, 433–434

Depression, **243–258**
 ADHD with, 326
 clinical course of, 253–254
 comorbid conditions with, 246–248
 diagnosis of, 244–246
 epidemiology of, 243–244
 protective factors in, 250–251
 referral in, 254–255
 risk factors for, 248–250
 suicidal ideation in, 264–265
 treatment of, 251–253

Developmental, individual-difference, relationship-based model, for autism spectrum disorders, 349

Developmental behavioral problems depression with, 247–248
 screening for, **177–201**
  barriers to, 181
  in internalizing child, 182–183
  in learning difficulties, 184

 information resources for, 184
 need for, 178–181
 referral after, 184–185, 200
 tests for, 179–199
 web sites for, 200

Diabetes mellitus
 depression with, 248
 type 2, prevention of, 207

Diagnostic Interview Schedule for Children and Adolescents, for posttraumatic stress disorder, 393, 398

Diarrhea, in autism spectrum disorders, 354

Diet
 for adult health promotion, 207, 209
 for autism spectrum disorders, 349–350

Dopamine dysregulation, in ADHD, 319–320

Down syndrome, depression with, 247

Doxepin, for depression, 253

Drug abuse. *See* Substance abuse.

Dyscalculia, 367

Dysgraphia, 367

Dyslexia, 365

Dysthymic disorder. *See* Depression.

E

Early and intensive behavioral intervention, for autism spectrum disorders, 348

Early Child Development Inventory, 186–187

Eating disorders, in autism spectrum disorders, 353

Electroconvulsive therapy, for depression, 252

Emotional self-regulation and expressiveness, development of, deafness impact on, 411–413

Empathy, as survival skill, 221–222

Environmental factors
 in ADHD, 318
 in depression, 249

Escitalopram, for depression, 253

Ethnic group, definition of, 227–229

Ethnicity, definition of, 227–229

Ethnocentric view, definition of, 229

Eurocentric view, definition of, 229
Exercise, for adult health promotion, 210
Exposure therapy, for posttraumatic stress disorder, 399–400
Eyberg Child Behavior Inventory, 190–191
Eye movement desensitization and reprocessing, for posttraumatic stress disorder, 398–399

F

Family Psychosocial Screening test, 194–195
Feeding disorders, in autism spectrum disorders, 353
Fluoxetine, for depression, 252–253
Fragile X syndrome, depression with, 247
Freud psychosexual stages of, 275–276

G

Gastrointestinal disorders, in autism spectrum disorders, 354
Gay, lesbian, bisexual, transgender, and questioning youth, **293–304**
　biosocial risk factors for, 297
　clinician reaction to, 296
　Clinician's Framework Guide Questions for, 300–304
　confidentiality for, 297
　electronic technology impact on, 293–295
　referral of, in case of personal issues with, 297
　respect of, 297
　statistics on, 293
　understanding of, 296
Genetic factors
　in ADHD, 318
　in depression, 248
Gluten-free diet, for autism spectrum disorders, 349–350
Grief work, in posttraumatic stress disorder, 401
Guanfacine
　for ADHD, 335
　for posttraumatic stress disorder, 395

H

Health promotion, for adult health starting in childhood. *See* Adult disease prevention.

Hearing
　assessment of, in intellectual disability, 383
　evaluation of, in learning disorders, 370
　loss of. *See* Deafness.
　normal development of, 363
Homeless youth, suicidal ideation in, 267
Homosexuality. *See* Gay, lesbian, bisexual, transgender, and questioning youth.
Human immunodeficiency virus infection, prevention of, 210–211
Hyperactivity. *See* Attention-deficit–hyperactivity disorder.
Hyperbaric oxygen therapy, for autism spectrum disorders, 351–352
Hypertension, high levels of, 204–206

I

Identity development, deafness impact on, 417–418
Imipramine, for depression, 253
Inattention. *See* Attention-deficit–hyperactivity disorder.
Individual Education Plan, 184, 371
Infant Development Inventory, 186–187
Infant-Toddler Checklist for Language and Communication, 189
Insomnia, **427–435**
　behavioral, of childhood, 431433
　behavioral sleep medicine for, 429–431
　delayed sleep phase disorder as, 433–434
　in autism spectrum disorders, 352–353
　interventions for, 428–429
　teaching sleep for, 434
　value of sleep and, 427–428
Integrative skills, assessment of, in intellectual disability, 384
Intellectual disability, **375–386,** 381
　definition of, 375
　diagnosis of, 376–378
　differential diagnosis of, 378–379
　domains of function in, 381–384
　etiology of, 376
　prevalence of, 376
　prognosis for, 379–380
　severity of, 378–380
　signs of, 376

Internalizing behavior, 182–183
Isocarboxazid, for depression, 253

L

Language
 development of, deafness impact on, 408–411
 disorders of, 365–367
 evaluation of
  in intellectual disability, 383–384
  in learning disorders, 367
 normal development of, 362–363

Learning disorders, **361–374**
 assessment of, 369–370
 behavioral assessment in, 184
 comorbid conditions with, 368–369
 definition of, 364–365
 diagnosis of, 365
 differential diagnosis of, 369
 etiology of, 367–368
 impact of, 364
 in deafness, 416–417, 420–421
 presentation of, 361–362
 prognosis for, 371–372
 treatment of, 370–371
 types of, 365–367
 versus normal learning ability development, 362–364

Legal issues, regarding sexual offenders, 307, 312–313

Leiter International Performance Scale, for intellectual disability, 377

Lesbians. *See* Gay, lesbian, bisexual, transgender, and questioning youth.

Lifestyle choices, for adult health promotion
 exercise, 210
 good dietary habits, 207, 209
 safe sexual behavior, 210–211
 smoking cessation, 209
 substance abuse avoidance, 211

Lis-amphetamine, for ADHD, 333–334

M

McCarthy Scales of Children's Abilities, for intellectual disability, 377

Magnesium supplementation, for autism spectrum disorders, 350

Magnetic stimulation, transcranial, for depression, 252–253

Major depression disorder. *See* Depression.

M-CHAT (Modified Checklist for Autism in Toddlers), 181–182, 198–199, 347

Mental retardation. *See* Intellectual disability.

Methylphenidate, for ADHD
 clinical trials of, 329–330
 formulations for, 330
 side effects of, 330–334
 titration of, 330–331

Mirtazapine
 for depression, 253
 for posttraumatic stress disorder, 395

Modafinil, for ADHD, 335

Modified Checklist for Autism in Toddlers (M-CHAT), 181–182, 198–199, 347

Monoamine oxidase inhibitors
 for ADHD, 335
 for depression, 253

Mood disorders, ADHD with, 325–326

Moral development, deafness impact on, 419–420

Mortality, leading causes of, 204

Motor skills
 disorders of, in learning disorders, 367
 evaluation of
  in intellectual disability, 383
  in learning disorders, 370

Multicultural relationship, definition of, 233

N

Naturalistic techniques, versus nonbiomedical techniques, 234–235

Nefazodone
 for depression, 253
 for posttraumatic stress disorder, 395

Negative life events, depression due to, 249–250

Neurofibromatosis type 1, depression with, 248

NICHQ Vanderbilt assessment of behavior, 182

Norepinephrine dysregulation, in ADHD, 319–320

Nortriptyline, for depression, 253

O

Obesity, health impact of, 204–206

Occupational therapy, for autism spectrum disorders, 349

Operant theory, in behavioral sleep medicine, 429–430

Oppositional defiant disorder
 ADHD with, 325
 depression with, 246

Osteoporosis, prevention of, 207

P

Paraphilias, 309

Parent education, for posttraumatic stress disorder, 400

Parents' Evaluation of Developmental Status (PEDS), 186, 188, 192
 Developmental Milestones, 190, 194

Paroxetine
 for depression, 253
 suicidal ideation and, 268

Pediatric patients
 as sexual offenders, **305–316**
 attention-deficit–hyperactivity disorder in, 246, **317–341**
 autism spectrum in, **343–359**
 cross-cultural assessment and management of, **227–242**
 deafness in, **407–426**
 depression in, **243–258**
 developmental behavioral problems in, screening for, **177–201**
 homosexuality in, **293–304**
 insomnia in, **427–435**
 intellectual disability in, **375–386**
 interventions in, for adult disease prevention, **203–217**
 learning disorders in, 184, **361–374**
 prosocial triad acquisition in, **219–225**
 sexuality in, **275–292**
 suicide in, **259–273**
 trauma in, psychologic impact of, **387–405**

Pediatric Symptom Checklist, 182, 191

Perceptual motor development, normal, 363–364

Personal competence, as protective factor, in depression, 251

Personalistic techniques, versus nonbiomedical techniques, 234–235

Personality development, deafness impact on, 418–420

Pervasive developmental disorders. See Autism spectrum disorder.

Pervasive Developmental Disorders Screening Test, 347

Phenelzine, for depression, 253

Phototherapy, for delayed sleep phase disorder, 433–434

Physical activity, for adult health promotion, 210

Posttraumatic stress disorder. See Trauma, psychologic impact of.

Prader-Willi syndrome, depression with, 247

Pregnancy, adolescent, 284, 290

Preschool Developmental Inventory, 186–187

Prison, youth in, suicidal ideation in, 267

Project TEACCH (Treatment and Education of Autistic and Related Communication-Handicapped Children), 348

Propranolol, for posttraumatic stress disorder, 396

Prosocial triad, 220–222

Psychoeducational treatment, for autism spectrum disorders, 348

Psychologic evaluation, in learning disorders, 370

Psychologic impact
 of deafness, **407–426**
 of trauma, **387–405**

Psychosocial skills, assessment of, in intellectual disability, 384

Psychosocial-emotional development, normal, 364

Psychotherapy, for depression, 251

PTSD (posttraumatic stress disorder). See Trauma, psychologic impact of.

Puberty
 anticipatory guidance for, 288–290
 precocious, 277–278
 sequential stages of, 277

Q

Quetiapine, for posttraumatic stress disorder, 396

R

Reading disorder, 365

Relationship development intervention model, for autism spectrum disorders, 349

Religion, as protective factor, in depression, 251

Repetitive behavior, in autism, 344

Resilient youth, qualities of, 224

Risperidone, for autism spectrum disorders, 350–351

Routines, reestablishing, in posttraumatic stress disorder, 401

S

Safety Word Inventory and Literacy Screen, 187, 198

Secretin, for autism spectrum disorders, 351

Selective serotonin reuptake inhibitors
 for depression, 252–253
 suicidal ideation and, 268

Selegiline, for depression, 253

Self-control, as survival skill, 222

Self-injury, behavioral assessment in, 183

Self-regulation, emotional, development of, deafness impact on, 411–413

Sensory integrative therapy, for autism spectrum disorders, 349

Sensory-perceptual development, normal, 363–364

Sertraline, for depression, 252–253

Sex education guidelines, 285–290

Sexual abuse, suicidal ideation in, 267

Sexual offenders, **305–316**
 assessment of, 311–312
 behavior of
  etiology of, 306
  incidence of, 306–307
  versus normal sexual developmental play, 309–311
 biologic factors in, 307
 comorbid disorders in, 308
 definition of, 307
 family of, characteristics of, 308
 individual characteristics of, 307–308
 interventions for, 305
 legal issues in, 307, 312–313
 presentation in office, 306

Sexuality, **275–292**. *See also* Gay, lesbian, bisexual, transgender, and questioning youth.
 anticipatory guidance for, 285–290
 latency period of, 276–277, 286–288
 normal sexual developmental play versus deviant behavior, 309–311
 of adolescents, 277–284, 289–290
  behaviors in, 283–284
  deviant behavior and, **305–316**
  pregnancy and, 284, 290
  psychosocial aspects of, 278–283
  stages of, 277–278
 of infants, 275, 285–286
 of preschoolers, 276, 286
 of toddlers, 275–276, 286

Sexually transmitted diseases, 210–211, 283–284

SIGECAPS mnemonic, for depression diagnosis, 244–245

Sleep
 disorders of. *See also* Insomnia.
  delayed sleep phase, 433–434
  in autism spectrum disorders, 352–353
 teaching, 434
 value of, 427–428

Smoking cessation, for adult health promotion, 209

Social behavior, in autism, 344

Social Communications Questionnaire, for autism spectrum disorders, 347

Social development, deafness impact on, 413–414

Social factors, in ADHD, 318

Social independence, deafness impact on, 417–418

Social support, as protective factor, in depression, 250–251

Speech, disorders of, 365–366

Spirituality, as protective factor, in depression, 251

Stimulants, for ADHD, 328–334
 clinical trials of, 328–330
 formulations for, 330
 side effects of, 330–334
 titration of, 330–331

Stress, depression due to, 249–250

Stroop test, in ADHD, 319

Substance abuse
 depression with, 247
 in ADHD, 326
 prevention of, 211

Suicide, **259–273**
 biologic factors in, 264

Suicide (*continued*)
  controversy over, 260
  epidemiology of, 259–264
  ideation for, management of, 269–270
  methods of, 264
  peer advice concerning, 270
  precipitants of, 265
  reasons for, 260
  repeat, 268
  risk factors for, 265–267
  selective serotonin reuptake inhibitors and, 268

Survival skills, promotion of, **219–225**
  altruism, 220–221
  defining skills for, 222–223
  empathy, 221–222
  interventions for, 223–224
  self-control, 222

Sutter-Eyberg Student Behavior Inventory, 190–191

T

Tanner stages, 277

TEACCH (Treatment and Education of Autistic and Related Communication-Handicapped Children) Project, 348

Tic disorders, in ADHD treatment, 332–333

Transcranial magnetic stimulation, for depression, 252–253

Transgender youth. *See* Gay, lesbian, bisexual, transgender, and questioning youth.

Tranylcypromine, for depression, 253

Trauma, psychologic impact of, **387–405**
  assessment of, 392–393, 397
  brain function and, 389
  clinical encounters with, 389–391
  in cognitive development, 388–389
  information resources for, 401
  physician-primary staff communication and, 392
  risk for, 387, 390–391
  suspicion of, 391–392
  symptoms of, 388, 393
  treatment of, 391–392, 394–396, 398–401
  types of trauma and, 387–388

Trazodone, for depression, 253

Treatment and Education of Autistic and Related Communication-Handicapped Children (TEACCH) project, 348

V

Velocardiofacial syndrome, depression with, 247

Venlafaxine
  for ADHD, 335
  for depression, 253

Vision evaluation, in learning disorders, 370

Visual-motor development, normal, 363

Vitamin supplementation, for autism spectrum disorders, 350

W

War experiences, suicidal ideation in, 267

Wechsler's Intelligence Scale for Children, for intellectual disability, 377

Wechsler's Pre-School and Primary Scale of Intelligence, for intellectual disability, 377

Writing disorders, 366–367

Y

Youth. *See* Pediatric patients.

Moving?

Make sure your subscription moves with you!

To notify us of your new address, find your **Clinics Account Number** (located on your mailing label above your name), and contact customer service at:

E-mail: elspcs@elsevier.com

800-654-2452 (subscribers in the U.S. & Canada)
407-345-4000 (subscribers outside of the U.S. & Canada)

Fax number: 407-363-9661

Elsevier Periodicals Customer Service
6277 Sea Harbor Drive
Orlando, FL 32887-4800

*To ensure uninterrupted delivery of your subscription, please notify us at least 4 weeks in advance of move.

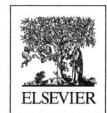